Clinical Anatomy

FOR

DUMMIES®

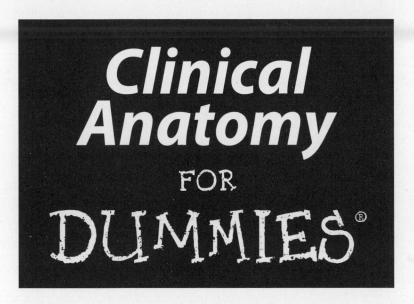

Clinical Anatomy

FOR

DUMMIES®

by David Terfera, PhD, and
Shereen Jegtvig, DC, MS

WILEY

John Wiley & Sons, Inc.

Clinical Anatomy For Dummies®

Published by
John Wiley & Sons, Inc.
111 River St.
Hoboken, NJ 07030-5774
www.wiley.com

Copyright © 2012 by John Wiley & Sons, Inc., Hoboken, New Jersey

Published simultaneously in Canada

For general information on our other products and services, please contact our Customer Care Department within the U.S. at 877-762-2974, outside the U.S. at 317-572-3993, or fax 317-572-4002.

For technical support, please visit www.wiley.com/techsupport.

Wiley publishes in a variety of print and electronic formats and by print-on-demand. Some material included with standard print versions of this book may not be included in e-books or in print-on-demand. If this book refers to media such as a CD or DVD that is not included in the version you purchased, you may download this material at http://booksupport.wiley.com. For more information about Wiley products, visit www.wiley.com.

Library of Congress Control Number: 2012933632

ISBN 978-1-118-11643-2 (pbk); ISBN 978-1-118-22436-6 (ebk); ISBN 978-1-118-23012-1 (ebk); ISBN 978-1-118-23018-3 (ebk)

Manufactured in the United States of America

10 9 8 7 6 5 4 3 2 1

WILEY

About the Authors

David Terfera, PhD, received his PhD in cell and developmental biology from SUNY Upstate Medical University and currently teaches biomedical sciences at the University of Bridgeport College of Naturopathic Medicine. In addition, he is an adjunct professor at Quinnipiac University, where he teaches undergraduate anatomy and physiology.

Shereen Jegtvig, DC, MS, is a health and nutrition writer who began her professional career as a chiropractor in western Wisconsin in 1990. Her chiropractic education included an extensive amount of coursework in human anatomy, physiology, physical diagnosis, and chiropractic care.

Shereen also has a master's degree in human nutrition and is a member of the Academy of Nutrition and Dietetics and the Association of Health Care Journalists. She writes about nutrition for the website About.com, is co-author of *Superfoods For Dummies* (Wiley), and teaches evidence-based nutrition to graduate students at the University of Bridgeport in Connecticut.

Dedication

David dedicates this book to Danielle, for her love and patience, and to his family, especially Raymond and Doris, for their never-ending encouragement.

Shereen dedicates this book to Dr. James Lehman, her partner in love and life, and to her daughter, Kendyl Reis, and son, John Reis, who both make it easy to be a happy mom. Special thanks to her parents, Virgil and Becky Jegtvig, who brought her into this world and bought her that first copy of *Gray's Anatomy* in 1978.

Authors' Acknowledgments

The authors thank the following people:

To our project editor, Georgette Beatty, for her patience and expertise, and special thanks to acquisitions editor Stacy Kennedy for getting us started.

To our agent, Barb Doyen, for her ideas and guidance.

To our illustrator, Kathryn Born, whose beautiful drawings bring our book to life.

We'd also like to thank our copy editor, Caitie Copple, and our technical reviewers, David Brzezinski and Steve Dougherty.

Publisher's Acknowledgments

We're proud of this book; please send us your comments at http://dummies.custhelp.com. For other comments, please contact our Customer Care Department within the U.S. at 877-762-2974, outside the U.S. at 317-572-3993, or fax 317-572-4002.

Some of the people who helped bring this book to market include the following:

Acquisitions, Editorial, and Vertical Websites

Senior Project Editor: Georgette Beatty

Acquisitions Editor: Stacy Kennedy

Copy Editor: Caitlin Copple

Assistant Editor: David Lutton

Editorial Program Coordinator: Joe Niesen

Technical Editors: David W. Brzezinski, MD, CGS; Steve Dougherty

Editorial Manager: Michelle Hacker

Editorial Assistant: Alexa Koschier

Art Coordinator: Alicia B. South

Cover Photo: © iStockphoto.com / Max Delson Martins Santos

Cartoons: Rich Tennant (www.the5thwave.com)

Composition Services

Project Coordinator: Katherine Crocker

Layout and Graphics: Corrie Niehaus, Jennifer Mayberry, Christin Swinford

Proofreaders: John Greenough, Susan Hobbs

Indexer: Valerie Haynes Perry

Illustrator: Kathryn Born, MA

Special Help Victoria M. Adang; Danielle Voirol

Publishing and Editorial for Consumer Dummies

Kathleen Nebenhaus, Vice President and Executive Publisher

Kristin Ferguson-Wagstaffe, Product Development Director

Ensley Eikenburg, Associate Publisher, Travel

Kelly Regan, Editorial Director, Travel

Publishing for Technology Dummies

Andy Cummings, Vice President and Publisher

Composition Services

Debbie Stailey, Director of Composition Services

Contents at a Glance

Table of Contents

Part IV: Moving to the Upper and Lower Extremities.... 257

Introduction

C linical anatomy is the study of the human body as it pertains to examination and treatment in a clinical setting, so it's a little different than your typical gross anatomy (which is learning about the body in a lab). We understand how much effort it takes to study anatomy of any kind — the body has a lot of working parts — but knowing where those parts are and how they work together is very important when you're examining a person who needs your help.

We wrote this book because we want to help you get comfortable with clinical anatomy. Whether you're a student who needs a study guide for the next test or a seasoned veteran who just wants a handy and practical reference, *Clinical Anatomy For Dummies* is just what the doctor ordered.

About This Book

If we tried to recreate an anatomical library, this book would weigh a ton and you'd have to buy a new bookshelf just for it. So in the interest of practicality, we give you just an overview of systemic anatomy before diving into the more popular regional approach. With each chapter we hit on the high points of clinical anatomy so you know exactly what's important from a clinical perspective, complete and succinct. You don't have to read this book from cover to cover (although we won't mind if you do); you can look up only the information you need and set this book aside until you need it again.

Conventions Used in This Book

We know this book contains a lot of information. The following conventions are used throughout the book to make things consistent and easy to understand:

- ✔ Important organs and structures (along with other new terms) are in *italics*.
- ✔ **Boldface** highlights key words in bulleted lists.
- ✔ Illustrations include callouts naming specific structures noted in the text.

What You're Not to Read

We've written this book so you can find the information you need easily and quickly. All the chapters provide you with important information, but some sections offer greater detail or tidbits of clinical information that you can skip if you'd like. We encourage you to read this information along with the main text, but if you want to focus on the main points of the chapters, you can always come back to these items another time:

- ✔ **Sidebars:** Sidebars are shaded boxes that give detailed examples or explore a tangent in more detail. Ignoring these boxes won't compromise your understanding of the rest of the material.

- ✔ **Text marked with the Technical Stuff icon:** Like sidebars, text highlighted with the Technical Stuff icon provides extra details on a given topic, but skipping these bits won't affect your overall understanding.

- ✔ **The stuff on the copyright page:** No kidding. You'll find nothing here of interest unless you're inexplicably enamored of legal language and Library of Congress numbers.

Foolish Assumptions

This book is for anyone who's learning about clinical anatomy or brushing up on what they've learned in the past. In writing this book, we assume that you, the reader, fall into one or more of the following categories:

- ✔ You're a student of medicine or an allied health field and you're looking for an easy-to-read study guide for a clinical anatomy course.

- ✔ You've been out of school for a while and you want to keep your anatomical knowledge sharp.

- ✔ You're comfortable with anatomical terminology or have a large anatomy textbook (or two) on hand.

- ✔ You're an anatomy teacher who wants a more clinical perspective.

How This Book Is Organized

Clinical Anatomy For Dummies is divided into five parts that are packed with important information to hone your knowledge of clinical anatomy. We organized these parts so you can easily navigate through the book to find whatever topic you're looking for. Here's a quick look at what each part covers.

Part I: Beginning with Clinical Anatomy Basics

Part I starts out with an explanation of clinical anatomy and how it compares to other types of anatomical study. We also cover the vocabulary that anatomists use to describe movements and locations of structures. Part I also sorts out the body's different anatomical systems.

Part II: Understanding the Thorax, Abdomen, and Pelvis

Part II focuses on the trunk, which is everything between the neck and the hips. Two chapters tell the story of the thorax — inside and out. Two more chapters cover the abdomen, and one final chapter gets into the very personal pelvic region.

Part III: Looking at the Head, Neck, and Back

Part III moves up and back to take a look at what's going on in your head, neck, and back. Two chapters describe the structures found in and on the head, while another chapter pokes into the neck. Finally, we've got your back with a chapter on spinal anatomy.

Part IV: Moving to the Upper and Lower Extremities

Part IV is all about the upper extremities that swing and the lower extremities that do all the heavy lifting. Three chapters cover the shoulder, arm, wrist, and hand; then three more chapters detail the anatomy of the hip, leg, ankle, and foot.

Part V: The Part of Tens

The Part of Tens is designed to present lots of information in quick, easy-to-read segments. We offer two top-ten lists in this part, starting with our favorite mnemonics, or memory devices, for remembering anatomy. Then we give you ten ways to look into the body without cutting it open. Which, most patients would agree, is a good thing.

Icons Used in This Book

This book uses icons — small graphics in the margins — to help you quickly recognize especially important information in the text. Here are the icons we use and what they mean:

Any time you see this icon, you know the information that follows is so important that it's worth reading more than once.

This icon provides interesting (yet nonessential) details on how a body part functions, or maybe how certain organs or structures work together.

This icon appears whenever an idea or example can help you understand how the structures being described are clinically relevant.

Where to Go from Here

For Dummies books are organized in such a way that you can surf through any of the chapters and find useful information without having to start at Chapter 1. We (naturally) encourage you to read the whole book, but this structure makes it very easy to start with the topics that interest you the most.

If you're new to clinical anatomy, we suggest you turn to Chapter 2 so you can get a handle on the descriptive terms used for location and movement. If you want to brush up on your systems, you can start with Chapters 3 through 6. No matter where you go in *Clinical Anatomy For Dummies,* you're sure to find out a lot!

Part I
Beginning with Clinical Anatomy Basics

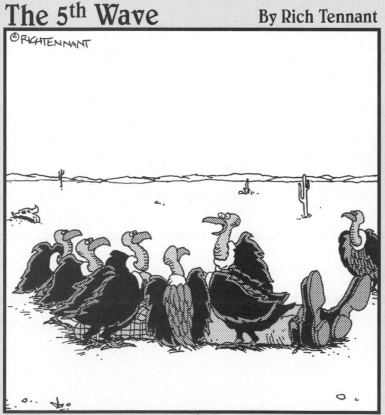

The 5th Wave   By Rich Tennant

"Can anyone tell me if I'm eating from the endocrine system or the nervous system? I always get those two mixed up."

In this part . . .

Clinical anatomy combines the best of regional and systemic anatomy, so before you dig into the details, you want to be sure you have a handle on a few basics. Part I introduces the terminology used in clinical anatomy and then moves on to a review of systemic anatomy, which is a look at the body as it's arranged by certain physiological functions (such as respiration, digestion, and the like).

Chapter 1

Entering the World of Clinical Anatomy

In This Chapter

▶ Looking at different types of anatomy

▶ Arranging anatomy by systems and regions

*Y*ou're reading this book, so you're probably embarking on a career in medicine and healthcare. That means you need to know how the human body works, and you also need to know how to find and examine the parts of the body. This chapter introduces you to the concept of clinical anatomy and how it compares with other ways to look at anatomy.

Studying the Body in Different Ways

Anatomy is the study of the tissues, organs, and other structures of the body, and it's often combined with *physiology,* which describes how the body parts function. We present the info in this book from a clinical perspective, but the following sections describe multiple ways that people in medical fields study and discuss the body.

Looking under the microscope or with your eyes

Bodies are made up of cells — lots and lots of little cells that have different shapes and functions. For example, skin cells provide a protective barrier for the tender parts inside, red blood cells carry oxygen, and brain cells let you think about things (including anatomy).

Histology, or microanatomy, is the study of the anatomy of tissues and the cells of which they're comprised. Because cells are ridiculously small, you can't look at them with unaided eyes, but a microscope gives you a close-up view of the cells. Understanding the anatomy of cells is important, especially in the laboratory, but you really can't examine patients under a microscope.

Gross anatomy, or macroscopic anatomy, is the study of the parts of the body you can see with your eyes. These parts include big structures like the pancreas, liver, bones, and muscles and smaller parts like little blood vessels and nerves. Of course, sometimes you need to use invasive methods to understand gross anatomy, which is fine when you're working with a cadaver. However, gross anatomy isn't always so helpful with a living, breathing patient.

Speaking clinically: Terms used in clinical anatomy

Anatomy has a lexicon of words that you'll need to know. Most of them help you locate structures or understand how those structures relate to other parts of the body. The terms also help you describe the locations of things you find during a physical examination. For example, if you see a contusion (bruise) on a patient's back, you'll need to be able to explain exactly where it is in words that other healthcare providers will understand.

Certain anatomical words describe how the body (or parts) of the body move. Don't worry, you don't need to learn a whole new language — we cover the basic terminology in Chapter 2.

Dividing the Body into Systems and Regions

Medical practitioners rarely look at only one organ or body part at a time. In clinical anatomy, body parts can be grouped together by the system they belong to or by the area or region where they're located. We describe both types of organization in the following sections.

Organizing the body by systems

Body parts don't work alone; they work in concert with other body parts and tissues in systems to perform certain functions. You can group the organs and other structures of the body by these interactions.

The integumentary, musculoskeletal, and nervous systems

The main organ of the *integumentary system* is the skin, which is also called the *integument.* This system also includes the various structures that accompany the skin, like hair, eyelashes, and nails. The integumentary system works together to protect the vital tissues underneath, which includes almost everything.

The *musculoskeletal system* includes the muscles and bones and the tendons and ligaments that connect them all together. The main purposes of the musculoskeletal system are to provide the main structural frame of the body and to produce movement, ranging from walking with long strides to making delicate maneuvers with your fingers.

The *nervous system* includes the brain, spinal cord, and the nerves that run throughout the body. The nervous system serves as a control center that interprets sensory information and sends back instructions so your various body parts know what to do next.

We take a closer look at all three systems in Chapter 3.

The cardiovascular and respiratory systems

The *cardiovascular system* includes the heart and blood vessels that convey blood throughout the body. The blood carries oxygen and nutrients to the cells of the body and carries away waste products.

The *respiratory system* includes the airways and lungs. *Ventilation,* or breathing, is the act of taking air into and out of the lungs so that *respiration,* or gas exchange, between the air and blood can occur. Along with the vocal cords and other structures, it also helps you speak.

These two systems are covered in Chapter 4.

The lymphatic and immune systems

The *lymphatic system* includes lymphatic vessels and lymph nodes that filter fluids from tissues and return them to the bloodstream. The *immune system* is made up of white blood cells and proteins that help fight off bacteria, viruses, and other unfriendly invaders. Many white blood cells of the immune system reside in the organs of the lymphatic system to provide the surveillance that protects you from foreign invaders.

These systems are described in Chapter 5.

The digestive, urinary, and endocrine systems

The *digestive system* is composed of the digestive tract and organs including the liver and pancreas. The function of the digestive system is to break the foods you eat into individual nutrients and to absorb them into the body. It also eliminates waste products.

The *urinary system* includes the kidneys, ureters, bladder, and urethra. Its function is to filter blood and remove waste products such as urine.

The *endocrine system* includes organs called *glands*. The glands secrete hormones that target specific tissues and regulate processes such as metabolism, development, and reproduction.

These systems are described in Chapter 6.

Organizing the body by regions

Another way to study clinical anatomy (other than by systems; see the preceding section) is by looking at all the parts that reside in a certain area. To keep everyone on the same page, the body is divided into specific regions for this purpose.

The thorax

The *thorax* includes the *thoracic cage* and the *thoracic cavity*.

- ✔ The thoracic cage includes the ribs and associated structures.
- ✔ The thoracic cavity includes everything in the thorax from just below the neck down to a muscle called the *diaphragm*. Important structures in the thoracic cavity include the heart, lungs, great blood vessels, and thymus gland.

We cover the thoracic cavity along with the thoracic cage and organs in Chapters 7 and 8.

The abdomen

The *abdomen* includes the *abdominal wall* and the *abdominal cavity*.

 ✔ The abdominal wall is made up of tissues and supporting structures that cover the abdominal cavity.
 ✔ The abdominal cavity includes everything from the diaphragm down to the pelvic cavity (see the next section).

The abdomen is home to much of the digestive tract as well as the liver, gallbladder, pancreas, kidneys, and spleen. We describe the abdomen in Chapters 9 and 10.

The pelvis and the perineum

The *pelvis* is the lowest portion of the trunk, found between the hip bones. It includes the urinary bladder, urethra, internal sex organs, and distal end of the digestive tract. The *perineum* is the region between the thighs. We describe the pelvis and perineum in Chapter 11.

The head

The *head* sits at the top of everything and includes the bones that form the skull. It also includes the structures that create the face. Housed inside these structures are the brain, eyes, ears, mouth, nose, and sinuses.

We discuss the bones of the skull and the brain in Chapter 12 and the eyes, ears, nose, and mouth in Chapter 13.

The neck

The *neck* sits atop the thorax and supports the head. It may not appear to be too complicated on the outside, but inside the neck are many blood vessels, the trachea and pharynx, lymph nodes, glands, and muscles. We cover all the parts of the neck in Chapter 14.

The back

The *back* is the posterior part of your trunk, and it includes the vertebral column, the spinal cord, and lots of muscles (among other things). The back is a major structural component of the trunk that allows you to stand straight or bend and twist in several directions. We break down the structures of the back in Chapter 15.

The upper extremities

The *upper extremities* include the shoulder, arm, forearm, wrist, and hand; their corresponding bones and muscles; and the blood vessels, lymphatics, and nerves in those regions. The shoulder and elbow allow your arm and forearm to move in many directions so you can put your hands where you want them. Your fingers are able to perform fine movements like playing a piano or turning the pages of this book.

We explain the anatomy of the shoulder and arm in Chapter 16, the elbow and forearm in Chapter 17, and the parts of the wrist and hand in Chapter 18.

The lower extremities

The *lower extremities* extend from the hips to the ground. They include the bones of the thigh, knee, leg, ankle, foot, and toes along with the corresponding muscles, blood vessels, lymphatic vessels, and nerves. The lower extremities let you walk around the block, run down a hill, kick a ball, sit down, and stand up again.

We talk about the hip and thigh in Chapter 19, the knee and leg in Chapter 20, and the ankle, foot, and toes in Chapter 21.

Chapter 2

Getting a Grip on Terms Used in Clinical Anatomy

- -

In This Chapter

▶ Locating and relating structures of the body

▶ Making sense of the ways the body moves

- -

Clinical anatomy uses a special vocabulary that helps you understand where certain body parts are in relation to other body parts. The terms in this vocabulary also include several ways to describe physical movement. You (and anyone else studying clinical anatomy) can use these terms and descriptions to ensure that your meaning is clear and errors aren't made in diagnosing and treating patients.

This chapter reviews the specific terminology you need to know, including the description of the anatomical position, the imaginary planes that intersect in that position, and the words that describe how the body moves.

Describing Anatomy by Position, Region, and Plane

How do you describe where one body part is in relation to another? For example, is the heart above the back or above the belly? Well, it depends on whether you're lying down or standing up. Describing location is even more difficult when you look at the arms and legs, because they can move all over the place. Is your hand above your wrist or below it?

In the following sections, we explain how to accurately describe the location of body parts in several different ways. First, you need to familiarize yourself with the anatomical position, and then you can talk about regions, specific positional terms, and planes.

Beginning with the anatomical position

Before you can find out about the various parts of the body, you need to have a reference so you can understand how any of those parts relate to each other. We use the *anatomical position* to describe the positions of the body parts. So as you read the rest of this book, imagine the body standing in the following anatomical position:

- ✔ The head faces forward with eyes looking straight ahead.

- ✔ Arms are down to the sides with the palms facing forward, and the fingers and thumbs are straight.

- ✔ Legs are straight and close together, the feet are flat on the floor, parallel, and the toes are pointing forward.

Take a look at Figure 2-1 to see what the anatomical position looks like.

The following terms also refer to general positions of the body:

- ✔ *Supine* means a person is lying on her back.

- ✔ *Prone* means a person is lying face down.

Figuring out what goes where in anatomical regions

The body is divided into eight separate regions, as described in Chapter 1. Here's a look at all of the major regions (from the outside of the body) and how they relate to each other in the anatomical position that we talk about in the preceding section. You can see these regions in Figure 2-1:

- ✔ The *cephalic region* (head) or *cranial region* (skull) is at the top of the body and visible from the front and rear.

- ✔ The *cervical region* (neck) starts below the head, ends at the thorax, and is visible from the front and rear from below the head to the shoulders.

- ✔ The *dorsal region* (back) runs from immediately below the neck down to the area below the waist. It doesn't include the shoulders. It's visible from the rear.

- ✔ The *thorax* starts immediately below the neck, at the clavicles, and ends along the bottom of the ribcage. It's visible from the front.

- ✔ The *abdomen* starts where the thorax ends (along the bottom of the ribcage) and includes the area down to the hips. It's visible from the front.

✔ The *pelvis* and *perineum* are between the hips and thighs. The pelvis starts where the abdomen ends and takes up the area between the hip bones. The perineum is between the thighs so very little is visible in the anatomical position.

✔ The *upper extremities* include the shoulders, arms, forearms, elbows, wrists, and hands and are visible from the front and the rear.

✔ The *lower extremities* include the hips, buttocks, thighs, knees, legs, ankles, and feet. The buttocks are visible only from the rear, but the rest of the lower extremities are visible from the front and the rear.

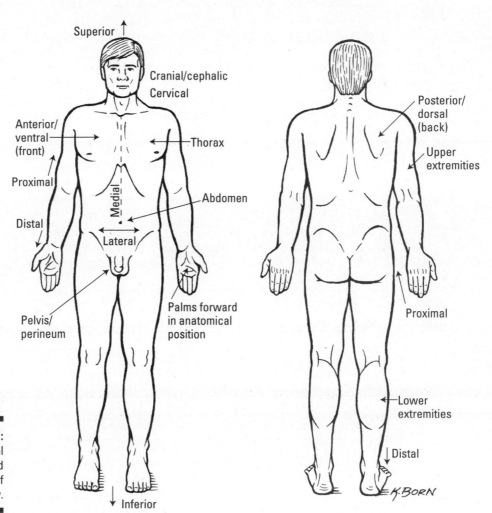

Figure 2-1:
Anatomical position and regions of the body.

Knowing what's up, down, back, and front in specific terms

Words like *up* or *down* and *back* or *front* are okay for some things, but for clinical anatomy, using words that are more specific is best to avoid confusion. That way if you're examining a body that's not in the anatomical position, your descriptions will make sense to anyone else.

Here we run down a list of common terms that help describe how structures relate to each other in the body, along with some examples (refer to Figure 2-1):

- ✔ **Superior:** Closer to the top of the head. For example, the nose is superior to the chin, and the lungs are superior to the stomach. *Cephalic* is similar, also meaning toward the head, but *superior* is used more often in human anatomy.

- ✔ **Inferior:** Closer to the feet. The chin is inferior to the nose, and the stomach is inferior to the lungs. *Caudal* is similar to inferior, but it refers to the "tail," or where the tail would be if people had them. *Inferior* is used more often in human anatomy.

- ✔ **Anterior:** Closer to the front of the body (in the anatomical position). For instance, the abdominal muscles are anterior to the spine, and the lips are anterior to the mouth. *Ventral* is similar to anterior; it means toward the abdomen.

- ✔ **Posterior:** Closer to the rear (in the anatomical position). The spine is posterior to the abdominal muscles, and the mouth is posterior to the lips. The term *dorsal* has a similar meaning as posterior; it means toward the back.

- ✔ **Median:** At the midline of the body. The nose is a median structure.

- ✔ **Medial:** Closer to the midline of the body. The big toe is medial to the little toe, and the nose is medial to the ear.

- ✔ **Lateral:** Farther away from the middle. For example, the little toe is lateral to the big toe, and the ear is lateral to the nose.

- ✔ **Proximal:** Closer to the trunk or closer to the point of origin. The shoulder is proximal to the elbow, and the proximal part of the small intestine is where it begins at the stomach.

- ✔ **Distal:** Farther from the trunk or from the point of origin. The elbow is distal to the shoulder, and the distal portion of the small intestine is where it ends at the large intestine.

- ✔ **Superficial:** Closer to the surface. For instance, the skin is superficial to the muscles, and the abdominal muscles are superficial to the small intestine.

✔ *Intermediate:* In between. The abdominal muscles are intermediate between the skin and the small intestines.

✔ *Deep:* Farther from the surface. The abdominal muscles are deep to the skin, and the small intestines are deep to the abdominal muscles.

✔ *Unilateral:* On only one side of the body, like the stomach and liver.

✔ *Bilateral:* On both the left and right sides of the body, such as the eyes, the kidneys, and the arms and legs.

✔ *Ipsilateral:* On the same side of the body. For example, the right ear and the right eye are ipsilateral.

✔ *Contralateral:* On opposite sides of the body. The right ear is contralateral to the left ear.

Slicing the body into anatomical planes

Four imaginary planes help locate organs and structures inside the body. You can see these planes in Figure 2-2:

✔ *Midsagittal plane:* This division is a vertical plane that goes through the center of the body. It divides the body into left and right halves.

✔ *Sagittal planes:* These vertical planes are parallel to the midsagittal plane and divide the body into unequal left and right portions. There are many possible sagittal planes, so you should always give a reference point where the plane passes through. For example, a sagittal plane running vertically through the middle of the right clavicle (called the *midclavicular line*) would divide the body into a small right portion and a larger left portion.

✔ *Frontal (coronal) planes:* These vertical planes pass through the body at right angles to the midsagittal plane, so they divide the body into front and back. Frontal (coronal) planes can divide the body at any point, so you need to use a reference point to know where exactly the plane passes. For example, you can divide the body into anterior and posterior sections by drawing a frontal (coronal) plane that runs through the body at the ears.

✔ *Transverse (cross-sectional/horizontal) planes:* These horizontal planes pass through the body at right angles to the midsagittal and the frontal planes. They divide the body into upper and lower portions, and like the sagittal and frontal planes, you need to have a reference point to know exactly where a transverse plane lies. For example, a transverse plane can run through the belly button, dividing the body into an upper part and a lower part.

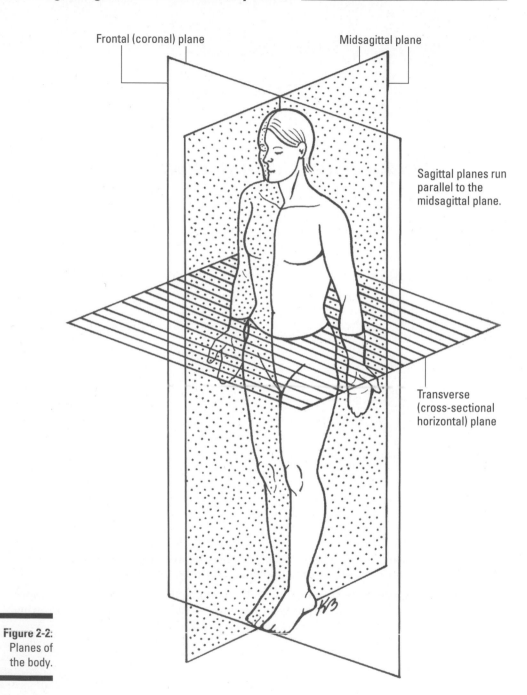

Frontal (coronal) plane

Midsagittal plane

Sagittal planes run parallel to the midsagittal plane.

Transverse (cross-sectional horizontal) plane

Figure 2-2: Planes of the body.

Labeling Anatomical Movement

The body isn't a static thing; it has lots of movement going on. You can use certain anatomical terms to describe how the parts of the body move, as you find out in the following sections.

Bending and straightening

Think of a hinge — it opens and closes; it bends and straightens. Many parts of the body can move in this fashion:

- *Flexion:* This movement is the bending of a part, or decreasing the angle between two parts. You flex your elbow when you bring your forearm up toward your upper arm, and you flex your spine when you bend your body forward.

- *Extension:* The opposite of flexion is extension, the straightening of a part, or increasing the angle between two parts. You extend your elbow when you move your forearm away from your arm to straighten your elbow, and you extend your back when you move from being in a flexed position back upright.

Going away and getting closer

Moving the body isn't always as simple as flexion and extension (see the preceding section). Some parts of the body move away and come closer:

- *Abduction:* Moving away from the midline. Think of a body in the anatomical position (refer to Figure 2-1) and imagine raising the upper extremities out to the sides — that's abduction. The fingers and toes are a little different because the hand and foot have their own midlines, so when you spread your fingers and toes you're abducting them (moving them away from the middle finger, or the third digit).

- *Adduction:* Moving toward the midline. Bringing the abducted upper extremities back down to the sides of the body is adduction. Drawing your fingers (or toes) close together is also adduction.

✔ *Protraction:* Moving a body part forward, like jutting your chin or sticking out your tongue.

✔ *Retraction:* Pulling backward, like retracting your chin back into its normal position.

Moving in circles

One common body movement is turning, as in a circle. Here's a look at some ways body parts can move in a circular fashion:

✔ *Circumduction:* Moving in a circular motion, like doing arm circles, is circumduction. It involves combining flexion, extension, abduction, and adduction all into one movement.

✔ *Medial rotation:* This movement is turning a body part around its long axis, with the anterior surface moving toward the midline, like when you turn your whole lower extremity so that your foot points inward. (*Anterior* means closer to the front of the body, as we explain in the earlier section "Knowing what's up, down, back, and front in specific terms.")

✔ *Lateral rotation:* You laterally rotate when you move a body part around its long axis with the anterior surface moving away from the midline, like turning your whole lower extremity so your foot points out toward the side.

✔ *Pronation:* Pronation is medial rotation of the forearm so that the palm faces posteriorly (toward the rear).

✔ *Supination:* This movement is lateral rotation of the forearm so the palm in the previous example faces anteriorly.

Surveying other ways to move

Here we wrap up with a few more types of movement. Sometimes you need to raise a body part up or lower it back down again, and of course clinical anatomy uses specific terms for those movements. The foot even has a couple of movements all its own.

- ✔ *Elevation:* You elevate when you move a part superiorly (closer to the top of the head), like shrugging your shoulders.

- ✔ *Depression:* Moving a part inferiorly (closer to the feet), like moving those raised shoulders back down again, is depression.

- ✔ *Inversion:* This foot-specific action is moving the foot so the sole (bottom of the foot) faces inward.

- ✔ *Eversion:* This term means moving your foot so the sole faces outward.

- ✔ *Dorsiflexion:* Elevating the foot, or moving the foot until the toes point upward, is dorsiflexion.

- ✔ *Plantarflexion:* This term is a specific kind of depression (see the earlier term) where you tilt the foot until the toes point down.

Chapter 3

Examining the Integumentary, Musculoskeletal, and Nervous Systems

....

....

Skin covers and protects the body and offers visual cues about a person's health. The skin covers the musculoskeletal system that allows you to move and protects the delicate internal organs. Movement is important for people, so the bones, muscles, nerves, and related anatomical features all work together to help you walk around the house and grab your coffee cup each morning. Understanding the systems that accomplish these tasks is important for examining a patient.

This chapter describes the different components and functions of the integumentary system, looks into the musculoskeletal system, and tells you what you need to know about the nervous system, including the brain, spinal cord, and nerves. (You can see all of these systems in the color section.)

Showing Interest in Integument

The largest organ of your body is your skin (known as *integument* in the world of clinical anatomy). It includes the outer covering that protects your inside parts from the elements and from viruses and bacteria. The skin is also necessary for heat regulation, sensation, and making vitamin D. In the following sections, we describe the skin's layers and structures as well as the tissues that lie right below the skin.

The skin can be a good indicator of health. A person who is in shock may have pale skin and goose bumps, and someone with a fever may feel warm to the touch.

Looking at the layers and structures of the skin

The skin has two layers, called the epidermis and the dermis:

✔ **Epidermis:** This tough layer of cells is the outermost layer of skin. It gets its toughness from a protein called *keratin*. The epidermis has five layers:

  • *Stratum corneum* is made up of dead, mature skin cells called *keratinocytes*. These cells are constantly shed and replaced by cells from the lower layers of the epidermis. These cells have lost most of their internal structures and organelles.

  • *Stratum lucidum* is found in thicker skin and helps reduce friction between the stratum corneum and the stratum granulosum. It's composed of dead, flattened cells.

    The skin is thicker in some areas (like the soles of your feet) and thinner in others; women also tend to have thinner skin than men do.

  • *Stratum granulosum* is where keratin is formed. The cells in this layer also produce materials that prevent evaporation, which helps waterproof the skin.

  • *Stratum spinosum* contains the keratin-producing cells that were formed in the stratum basale. Keratin is a major structural component of the outer layers of skin.

  • *Stratum basale* forms the deepest layer. The cells of this layer continuously divide and form new keratinocytes to replace the ones that are constantly shed. This layer also contains *melanocytes*, which are the cells that produce skin coloring.

✔ **Dermis:** This lower layer of the skin contains collagen and elastic fibers that give strength to the skin. This layer is also where the vasculature and nerves live.

Together the epidermis and dermis form the cutaneous layer. The *subcutaneous layer* (area below the skin) lies underneath the cutaneous layer and is sometimes called the *hypodermis* or *superficial fascia*. It holds most of the body's fat, so it varies in thickness from one person to another.

Creases form over joints because the skin always folds the same way as the joints bend. The skin is thinner in those areas and is firmly attached to the underlying structures by connective tissue.

Identifying problems in the stratum basale

Melanoma is a type skin cancer that affects the melanocytes, which are located in the stratum basale layer of the epidermis. Melanomas appear on the skin; they're usually irregular in shape and may have unusual coloring compared to moles. Assessing the physical characteristics of a mole (pigmented spot on the skin) is an important part of a skin inspection. Melanomas are commonly identified using the "ABCDs of melanoma":

✔ A = asymmetry. Melanomas are usually asymmetrical, whereas benign (noncancerous) moles are symmetrical.

✔ B = border. Melanomas usually have irregular, blurry, or uneven borders, whereas moles have typically have sharp, distinct borders.

✔ C = color. Melanomas often have different colors or different shades of a color. Moles are usually one uniform color throughout.

✔ D = diameter. Melanomas are about the size of the tip of a pencil eraser (about one-quarter inch in diameter) or larger, and moles are smaller.

The integument also includes the structures that grow out of the skin, plus a couple of glands:

✔ *Hair:* The protein keratin forms hair. Hair has an inner layer (the cortex), which contains pigments that give it color, and an outer layer (the cuticle). It grows out of *follicles,* which are little pockets of epidermis in the dermis. The shape of the follicle determines whether hair is curly or straight. Each follicle contains a *hair bulb* from which the hair develops. *Arrector pili* muscles connect the hair follicle to the skin.

Have you ever wondered how you develop goose bumps? When you're cold or frightened, the arrector pili muscles cause your skin to dimple and the hair to move vertically (stand on end).

✔ *Nails:* Keratin shows up again in the form of plates found on ends of the fingers and toes. Underneath each nail is a nail bed with a root at the *proximal* end (closer to the rest of the body).

✔ *Sebaceous glands:* These glands are connected to the hair follicles. They produce *sebum,* which is an oily substance that helps keeps the hair flexible.

✔ *Sweat glands:* Sweat glands are coiled tubular glands found in most of the skin. The secretory portion (the part that secretes the sweat) of each gland lies in the fascia with a duct that runs up to the surface of the skin. (Check out the next section for details on fascia.)

Going in farther to the fascia

The fascia is divided into two types: the superficial fascia (described in the previous section) and the deep fascia, which forms the following structures:

- *Investing fascia:* This part of the fascia covers deeper structures, such as muscles and ligaments.

- *Intermuscular septa:* The septa divide muscles into various groups.

- *Subserous fascia:* This part of the fascia lies between the body walls such as the thoracic wall (see Chapter 7) or abdominal wall (see Chapter 9) and the membranes that line corresponding body cavities.

- *Retinacula:* These band-like structures hold tendons in place while joints move.

- *Bursae:* These fluid-filled sacs are made of fibrous tissue; they're lined with membranes and contain a bit of viscous fluid. They reduce friction between body tissues. Major bursae are located near joints between the tendons and bone.

Bursitis is an inflammation of a bursa, which is usually the result of repetitive motion injuries.

Fasciitis is pain and inflammation of the fascial tissues. *Plantar fasciitis* occurs in the fascia that runs along the bottom of the foot from the heel bone to the toes (see Chapter 21 for more about foot fascia). It's a common cause of heel pain.

Boning Up on the Skeleton

The skeleton forms the basic framework of the body. The skeleton can be divided into two parts: the axial skeleton and the appendicular skeleton.

- The *axial skeleton* includes the bones of the head (the skull), neck, and trunk (vertebrae, ribs, and sternum).

- The *appendicular skeleton* includes the bones of the upper extremities and lower extremities.

In the following sections, we tell you about the makeup, shapes, and markings of bones.

Figuring out what makes a bone

Bones contain a *matrix* (a structural component made of water, collagen fibers, and crystallized calcium salts), cells called *osteoblasts* that build up bone, cells called *osteoclasts* that break down bone, cells called *osteocytes* that maintain bone, and collagen fibers. Bones are hard structures because of the calcium that builds up in the matrix, but they retain a slight amount of elasticity due to the fibers. Repeated stress on a bone from physical activity can stimulate the bone to increase *calcification* (calcium storage), and inactivity can lead to calcium loss.

On the exterior, all bones are covered with *periosteum,* a covering of fibrous connective tissue. Bones themselves are actually composed of two types of bone material:

✔ *Compact bone:* The "shell" of each bone is made up of *compact bone,* which looks like a solid mass.

✔ *Cancellous (spongy) bone:* Some bones have an interior mass of *cancellous bone,* which is a network of *trabeculae* (columns) arranged in such a way to reduce stress and pressure on the bone. The outer layer of cancellous bone is composed of compact bone.

Bones without an interior mass of cancellous bone have a *medullary cavity* (open space inside the bone) instead. The shaft of the long bones (such as the humerus of the arm or the femur of the thigh) are hollow. This space is filled with adipose (fat) tissue and/or red marrow, which forms blood cells. The medullary cavity is lined with *endosteum,* a thin layer of connective tissue.

At birth, the marrow of all your bones created blood cells. By the time you're an adult, though, blood cells are only produced in the bones of the skull, thoracic cage, spinal column, pelvic and shoulder girdles, and heads of the humerus and femur.

Surveying the shapes of bones

Bones can be classified by their general shape. Some are long, some are short, some are flat, and a few don't really match any specific shape. Here's a look at the shapes of the bones in the body:

✔ *Long bones: Long bones* are found in both upper and lower extremities (see Part IV for the scoop on those regions). The longest long bone is the thigh bone, the *femur.* It's substantially longer than the phalanges in the hands and feet, which aren't very long but are still called long bones. Each long bone has the following parts:

• The *diaphysis* is the shaft of the bone, made of compact bone.

• The *epiphysis,* the part that forms the enlarged ends of the bone, is made of cancellous bone and is covered with compact bone and hyaline cartilage (see the later section "Catching Up to Cartilage" for details).

- The *epiphyseal cartilage* is between the diaphysis and epiphysis. It's the site of bone elongation during the growing years, but after you're done growing, the cartilage is replaced by compact bone.

✔ **Short bones:** *Short bones* are found in the wrist and the ankle (see Chapters 18 and 21). They're cube-shaped and made from cancelleous bone with a thin layer of compact bone. They're also covered with a periosteum and hyaline cartilage.

✔ **Flat bones:** These types of bones resemble a bone sandwich made of two *tables,* which are thin layers of the compact bone, enclosing a layer of cancellous bone called the *diploe.* The frontal and parietal bones in the skull (see Chapter 12) are flat, as are the scapulae (or shoulder blades; see Chapter 16).

✔ **Sesamoid bones:** These small, round bones form in tendons. The biggest one is the *patella* (or kneecap) in the quadriceps tendon of the knee (see Chapter 20).

✔ **Irregular bones:** This category includes any named bones that just don't fit into the long, short, flat, or sesamoid categories. The rest of the bones of the skull, the vertebrae, and the pelvic bones (see Chapters 11, 12, and 15) fall into this group. These bones are made up of an irregularly shaped mass of cancellous bone covered in a thin layer of compact bone.

Feeling out bumps, ridges, and indentations

The surfaces of bones have all kinds of bumps, lumps, dips, and ridges. Here's a list of the different bone markings you may encounter:

✔ Raised lines are called *lines* or *ridges. Crests* are larger ridges.

✔ Rounded projections include (from smaller to larger in size) *tubercles, protuberances, tuberosities, malleoli,* and *trochanters.*

✔ Sharp points may be called *spines* or *processes.*

✔ Joint expansions at the ends of bones include *heads* (just one expansion on the end), *condyles* (two expansions; one on each side), and *epicondyles* (smaller expansions located just above condyles).

✔ *Facets* are small flat areas found on bones that form joint (articular) surfaces.

✔ Depressions include (from smaller to larger) *notches, grooves, sulci,* and *fossae.*

✔ Holes and openings may be called *fissures, foramens, canals, and meatuses* (the name of the marking depends on the bone where it's located).

Catching Up to Cartilage

Cartilage is a form of connective tissue made up of cells and fibers in a flexible matrix. It's found in joints (see the next section) as well as in your nose and ears. You'll run into three types of cartilage:

- ✔ *Hyaline cartilage:* This durable type covers most of the bone surfaces in synovial joints. It's also found in the nasal septum (see Chapter 13), rings of the trachea (see Chapter 14), and costal cartilages of the ribs (see Chapter 7), and it forms the epiphyseal plates of growing bones.

- ✔ *Fibrocartilage:* This cartilage has a larger number of collagen fibers and less matrix. It's found in the discs in joint spaces including the temporomandibular joint, knee joint, and joints between the bodies of the vertebrae (see Chapters 13, 15, and 20).

- ✔ *Elastic cartilage:* This type contains elastic fibers in the matrix, so it's more flexible than either hyaline or fibrocartilage. Your ear has elastic cartilage (see Chapter 13), and your epiglottis (see Chapter 13) is also formed from elastic cartilage.

Joining the Joints

A *joint* is the spot where two or more bones come together. Most joints allow for mobility, although several are fixed in their position. Joints are stabilized by *ligaments and cartilage.*

Joints are classified as fibrous, cartilaginous, or synovial based on their structures.

- ✔ *Fibrous joints:* The bones of a fibrous joint are connected by fibrous tissue. They range from being immovable (like joints between the bones of the skull) to being slightly moveable (joints between the tibia and fibula in the legs).

- ✔ *Cartilaginous joints:* The joint surfaces in cartilaginous joints are covered with hyaline cartilage and have fibrocartilaginous discs between them. Like the fibrous joints, the cartilaginous joints can be immoveable (for example, the epiphyseal plate, or growth plate of the bones) or slightly moveable, like the joints between vertebral bodies.

- ✔ *Synovial joints:* Synovial joints allow for the most movement. A typical synovial joint includes bones covered in hyaline cartilage and a joint cavity lined with a *synovial membrane* and filled with *synovial fluid.* A durable fibrous joint capsule surrounds the joint. Some synovial joints also have fibrocartilaginous discs between the bones.

The joints' adversary: Arthritis

Arthritis is an umbrella term for more than 100 diseases that affect the joints in people of all ages. Two noteworthy types of arthritis include osteoarthritis and rheumatoid arthritis:

✔ *Osteoarthritis* is the most common type of arthritis. It's more likely to occur after the age of 60, generally due to wear and tear on the joints that normally happens during the aging process. The damage occurs when the joint cartilage wears thin and eventually breaks down. Without the cushioning effect of cartilage, the joint just doesn't function like it should. Symptoms of osteoarthritis include joint pain and stiffness. Osteoarthritis is more likely to occur in joints that have been previously injured and in people who are obese. It can affect any joint but usually shows up in the hands, wrists, neck, back, knees, and hips. Osteoarthritis can't be cured, but it can be treated with nonsteroidal anti-inflammatory medication, exercise, and sometimes surgery.

✔ *Rheumatoid arthritis* is an inflammatory chronic joint condition that can occur much earlier than osteoarthritis (as early as childhood in some cases). It's an auto-immune disease, but the actual cause isn't always known. Patients with rheumatoid arthritis suffer from joint pain and stiffness along with fatigue and flu-like symptoms. Without treatment, rheumatoid arthritis can do a great deal of damage to the joints. Rheumatoid arthritis can't be cured either, but medications such as nonsteroidal anti-inflammatory drugs, steroid medications, and immunosuppressants may slow down progression of the disease.

The shapes of the bones determine what types of movements can occur in synovial joints. They're categorized and described by these shapes:

- *Plane joints,* such as the acromioclavicular joint of the shoulder (see Chapter 16), have flat articular surfaces that allow for a sliding motion.

- *Hinge joints* allow flexion and extension (bending and straightening) of joints like the elbow (see Chapter 17) and the knee (see Chapter 20).

- *Pivot joints* include a bone shaped like a pivot and a ring made of bone or ligament. Pivot joints, such as the atlantoaxial joint of the cervical spine, have rotational movements.

- *Condyloid joints* have an oval surface on one bone that articulates with an oval-shaped depression in another bone. This configuration allows for flexion, extension, abduction, adduction, and circumduction (flip to Chapter 2 for details on these and other types of movements). The metacarpophalangeal joints in the fingers are examples of condyloid joints (see Chapter 18).

- *Ball-and-socket joints* involve a ball-shaped head that fits into a bony socket. The shoulder and hip (see Chapters 15 and 19) are ball-and-socket joints. This type of joint allows for free movement in several directions, including flexion, extension, abduction, adduction, medial and lateral rotation, and circumduction.

- *Saddle joints* have the appearance of a saddle and allow for flexion, extension, abduction, adduction, and circumduction. The carpo-metacarpal joint at the base of the thumb is an example of a saddle joint.

Making the Body Move with Muscles

More than 600 muscles provide movement throughout the body. Some muscle movements require a bit of thought on your part, whereas others happen automatically. In general, muscles are made out of similar types of contractile cells. In the following sections, we describe the three different types of muscle: skeletal muscle, cardiac muscle, and smooth muscle (check 'em out in Figure 3-1).

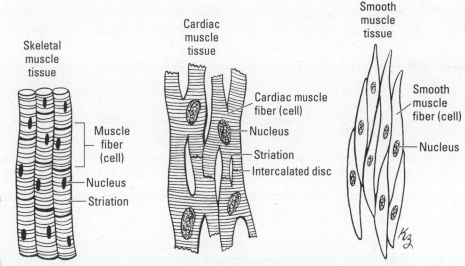

Skeletal muscle tissue

Muscle fiber (cell)

Nucleus

Striation

Cardiac muscle tissue

Cardiac muscle fiber (cell)

Nucleus

Striation

Intercalated disc

Smooth muscle tissue

Smooth muscle fiber (cell)

Nucleus

Figure 3-1: Type of muscles.

Moving the bones with skeletal muscle

Skeletal muscles are responsible for making the skeleton move. They're *voluntary muscles* because you can decide whether the muscles move or not — at least most of the time. Skeletal muscle is also subject to reflex actions.

Skeletal muscles have some basic roles when it comes to moving and positioning the body:

✔ A *prime mover* or *agonist* is the muscle that's mainly responsible for the movement.

✔ A *fixator* is a muscle that holds the proximal part down so the movement can occur distally (farther from the rest of the body).

✔ A *synergist* muscle helps the agonist.

✔ An *antagonist* muscle opposes the contraction of the agonist.

Each muscle has at least two attachments. The attachment that stays in place during movement is called the *origin*. The attachment that moves the most is called the *insertion*. The origin is usually proximal to the insertion.

During development, individual myoblasts (embryonic muscle cells) fuse together to form long, cylindrical, multinucleated (containing more than one nucleus) skeletal muscle fiber. You can see the nucleus and muscle fiber cell in Figure 3-1.

Each skeletal muscle is comprised of a contractile portion made up of muscle fiber bundles called *fascicles* (the fibers have a striped appearance, so sometimes these muscles are called *striated* muscles; refer to Figure 3-1). This part is called a *head* or *belly* of the muscle. Each muscle also has a portion that doesn't contract, which is made up of collagen fibers. The noncontractile portions are called *tendons* when they're rounded or *aponeuroses* when they're flat.

Skeletal muscles come in the following different shapes:

✔ *Circular muscles:* These muscles surround an orifice that is constricted when the muscle contracts.

✔ *Convergent muscles:* Muscles of this type have a wide attachment at one end. The fascicles start at that attachment and converge into a single tendon.

✔ *Digastric muscles:* These muscles have two heads in series that share a tendon.

✔ *Fusiform muscles:* These muscles are shaped like spindles — thicker in the middle with tapered ends.

✔ *Parallel muscles:* In these muscles, the fascicles lie parallel to the long axis of the muscle.

✔ *Pennate muscles:* This type of muscle resembles a feather because the fibers run obliquely to the tendon (in other words, at an angle to the tendon). *Unipennate muscles* have fibers running only on one side of the tendon, and *bipennate muscles* have two sets of fibers, one on each side of the tendon. *Multipennate muscles* are groupings of several bipennate muscles.

Powering through different types of muscle contraction

When a muscle contracts, the fibers may shorten, lengthen, or remain the same length. The three types of muscle contractions are reflexive, tonic, and phasic.

✔ *Reflexive contractions* are automatic. Tapping a reflex hammer on a tendon causes a reflexive contraction.

✔ *Tonic contractions* are just slight contractions that give the muscle tone, or firmness. Tonic contractions don't cause any actual movement, nor do they put up any resistance to a force.

✔ *Phasic contractions* include isometric contractions where the muscle length stays the same but the muscle resists some force, like gravity. Isotonic contractions involve either shortening or lengthening of a muscle to produce movement. Concentric phasic contractions produce movement by shortening the muscle while eccentric contractions produce the movement by lengthening the muscle.

Skeletal muscle can *atrophy* (waste away) when a limb isn't able to move for a long period of time, like when a person is wearing a cast while a bone heals. Some disorders of the nervous system can result in atrophy as well. *Hypertrophy,* the opposite of atrophy, refers to muscles increasing in size. That may sound like a good thing, but in the case of the heart muscle, it most definitely is not good because it reduces the size of the chambers of the heart. But next time you head to the gym to pump iron, feel free to tell everyone you're hypertrophying.

Keeping the heart ticking with cardiac muscle

The muscle of the heart, or *myocardium,* is similar to skeletal muscle because it also has a striated appearance (refer to Figure 3-1). But unlike skeletal muscle, you have no voluntary control over the heart muscle; it's all controlled by the autonomic nervous system (more about that later in this chapter).

Cardiac muscle also has *intercalated discs,* which are regions where the muscle cells connect. These connections help maintain the structure of the muscle and provide electrical connections between the cells so impulses can travel rapidly throughout the heart. We cover the heart and what makes it tick in Chapter 8.

Ouch! Separating sprains from strains

A slip and fall, auto accidents, or athletic injuries can result in either sprains or strains.

✔ *Sprains* occur when a ligament is damaged. They can be mild, moderate, or severe, depending on whether the ligament is stretched or torn.

✔ *Strains* happen to muscles. They can be mild with a little achiness (a "pulled" muscle) or worse, even to the point of the muscle tearing.

Having no control over smooth muscle

Smooth muscle doesn't have the striated appearance of the other types of muscle; instead, it has a smooth-looking surface (refer to Figure 3-1). The fibers are spindle shaped and form sheets of closely apposed cells. Smooth muscle is found in the walls of blood vessels and the digestive tract, in ducts, in the iris of the eyeball, and attached to the hair follicles in the skin.

Like cardiac muscle, smooth muscle is under the control of the autonomic nervous system that we describe later in this chapter, so it isn't under voluntary control. Smooth muscle doesn't tire out like your arm and leg muscles do; it can stay partially contracted for long time periods.

Getting on Your Nerves

The nervous system is the control center for your body. It interprets the things your body senses, and it sends information to the muscles and glands, telling them what to do. It also runs the systems you don't have to think about, like the digestive and cardiovascular systems. The nervous system is also responsible for your moods and your thoughts.

The structures of the nervous system include your brain, spinal cord, and nerves that reach to every part of your body. Following are the two common ways to divide up the nervous system:

✔ **Central and peripheral:** The *central nervous system* (CNS) includes the brain and spinal cord, and the *peripheral nervous system* (PNS) is all the nerves that branch out from the spinal cord and the brain and travel throughout the body.

✔ **Somatic and autonomic:** The *somatic nervous system* regulates the movement of skeletal muscles, and the *autonomic nervous system* controls involuntary actions such as heart rate, digestion, and perspiration.

In the following sections, we compare the different systems, but first, we describe the basic nerve cell, which is called a *neuron.*

Determining what's in (and on) a neuron

Neurons are the building blocks of the nervous system. Each neuron has a cell body with extensions called *dendrites* and an *axon. Dendrites* are the receiving part of a neuron. The signal received at the dendrite is transmitted toward the cell body of the neuron in the form of an electrical impulse. The impulse is transmitted away from the cell body to another neuron, muscle, or gland by the *axon,* which terminates at a synaptic bouton.

Some axons are surrounded in a *myelin sheath.* In the peripheral nervous system, the myelin sheath is formed by Schwann cells that wrap themselves around the axons. The myelin sheath is rich in fat and protein and insulates the axon to increase the speed that the impulse travels in the axon.

Figure 3-2 shows the structure of a *motor neuron,* which carries signals away from the central nervous system, and a *sensory neuron,* which carries sensory signals toward the central nervous system.

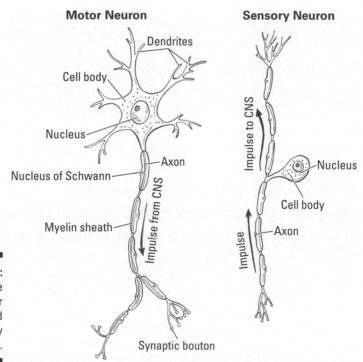

Figure 3-2:
Structure
of a motor
neuron and
a sensory
neuron.

Multiple sclerosis is a disease in which the immune system destroys the myelin that covers some of the nerves. Symptoms vary greatly depending on which of the nerves are affected, but people with severe cases may not be able to walk or talk.

Neuroglia are cells that form the primary structure of nerve tissues (*glia* means "glue"). Their function is to support and insulate the neurons, but they don't relay electrochemical impulses like neurons.

Coordinating input and signals with the central nervous system

The central nervous system (CNS) includes the brain (which we discuss in Chapter 12) and the spinal cord (which we discuss in Chapter 15). The focus of the central nervous system is on coordinating incoming and outgoing neural impulses. It's also responsible for your thought processes.

The CNS receives sensory input and produces motor responses via nerves. A nerve is composed of a bundle of neurons. Most nerves of the peripheral nervous system (discussed in the next section) contain both sensory neurons and motor neurons. The sensory neurons in the peripheral nerve carry sensory impulses to the CNS. The CNS processes this information and sends the appropriate *motor signals* (basically, the info about what should be done) back out to the nerves via the motor neurons.

Disorders of the central nervous system can affect either the brain or the spinal cord and can be due to trauma, infection, autoimmune disorders, tissue degeneration, strokes, or tumors. Examples of nervous-system disorders include Alzheimer's disease and other forms of dementia, multiple sclerosis, Parkinson's disease, and meningitis.

Touching and moving with the peripheral nervous system

The peripheral nervous system (PNS) connects the central nervous system (see the previous section) with the peripheral parts of the body. Peripheral nerves are made up of bundles of *nerve fibers* (axons of neurons), and they're categorized as either cranial nerves that arise from the brain or spinal nerves that arise from the spinal cord.

Peripheral nerves are protected by three layers of connective tissue:

- ✔ *Endoneurium:* This delicate layer surrounds each individual nerve fiber.

- ✔ *Perineurium:* This dense connective tissue surrounds a bundle of nerve fibers called a *fascicle* (see the earlier section "Moving the bones with skeletal muscle" for an introduction to fascicles).

- ✔ *Epineurium:* This thick layer of connective tissue surrounds a bundle of fascicles. The epineurium includes lymphatics, fat, and blood vessels that supply the nerve.

Nerve fibers that carry general sensory information from the body to the spinal cord are called *afferent* (sensory) *fibers*. They bring sensory information such as touch, pain, vibration, and temperature from the peripheral nervous system to the central nervous system for processing. *Efferent* (motor) *fibers* in the peripheral nervous system carry neural impulses to the muscles and other target organs.

Feeling and reacting with the somatic nervous system

The somatic nervous system includes the sensory input and the motor innervation to most of the body, except for the organs, smooth muscles, and glands. It deals with the parts of the body you can move voluntarily.

The part of the skin that's innervated by the general sensory fibers of a single spinal nerve is called a *dermatome*. All the spinal nerves have matching dermatomes on each side of the body. A muscle mass that receives innervation from the motor fibers of a single spinal nerve is called a *myotome*. Each side of the body also has matching myotomes.

Taking control with the autonomic nervous system

The autonomic nervous system works with the involuntary parts of the body, including the muscles of the heart, the digestive system, and the glands. The autonomic nervous system includes both *visceral afferent fibers* and the *visceral efferent fibers*. (The word *visceral* refers to organs.)

- ✔ *Afferent fibers:* These fibers carry pain and other impulses from the internal organs and help regulate visceral functions.

- ✔ *Efferent fibers:* These nerve fibers stimulate smooth muscles, glands, and the heart. Two efferent neurons are needed for the conduction of a nerve impulse to an organ. The cell body of the first neuron, also called the *preganglionic neuron,* is found in the gray matter of the central nervous system. The axon synapses (meets with) the cell body of the second neuron, called the *postganglionic neuron.*

These cell bodies are found in ganglia. A *ganglion* is a collection of nerve-cell bodies similar to the nuclei of the central nervous system, except that these ganglia are only found in the peripheral nervous system.

The autonomic nervous system has two divisions: the sympathetic and parasympathetic nervous systems. You can find out more about them in the following sections (and see them in the color section).

The sympathetic nervous system

The *sympathetic part* of the autonomic system (or the *thoracolumbar division*) prepares the body for emergency situations, also known as fight-or-flight reactions. It increases the heart rate, constricts blood flow to the most peripheral arteries, and raises blood pressure. The point is to supply more blood to the brain, heart, and muscles by reducing blood flow to the skin and to the digestive system.

The site where two neurons communicate is called a *synapse*. The neuron that carries the information is the *presynaptic neuron,* and the neuron that receives the information is the *postsynaptic neuron.*

The presynaptic neuron cell bodies are located in the *intermediolateral cell columns* of the spinal cord, which are part of the gray matter located between the first thoracic and the second or third lumbar segments of the spinal cord.

The postsynaptic neuron cell bodies are found in either the *paravertebral* or *prevertebral ganglia.* The paravertebral ganglia lie along the side of the vertebral column, whereas the prevertebral ganglia are near the aorta (see Chapter 8).

The parasympathetic nervous system

The *parasympathetic part* (or the *craniosacral division*) of the autonomic system is active during times of rest and normal conditions by decreasing the heart rate and stimulating the digestive system. This part of the autonomic system helps you rest and digest.

The presynaptic neuron cell bodies are located in the gray matter of either the brainstem or in the sacral segments of the spinal cord. The postsynaptic cell bodies occur in one of four pairs of *parasympathetic* (terminal) *ganglia,* which are found in the head, or in ganglia located intramurally or near the target organs being innervated.

Splanchnic nerves convey both visceral efferent and afferent fibers back and forth from the viscera.

Chapter 4

Moving Along with the Cardiovascular and Respiratory Systems

The cardiovascular and respiratory systems are all about moving stuff around. The cardiovascular system brings blood to every part of the body while the respiratory system focuses on the air you breathe in and out. This chapter reviews the cardiovascular system and why blood circulation is important; it then moves on to the respiratory system and how you breathe. (Check out both of these systems in the color section.)

Tracing Circulatory Pathways in the Cardiovascular System

The cardiovascular system is part of the larger circulatory system, which circulates fluids throughout the body. The circulatory system includes both the cardiovascular system and the lymphatic system, which is described in Chapter 5. The cardiovascular system moves blood throughout the body, and the lymphatic system moves *lymph,* which is a clear fluid that's similar to the plasma in blood.

Blood contains nutrients from the foods we eat and oxygen from the air we breathe. It also contains hormones (see Chapter 6 on the endocrine system) and cells that fight infection (see Chapter 5 for more about the immune system). The blood also transports waste products to various places that then promptly remove the waste from the body.

The parts of the cardiovascular system include the *heart,* which is the organ that pumps the blood, and a network of blood vessels (all of which we discuss in more detail later in this chapter):

- *Arteries:* The blood vessels that take blood away from the heart
- *Veins:* Blood vessels that return blood to the heart
- *Capillaries:* Very small vessels that lie between the arteries and veins

The *portal vein* and its tributaries carry blood from parts of the digestive system to the liver before reaching the heart. You can read more about the digestive system in Chapter 6.

The heart is a muscular pump with four chambers inside: the *right* and *left atria* and the *right* and *left ventricles* (see Chapter 8 for the details of cardiac anatomy). Those four chambers allow the heart to pump blood through the following two circulatory pathways, which we discuss in more detail in the following sections:

- *Systemic circulation:* Takes oxygen-rich blood to the tissues and organs of the body
- *Pulmonary circulation:* Takes oxygen-depleted blood to the lungs and oxygen-rich blood back to the heart again

Making the rounds: Systemic circulation

Here's the pathway taken by the blood while it's in systemic circulation, delivering oxygen-rich blood throughout the body:

1. The left ventricle of the heart receives oxygenated blood from the left atrium.

2. Blood is ejected from the left ventricle into the *aorta,* a large artery.

   - The *ascending aorta* sends blood to the upper thorax, upper extremities, neck, and head.

   - The *descending aorta* sends blood to the lower thorax, the abdomen, the pelvis, and the lower extremities.

3. The blood leaves the ascending and descending parts of the aorta and enters a network of systemic arteries that run to all places of the body.

4. Blood passes from the smallest arteries (called arterioles) into the *capillary beds.* In the capillary beds, blood exchanges oxygen, nutrients, and waste products with the tissues.

5. The oxygen-poor blood leaves the capillary beds via small veins (called *venules*) and drains into a network of systemic veins that eventually lead to the *venae cavae* (either of the two large veins leading into the heart).

   • The *superior vena cava* receives blood from the upper thorax, head, neck, and upper extremities.

   • The *inferior vena cava* receives blood from the lower thorax, the abdomen, the pelvis, and the lower extremities.

6. The venae cavae empty the oxygen-poor blood into the right atrium of the heart.

Fueling up: Pulmonary circulation

After systemic circulation, the blood in the right atrium is depleted of oxygen, so it needs to go to the lungs to exchange carbon dioxide for oxygen. The pathway from the heart to the lungs and back to the heart is called pulmonary circulation, and it takes the following path:

1. The right ventricle receives the oxygen-depleted blood from the right atrium.

2. The blood leaves the right ventricle and enters the *pulmonary trunk,* which splits into two *pulmonary arteries.*

   Like other arteries, the pulmonary artery carries blood away from the heart, but unlike the systemic arteries, it carries oxygen-poor blood (not oxygen-rich blood) away from the heart.

3. The pulmonary arteries lead to the *lungs,* where exchange of gases takes place. Carbon dioxide is removed from the blood, and oxygen enters the blood. (Turn to Chapter 8 for a discussion of the anatomy of the lungs.)

4. Blood leaves the lungs via the *pulmonary veins.*

   The pulmonary veins carry freshly oxygenated blood to the heart while the systemic veins carry oxygen-poor blood to the heart.

5. The oxygenated blood enters the left atrium of the heart.

The blood in the left atrium moves into the left ventricle and enters the systemic circulation that we describe in the preceding section.

What is cardiovascular disease?

A number of problems can be classified as *cardiovascular disease,* which refers to diseases of the heart and blood vessels. The problems often occur after a person has developed atherosclerosis, also known as "hardening of the arteries," which results in decreased blood flow because the blood vessels are plugged. It occurs when fat, cholesterol, and calcium build up within the walls of the arteries. These build-ups, called *plaques,* can block the arteries and reduce the flexibility of the arterial walls. Atherosclerosis is common in older people, especially in those who have high blood pressure, are diabetic, have high cholesterol, eat too much saturated fat, drink too much alcohol, smoke, don't get enough exercise, and are overweight or obese. Blood clots can also form in the diseased vessels and stop blood flow completely, depriving tissues of oxygen.

Heart attacks (myocardial infarcts) occur when blood flow to some part of the heart is blocked, causing damage to part of the heart. Sometimes heart-valve problems occur when they don't close or open properly. Heart failure occurs when the heart isn't able to pump blood properly to the rest of the body. *Arrhythmia* is a problem with the heart rhythm; the heart may beat too slow, too fast, or irregularly.

Cardiovascular disease can affect the brain as well. *Ischemic strokes* happen when a blood vessel in the brain is blocked. *Hemorrhagic strokes* occur when a blood vessel in the brain breaks open. Either type of stroke can result in damage to a part of the brain.

Symptoms of a stroke may include sudden numbness or weakness of the face or the extremities on one side of the body, confusion, trouble speaking or seeing, loss of balance, loss of consciousness, or a severe headache. A stroke can be diagnosed by imagining with CT scan or MRI (see Chapter 23 to learn more about ways to look into the body without cutting your patient open). Treatment for stroke depends upon the cause. Surgery is used to stop the bleeding of a hemorrhagic stroke. Medication to dissolve blood clots can be used to quickly restore blood flow to the affected part of the brain after an ischemic stroke.

*Pulmonary hypertensi*on is increased blood pressure in the pulmonary vessels when they become constricted. The heart has to work harder to pump blood to the lungs, which can damage the heart and cause fluid to build up in the liver and other places, like the legs. Early symptoms include feelings of dizziness, breathing problems, and fainting. As the disease progresses, the patient may have swelling of the legs and *angina* (chest pain caused by lack of oxygen to the heart muscle). Pulmonary hypertension is usually diagnosed by right heart catheterization, an invasive procedure in which a catheter is inserted into the femoral vein and guided into the right side of heart with the help of an X-ray. The catheter is connected to a monitor that measures the blood pressure in the heart and pulmonary arteries. Therapy involves treating any underlying disorders causing the problem or prescribing medications that dilate the pulmonary arteries.

Moving Blood Away from the Heart with Arteries

The aorta and pulmonary arteries are large vessels, but their branches (and branches of those branches) gradually get smaller in diameter until they reach the tiny capillaries. No matter their size, all arteries are hollow tubes with walls made up of three layers called *tunics* (see Figure 4-1):

✔ ***Tunica intima:*** The thin innermost lining of the arteries, containing endothelium and connective tissue

✔ ***Tunica media:*** A middle layer of smooth muscle

✔ ***Tunica adventitia:*** The outer layer of connective tissue, made of collagen fibers

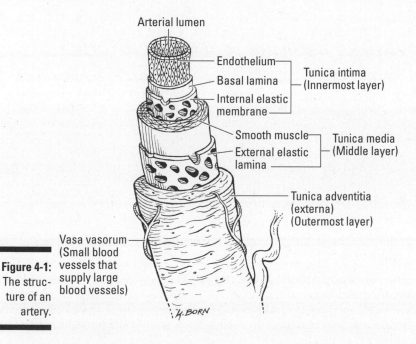

Figure 4-1: The structure of an artery.

Arterial lumen

Endothelium — Tunica intima (Innermost layer)
Basal lamina
Internal elastic membrane

Smooth muscle — Tunica media (Middle layer)
External elastic lamina

Tunica adventitia (externa) (Outermost layer)

Vasa vasorum (Small blood vessels that supply large blood vessels)

4. BORN

In the following sections, we describe all sizes of arteries, from large to small.

Looking inside large elastic arteries

The thick tunica media of the *large elastic arteries* contains smooth muscle and several sheets of elastic layers that give the large arteries plenty of flexibility to expand each time the heart beats. This expansion helps to maintain fairly even blood pressure and blood flow. Following are examples of large elastic arteries:

- ✔ *Aorta:* This artery leaves the left ventricle of the heart (covered in Chapter 8).

- ✔ *Pulmonary artery:* This artery runs from the heart to the lung (covered in Chapter 8).

- ✔ *Common carotid artery:* This artery travels through the neck (covered in Chapter 14).

- ✔ *Right subclavian artery:* This artery is also in the neck.

Moving to medium muscular arteries

The *medium muscular* (or *distributing*) *arteries* have less elastic tissue than the large elastic arteries because the main component of the tunica media is smooth muscle. The body has many medium muscular arteries (most of the arteries named in this book are medium muscular arteries), including the following:

- ✔ *Radial and ulnar arteries:* These arteries are in the forearm and wrist (see Chapter 18).

- ✔ *Brachial artery:* This artery travels through the arm (discussed in Chapter 16).

- ✔ *Femoral artery:* The femoral is the major artery of the thigh (see Chapter 19).

- ✔ *Anterior tibial and fibular arteries:* These arteries course through the leg (see Chapter 20).

- ✔ *Dorsalis pedis artery:* This artery is in the foot (look in Chapter 21).

Surveying small arteries and arterioles

The walls of the small arteries and arterioles are thick because they have a lot of smooth muscle, but they have small *lumen* (the open part inside the arteries). These little blood vessels regulate the amount of pressure in the arteries (blood pressure). When the smooth muscles contract, the blood flow is restricted and blood pressure goes up. When they relax, the blood pressure goes down.

Hypertension (high blood pressure) is a condition in which blood pressure remains elevated over time. Having high blood pressure increases the risk of heart disease, stroke, and kidney disease. Hypertension is referred to as the *silent killer* because high blood pressure has no symptoms and damage can be done to the heart, kidneys, and blood vessels before the person notices anything. Hypertension is treated in a variety of ways, including lifestyle changes (diet and exercise) and medication.

Anastomoses are connections formed between the branches of an artery. This type of connection allows for collateral circulation that ensures blood will reach the desired destination even if one of the branches is blocked or *occluded.* The *circle of Willis* (which is in the brain; see Chapter 12) is an arterial anastomosis.

Taking Blood Back to the Heart with Capillaries and Veins

Capillaries are the tiniest vessels that bridge the smallest arteries to small veins called *venules.* From there, blood passes into veins that serve as tributaries to larger veins before entering the heart. In the following sections, we describe capillaries and veins in more detail.

Exchanging gases, nutrients, and wastes in capillaries

Capillaries are the smallest, thinnest blood vessels in the whole body. They receive blood from the arterioles and form networks called *capillary beds,* which are the locations where gases are exchanged and nutrients and other substances are exchanged for waste products with the tissues (as we note in the earlier section "Making the rounds: Systemic circulation"). White blood cells may also leave the circulatory system through the capillary walls during immune-system responses (see Chapter 5 for the scoop on the immune system).

Peeking into veins and venules

Venules are the smallest, thinnest veins. They receive blood from the capillaries and deliver that blood into larger veins. The walls of the veins have the same three layers as the arteries: the tunica intima, the tunica media, and the tunica adventitia (refer to Figure 4-1 and "Moving Blood Away from the Heart with Arteries").

Veins differ from arteries in that veins may have valves that project into their lumens to prevent the backflow of blood, they have larger lumens, and they have less smooth muscle. Also, the blood pressure in veins is lower than that in the arteries.

Veins can be classified as deep or superficial.

- **Deep veins:** The *deep veins* usually run alongside arteries and frequently share the same names as those arteries. Examples of some deep veins include

  - The *posterior tibial vein* of the ankle and leg (see Chapter 20)

  - The *external* and *internal iliac veins* of the pelvis (see Chapter 11)

  - The *brachial vein* of the arm (see Chapter 16)

Deep venous thrombosis is a blood clot (thickened clump of blood) that forms in a vein. It can break loose and form an embolus (a blood clot that isn't attached to the walls and can travel through the vein), which can be life threatening if it reaches the lungs, causing a pulmonary embolism (a blood clot lodged in an artery of the lung).

- **Superficial veins:** The *superficial veins* are closer to the surface of the body and are often visible through the skin. They include

  - The *great saphenous vein* of the lower extremity (see Chapters 19 and 20)

  - The *cephalic vein* of the upper extremity (see Chapter 16)

  - The *median cubital vein* just anterior to the elbow (see Chapter 17)

Varicose veins are swollen veins that may have a tortuous appearance and may become painful. They're often visible in the lower extremities and are more likely to affect women who stand for long periods of time. Compression stockings that squeeze the leg and assist in moving the blood through the veins may be prescribed to treat varicose veins. Other treatments include laser surgery that closes the vein or vein stripping (a surgical procedure that removes the vein).

Breathing In and Out: The Respiratory System

Before it can find its way into the bloodstream, oxygen has to get into the lungs; plus the carbon dioxide has to find its way out. You accomplish these tasks by breathing air in and out via the respiratory system. This system is divided into two parts: the upper respiratory tract and the lower respiratory tract.

The *upper respiratory tract* includes the structures that bring air into the body and down to the lower respiratory tract:

- ✔ *Nose:* The nose draws in air through the nostrils and into the nasal cavity (see Chapter 13). The nasal cavity opens into the pharynx (throat) at the nasopharynx.
- ✔ *Mouth:* The mouth (see Chapter 13) also draws in air, especially during times of physical exertion or when the nose is "stuffy." The oral cavity opens into the pharynx at the oropharynx.
- ✔ *Laryngopharynx:* Air passes through the nasopharynx and oropharynx toward the laryngopharynx, which is the opening to the larynx (or voice box), which is described in Chapter 14.

The *lower respiratory tract* includes the lungs and the tubes that bring air to them:

- ✔ *Trachea:* The trachea (or windpipe) continues from the larynx. It's described in Chapter 14.
- ✔ *Bronchi:* The trachea splits into two bronchi that each lead to a lung (see Chapter 8).
- ✔ *Lungs:* Each lung is divided into lobes. The right lung has three lobes and the left lung has two.
- ✔ *Alveoli:* The bronchi branch into smaller bronchioles that lead to the alveoli, which are small air sacs surrounded by capillaries (see Chapter 8). Gas exchange between the air and blood occurs across the alveolar and capillary walls.

As you inhale, the diaphragm lowers, the chest wall expands, and air is drawn into the lungs. As you exhale, the diaphragm moves upward and the chest wall contracts, forcing air out of the lungs, through the trachea, and out the nose or mouth. (See Chapter 7 for more on the diaphragm.)

Pulmonary disorders refer to diseases involving the lungs. The airways (bronchi, bronchioles, and alveoli) can be affected, the lung tissues can become inflamed, and circulatory diseases can affect the blood vessels. Common pulmonary disorders include asthma, bronchitis, emphysema, and lung cancer.

Chapter 5

Looking at the Immune and Lymphatic Systems

In This Chapter

▶ Finding out how leukocytes fight invaders

▶ Discovering the purpose and setup of the lymphatic system

▶ Broadening your view to look at the lymphoid organs

*T*he immune system works hard to defend you from pathogens, including bacteria and viruses. It's made up of *leukocytes* (white blood cells), proteins, and other tissues, including the lymphatic system. When it's not fighting infection, the lymphatic system is busy draining excess fluid from the body's tissues and removing debris from that fluid.

This chapter starts with a look at the components of the immune system and the lymphatic system. Then we show you a few additional lymphoid organs. (You can flip to the color section for a view of the lymphatic system.)

Beginning with Red Bone Marrow and Leukocytes

Red bone marrow is the soft part inside certain bones (see Chapter 3 for more about the skeletal system). Red bone marrow makes red blood cells and platelets that are important for the cardiovascular system (see Chapter 4 for details), and it also makes leukocytes, which are part of the immune system.

As you find out in the following sections, different types of leukocytes exist: *lymphocytes,* which identify and remember enemy microorganisms to help the body destroy them, *phagocytes,* which chew up those microorganisms, and *basophils,* which are involved with allergies and inflammation.

Fighting infection with lymphocytes

One group of leukocytes consists of lymphocytes, and you can break them down into two types: B cells and T cells. After they're born in the red bone marrow, some lymphocytes stay in the bone and others leave to seek out the thymus (find out more about the thymus later in this chapter).

- ✔ **B cells:** Cells that stay in the bone marrow to fully mature
- ✔ **T cells:** Cells that travel to the thymus

So what exactly do B cells and T cells do? They start the war against *antigens*, foreign invaders such as bacteria or viruses in the body. When antigens are detected by any of the lymphocytes, the B cells are stimulated to produce *antibodies*, which are proteins that attach themselves to those antigens. Together they form complexes called the *antigen-antibody complexes.* Although the antibodies find the antigens, they can't kill them, so the T cells come in to help. The T cells call in phagocytes (see the next section) to help finish off the invaders, and then the phagocytes help clean up.

The antibodies stay in your body, so if the antigens they're specifically targeted for return, they're ready to destroy them as soon as they show up. You become immune to diseases such as chicken pox and measles through this *sensitization.*

Binging on bacteria with phagocytes

Phagocyte means a cell that eats. Phagocytes, a type of white blood cell, engulf foreign particles such as bacteria by a process called *phagocytosis.*

Phagocytes come in three types: neutrophils, eosinophils, and monocytes.

- ✔ **Neutrophils:** This type of phagocyte is the most common. They're small and contain granules, so they're sometimes referred to as *neutrophil granulocytes.* They eat up (or in other words, *phagocytize*) bacteria.
- ✔ **Eosinophils:** These phagocytes are also granulocytes. They destroy the complexes formed by antigens and antibodies (see the previous section). Eosinophils are also important in fighting foreign invades like parasites that may hitch a ride on your sushi, which is why they're located in the lining of your gut. They're also active during allergic reactions.
- ✔ **Monocytes:** These cells are immature *macrophages* (large cells that eat). A large number of monocytes are stored in the spleen (which we talk about later in this chapter). The macrophages phagocytize enemy cells

and produce *cytokines* (cell-signaling proteins) that communicate with other cells. They also help T cells recognize antigens (see the previous section).

Controlling histamines with basophils

One other type of white blood cell isn't a phagocyte or lymphocyte (but is a granulocyte). It's called the *basophil,* and it's involved in inflammatory reactions, allergies, and parasitic infections. Basophils release histamines that increase blood flow to tissues, but they're also responsible for some of the symptoms of allergies.

Allergies are an exaggerated immune response to allergens. Allergens, like antigens, are foreign substances, but they're generally not harmful. In a person with allergies, the allergen stimulates an immune response that is triggered by the release of the histamine from basophils and eosinophils (a type of phagocyte). Histamine causes the symptoms associated with allergies, including itchy, watery eyes and a runny nose. Antihistamine drugs attempt to block the effects of histamines.

Surveying the Lymphatic System

The lymphatic system, as you find out in the following sections, includes a system of lymphatic capillaries, vessels, nodes, and ducts that collects and transports *lymph,* which is a clear to slightly yellowish fluid, similar to the plasma in blood (see Chapter 4 for more about plasma). The lymphatic system is important for maintaining your body's fluid balance, and it helps transport some fats. It also works along with the rest of the immune system (namely, the leukocytes) to fight infections.

The lymphatic system is really a one-way street; lymph doesn't circulate the way blood does through both veins and arteries.

Networking with lymphatic capillaries and vessels

Lymphatic plexuses (networks) are made up of tiny *lymphatic capillaries,* which are located in most of the tissues of the body. The capillaries collect extra cellular fluid (lymph) from the tissues. The lymph comes from blood plasma that leaks out of small blood vessels called capillaries (see Chapter 4). The lymph enters into small tubes called *lymphatic vessels,* which come together to form larger and longer lymphatic vessels as they carry the lymph away from the tissues and return it to the blood at the subclavian veins (see Chapter 8).

Lymphatic vessels are both superficial and deep. The superficial vessels start in the tissue just below the skin and drain into the deep vessels that usually run alongside the blood vessels.

Special lymphatic capillaries called *lacteals* receive fat that has been absorbed from the small intestine. The fat is transported to the lymphatic ducts and then to the venous system.

Lymphatic vessels that carry lymph toward a lymph node (see the next section) are called *afferent lymphatic vessels.* The ones that carry lymph away from lymph nodes are called *efferent lymphatic vessels.*

Lymphatic vessels are similar to veins (see Chapter 4 for more about veins), but they have a bumpier appearance due to a large number of valves found in the vessels. The valves keep lymph from flowing backward.

Lymphatic vessels are found in most of the organs and tissues of the body, but they're not found in the eyeball, the epidermis (outer layer of the skin), the cartilage, or the bone marrow. The central nervous system has no lymphatic vessels, either — extra fluid drains into the cerebral spinal fluid (see Chapter 3 to learn more about the central nervous system).

Filtering lymph through nodes

Afferent lymphatic vessels carry lymph to small, bean-shaped masses of lymphatic tissue called *lymph nodes* (see Figure 5-1). They're found mostly around the neck, armpits, groin, thorax, knees, and elbows, and their function is to filter and monitor the lymph for foreign particles such as pathogens (bacterial and viruses) and cancerous cells before it returns to the blood. As the lymph enters the node, it flows through spaces called *sinuses* on its way toward the efferent vessels. The cortex houses the lymphocytes that participate in the monitoring of the lymph.

After the lymph is filtered, it leaves the lymph node via an efferent lymphatic vessel, traveling toward even larger vessels called *lymphatic trunks* that are formed by the confluence of lymphatic vessels. It finally travels to the lymphatic ducts.

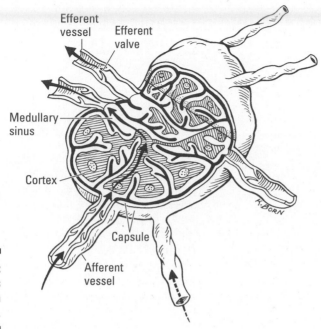

Efferent vessel

Efferent valve

Medullary sinus

Cortex

Capsule

Afferent vessel

K. BORN

Figure 5-1:
The parts
of a lymph
node.

Collecting lymph in ducts

REMEMBER

The *lymphatic ducts* are the final step along the lymphatic pathway. From there, the lymph joins the blood in the venous system that we describe in Chapter 4. Here are the major lymphatic ducts you should know:

✔ *Right lymphatic duct:* This duct drains lymph from the upper-right side of the body, including the right sides of the head, neck, and thorax and the entire right upper extremity. It ends at the right subclavian vein at the junction of the right internal jugular vein (see Chapter 14 for more about these veins).

✔ *Thoracic duct:* This duct receives lymph from the rest of the body. It starts off in the abdomen as a sack called the *cisterna chyli* and runs upward through the thorax and enters the left subclavian vein at the junction of the left internal jugular vein (see Chapter 14).

Delving into a few disorders of the lymphatic system

Lymphedema is a disorder where lymph accumulates in the tissues because it isn't removed properly by the lymphatic system. The accumulation causes swelling (the technical term is *edema*) and can occur when part of the lymphatic system is damaged or blocked. Lymphedema can be caused by infections, cancer, surgical removal of lymph nodes, damage of lymph nodes due to radiation therapy, or certain inherited conditions.

Lymph nodes may become swollen, usually due to exposure to bacteria or viruses, but they can also swell as a result of cancer. Swollen lymph nodes can become infected as a complication of bacterial exposure. This condition is called *lymphadenitis,* and the swollen lymph nodes may become inflamed, red, and tender.

Lymphoma is a cancer that originates in the lymphatic system. It occurs when the T cells or B cells become abnormal and then those abnormal cells continue to divide and reproduce. Lymphoma can spread throughout the body. Other types of cancer, such as breast, lung, or colon cancer, can also spread through the lymphatic system.

Assessing Additional Lymphoid Organs

In addition to being present in the lymph nodes, lymphatic tissue is also found in a few additional spaces of your body. The *lymphoid organs* assist the lymphatic system that we describe in the previous section. They include the thymus, spleen, tonsils, and appendix, along with some special tissue in the gut.

The thymus

The *thymus* is located in the thoracic cavity, just under the neck (see Chapter 8 for more specifics). It's made up of two lobes of lymphoid tissue. Each lobe has a *medulla* surrounded by a *cortex.* The cortex is where immature lymphocytes first go to become T cells, but their maturation finishes in the medulla. (See the earlier section "Fighting infection with lymphocytes" for the scoop on T cells.)

The thymus is large during childhood, but during the early teen years it starts to decrease in size. Why does it get smaller (or to be more clinical, *involute*)? No one knows — it's still a mystery.

The spleen

The *spleen* is located in the upper-left part of the abdomen. It's tucked up under the ribs, so you generally can't *palpate* it (medically examine by touch) unless it's enlarged (turn to Chapter 10 for more anatomical details about the spleen).

The spleen's main function is to filter the blood. It removes old or damaged red blood cells, which are phagocytized by macrophages. The spleen also detects viruses and bacteria and triggers the release of lymphocytes.

The tonsils, the appendix, and the gut

The *tonsils* are masses of lymphoid tissue found in the back of the throat and nasal cavity. They're part of the immune system, so they help fight infections, but removing the tonsils doesn't appear to increase your risk of infections.

Tonsillitis occurs when the tonsils become infected. They're usually easy to see by shining a light into your patient's mouth. Infected tonsils are usually red and swollen, or they may have a whitish coating on them. Sometimes tonsils are enlarged but not actually infected.

The appendix is a pouch of lymphatic tissue that's attached to the large intestine. It's located in the lower-right area of the abdomen (take a look at Chapter 10 for more information). Although it's made of lymphatic tissue, the appendix doesn't appear to have much lymphatic function in humans, but it does release some mucus into the large intestine.

An obstructed appendiceal *lumen* (opening) can cause appendicitis when bacteria start to multiply. The result is abdominal pain and tenderness over the appendix.

Some lymphatic tissue similar to the tonsils is also located in the digestive tract. Called *gut associated lymphoid tissue (GALT),* it comes in the following three varieties:

- **Peyer's patches:** These patches of lymphoid tissue are located in the mucosa and submucosa throughout the small intestine, although they're more concentrated in the ileum. Peyer's patches contain mostly B cells.

- **Lamina propria lymphocytes:** This type of GALT is located in the mucosa of the small intestine. It also contains mostly B cells.

- **Intraepithelial lymphocytes:** These tissues are located between the cells of the epithelial layer of the small intestine, between the tight junctions.

Flip to Chapter 10 for full details on the anatomy of the digestive tract.

Chapter 6

Delving into the Digestive, Urinary, and Endocrine Systems

When you eat a meal, your digestive system is responsible for getting the nutrients into your bloodstream and for eliminating the leftover waste products. The urinary system includes the structures that produce, store, and eliminate urine. The endocrine system produces hormones that regulate a number of functions. This chapter takes a closer look at the digestive, urinary, and endocrine systems (all of which you can check out in the color section).

Breaking Down and Absorbing Your Food: The Digestive System

The function of the digestive system is to take food into your body, break it down into individual macronutrients (proteins, fats, and carbohydrates) and micronutrients (vitamins and minerals), and then absorb those small bits and pieces of nutrients so the rest of your body can use them as fuel and raw materials for building tissues and structures.

Of course, you don't absorb everything you eat, and some of it has to leave the body as waste. The digestive system takes care of that, too.

As you find out in the following sections, the digestive system includes a very long tube called the digestive tract and a couple additional organs that lend a little help along the way.

Starting in the mouth

Digestion begins in the mouth where the salivary glands make saliva (often before you start eating — just smelling a pumpkin pie can make your mouth water).

Saliva is a fluid that contains mucin to lubricate foods, buffering agents that help to reduce acidity, antibacterial agents to kill germs, and a digestive enzyme called *salivary amylase* that begins the job of digesting complex carbohydrates. Who knew saliva contained so much stuff?

The mouth also contains teeth, which are used to chew food into smaller bits that make the process of digestion easier later on, and a tongue, which helps move foods around in your mouth. We describe all these structures in Chapter 13.

Continuing through the esophagus and into the stomach

After chewing food in the mouth, the next step of digestion is to move the food down into the stomach, so it travels through the *esophagus,* a simple tube that connects the pharynx (throat) with the stomach. (Flip to Chapter 10 for details on the esophagus.)

Between the esophagus and the stomach is a sphincter (a ring-like muscle that surrounds an opening or passageway) called the *lower esophageal sphincter* that only opens when you swallow foods or liquids or when you need to belch. The rest of the time it stays shut so the delicate lining of the esophagus isn't damaged by the strong acid found in the digestive juices of the stomach.

Gastroesophageal reflux disease (GERD) occurs when stomach acid backs up into the esophagus often enough to cause damage to the lining.

The *stomach* is a muscular bag located in the upper part of the abdomen, toward the left side. It squeezes and mixes food with digestive juices that are released from specialized cells in the wall of the stomach. Digestive juices include *hydrochloric acid,* which kills microorganisms and activates an enzyme called *pepsin* that helps break down proteins, and *intrinsic factor,* which is a substance that helps the small intestine absorb vitamin B12. Its lining contains cells that produce mucus to help protect the walls of the stomach from damage due to the acid. We give the details on stomach anatomy in Chapter 10.

Finishing in the small intestine with help from the pancreas, gallbladder, and liver

The stomach slowly empties its contents into the small intestine, which is the longest portion of the digestive tract. It's divided into three sections: the *duodenum,* the *jejunum,* and the *ileum,* which are described in Chapter 10. Digestion finishes in the small intestine, and absorption of nutrients begins with a little assistance from a few other organs.

- ✔ **Pancreas:** This organ is located behind the stomach. It produces digestive enzymes and releases them into the duodenum. These enzymes include
  - *Lipase,* which breaks down fats
  - *Pancreatic amylase,* which breaks down carbohydrates
  - *Proteases,* which break down proteins
- ✔ **Gallbladder:** This sac-like organ is located near the liver and stores *bile,* a substance that helps emulsify fats so the lipases have an easier time digesting them.
- ✔ **Liver:** The liver is located on the right side of the abdomen. It makes the bile that helps emulsify fats, and it processes the nutrients that are absorbed in the small intestine.

Need more info on any of these structures? We break down the anatomy of the pancreas, gallbladder, and liver in Chapter 10.

After the nutrients are digested, they're absorbed into the cells of the small intestine. From there, they're absorbed into the blood and carried away to be processed and metabolized or stored.

Forming and removing bulk in the large intestine

The material that's left after digestion and absorption in the small intestine travels into the large intestine, or colon. It travels up the right side of the abdomen, across the top, and down again on the left. From there it moves toward the midline of the body and terminates at the rectum with the anus that opens to the outside.

The main function of the colon is to absorb water, leaving more solid material that's passed through the rectum as stool. The anatomy of the colon, rectum, and anus is described in Chapters 10 and 11.

The *appendix* is a tube-like pouch of lymphoid tissue that hangs from the large intestine in the right lower quadrant of the abdomen. We're not sure what it does, and you can be perfectly healthy without it. We discuss the appendix in Chapter 10.

Removing Wastes: The Urinary System

The urinary system filters waste from the blood and produces urine in the kidneys; then it removes the urine from the body. Adults produce about a quart and a half of urine every day, but that amount can vary greatly depending on how much fluid and what types of foods are consumed and how much fluid is lost by sweating or breathing.

Two bean-shaped organs called the kidneys are found in the abdomen, near the back and just below the ribs. The kidneys are responsible for filtering the blood. The filtrate, as it moves through the kidney tubules, is modified to produce urine. (Turn to Chapter 10 to find out about the anatomy of the kidneys.)

The body needs a way to store the urine until you have a convenient time to urinate (remove urine from the body). Urine leaves the kidneys and travels down the *ureters,* which are two long tubes that lead to the urinary bladder. The *bladder* is a thin-walled, bag-like organ that can hold up to two cups of urine.

The bladder is connected to the urethra, which is a tube that opens externally through an opening called the *external meatus.* Sphincter muscles keep urine from leaving the bladder until the person is ready to urinate. The female urethra is quite short, whereas the male urethra is longer and runs through the penis.

Sometimes in the process of filtering blood and forming urine, salt-and-mineral crystals form in the kidneys. These *kidney stones* can travel down the ureters and into the bladder. The stones vary in size, and in some cases passing kidney stones can be extremely painful. The stones can become lodged in the ureter, blocking the flow of urine and causing a back-up of urine in the kidney. Treatments include medications and the use of lithotripsy (shock waves) to reduce the size of the stone so that it is more easily passed.

Handling Hormones: The Endocrine System

The endocrine system is made up of glands, which are organs that produce hormones and release them into the blood. The hormones cause certain reactions to occur in specific tissues. The endocrine system affects a large number of the body's functions, including temperature, metabolism, sexual function, reproduction, moods, and growth and development. The following sections describe the major glands of the endocrine system.

The master gland: The pituitary

The pituitary gland controls the functions of several other endocrine glands. It's not very big, though — only about the size of a pea. The pituitary gland is located at the base of the brain, and it secretes several different hormones:

- **Adrenocorticotropic hormone:** Stimulates the suprarenal glands to produce cortisol, which is a stress hormone (meaning production of this hormone is triggered by stressful situations)

- **Antidiuretic hormone:** Regulates fluid balance in the body

- **Follicle-stimulating hormone:** Stimulates the ovaries to produce eggs, or *ova,* in women and sperm production in men

- **Growth hormone:** Stimulates growth during childhood and helps to maintain bone and muscle mass in adults

- **Luteinizing hormone:** Helps regulate testosterone in males and estrogen in women

- **Melanocyte-stimulating hormone:** Stimulates the production of melanin (skin pigment) by the melanocytes in the skin and hair

- **Oxytocin:** Stimulates lactation (milk production) in the breasts and contraction of the smooth muscles of the uterus during birth

- **Prolactin:** Stimulates milk production after the birth of a baby

- **Thyroid-stimulating hormone:** Stimulates the thyroid gland to produce the thyroid hormones that regulate metabolism and blood calcium levels

The anatomy of the pituitary gland is described in Chapter 12.

Pituitary tumors can cause the gland to secrete too much or too little of the pituitary hormones.

The pituitary's assistants: The hypothalamus and pineal glands

The *hypothalamus* is a part of the brain located near the pituitary gland. It assists the pituitary gland in regulating other glands by releasing hormones that communicate with it:

- **Corticotropin-releasing hormone:** Tells the pituitary gland to secrete adrenocorticotropic hormone

- **Dopamine:** Tells the pituitary gland to produce less prolactin

- **Gonadotropin-releasing hormone:** Tells the pituitary to secrete follicle-stimulating hormone and luteinizing hormone

- **Growth-hormone-releasing hormone:** Tells the pituitary gland to secrete growth hormone

- **Somatostatin:** Tells the pituitary gland to release less growth hormone and thyroid-stimulating hormone

- **Thyrotropin-releasing hormone:** Tells the pituitary gland to release thyroid-stimulating hormone and prolactin

The *pineal gland* is also located in the brain (see Chapter 12). It secretes *melatonin,* which is a hormone that helps regulate sleep cycles and influences sexual development.

The body's metabolism booster: The thyroid gland

The *thyroid gland* is located in the anterior (front) part of the neck, just in front of the trachea below the larynx. It helps regulate the body's metabolism (how the body gets energy from food) and blood-calcium levels by secreting three hormones:

- **Calcitonin:** Regulates blood calcium levels by slowing down the amount of calcium lost from bones

- **Thyroxine:** Stimulates your body to use more oxygen and increases metabolism

- **Triiodothyronine:** Affects metabolism, growth and development, body temperature, and heart rate

Too much or too little: Thyroid disorders

The following thyroid disorders can cause the thyroid gland to secrete too much or too little thyroid hormone:

✔ *Hyperthyroidism* is the condition when the thyroid gland produces too much of the hormones. It can be caused by getting too much iodine, as a result of Graves' disease (an immune-system disorder), inflammation of the thyroid due to infections, or tumors. Symptoms of hyperthyroidism include increased sweating, weight loss, feeling too hot, feeling nervous and restless, goiter (visibly enlarged thyroid gland), and difficulty concentrating. It's diagnosed by blood tests that measure the thyroid hormones and thyroid-stimulating hormone that's produced by the pituitary gland. Hyperthyroidism can be treated by surgery or medications that slow the thyroid down.

✔ *Hypothyroidism* is the opposite condition, in which the thyroid gland doesn't secrete enough of the hormones. It's usually due to low levels of iodine and inflammation of the thyroid gland due to autoimmune reactions. It can also be due to radiation exposure, thyroiditis, or pregnancy.

Four small *parathyroid glands* are located on the thyroid gland. They secrete *parathyroid hormone*, which raises calcium levels in the blood. They work together with the thyroid gland to keep blood calcium at just the right level. (Turn to Chapter 14 for more about the thyroid and parathyroid glands.)

Fighting infection: The thymus

The *thymus gland* is located in the thoracic cavity, posterior to the sternum (the breastbone). It's part of the immune system and is made of lymphoid tissue (see Chapter 5 for more on the lymphatic system).

The function of the thymus gland is to take immature T cells (a type of white blood cells) and develop them into mature T cells that are capable of recognizing foreign substances that may cause damage to the body.

Stressing out: The suprarenals

The suprarenal glands sit atop the kidneys. They respond to stress, affect fluid balance in the body, and make a small amount of sex hormones:

- **Aldosterone:** Decreases sodium loss in the blood to regulate blood volume and blood pressure

- **Cortisol:** Helps regulate the body's use of proteins, fats, and carbohydrates and helps regulate blood pressure and heart function (see Chapter 4 for more information on the cardiovascular system)

- **Epinephrine (adrenaline):** Increases heart rate, increases blood flow to the brain and muscles, and takes glucose out of storage for use as fuel

- **Norepinephrine (noradrenaline):** Constricts blood vessels and increases blood pressure; also takes glucose out of storage to fuel the muscles and brain

- **Sex hormones:** Involved with the development of sex organs at the beginning of puberty

Flip to Chapter 10 for more about the suprarenals.

Digestive aid: The pancreas

Part of the pancreas makes digestive enzymes (as we explain earlier in this chapter), but another part makes *insulin,* which is a hormone that helps regulate carbohydrate metabolism and fat storage. It's secreted after a person consumes carbohydrates (starches or sugars).

People who can't make insulin have a condition called *type 1 diabetes mellitus.* People with *type 2 diabetes mellitus* either don't make enough insulin or can't use insulin properly. *Gestational diabetes* occurs during pregnancy. Diabetes results in elevated blood-sugar levels and can cause the person to feel thirsty or hungry more frequently than usual and urinate more frequently. Diabetes is diagnosed by urine tests that detect glucose (blood sugar) in the urine and blood tests that measure levels of blood glucose after a 12-hour fast. Treatment depends on the type and severity of the disease and includes insulin injections, medications that regulate glucose levels, and dietary interventions.

Considering cortisol conditions

The body responds differently when it has too much or too little cortisol:

✔ *Cushing's syndrome* is a condition where the body makes too much cortisol (or is exposed to corticosteroid medications). It causes weight gain, especially in the face, between the shoulders, and around the abdomen. It also causes thin skin and acne and can result in lower healing time from other health problems. Cushing's syndrome can be detected by measuring the levels of cortisol in the blood, saliva, and urine. Other tests, such as MRI or CT scans, may need to be performed to determine if the cause is due to a pituitary or suprarenal tumor. Treatment depends on the cause. Tumors may require surgery, and corticosteroid medications may require a slow decrease of the dosage.

✔ *Addison's disease* occurs when the body makes too little cortisol. People with Addison's disease suffer from weakness, fatigue, weight loss, darkened skin, salt cravings, depression, and low blood pressure. Addison's disease is diagnosed by the ACTH stimulation test, which involves measuring levels of cortisol in the blood, saliva, and urine before and after a synthetic version of ACTH (adrenocorticotropic hormone) is injected into the body. Normally the ACTH causes the cortisol levels to rise, but in Addison's disease, the levels remain low. Treatment involves taking synthetic forms of cortisol every day.

Mars and Venus: The testes and the ovaries

The testes and ovaries both produce male and female hormones. The testes are found in males, and the ovaries are found in females:

✔ **Testes:** The testes are two oval-shaped organs located in the scrotum, which is described in Chapter 9. The testes produce large amounts of *testosterone,* a male hormone that promotes development of male reproductive organs and masculine physical characteristics. It also stimulates production of sperm that's needed to fertilize an ovum. The testes also produce small amounts of estrogen and progesterone.

✔ **Ovaries:** The ovaries are in the female pelvis. They produce ova, which are the eggs needed to have babies. They also produce a little bit of testosterone and much more of the female hormones:

   • The *estrogens* affect sexual function and are responsible for development of female characteristics.

   • *Progesterone* prepares the lining of the uterus for receiving a fertilized ovum.

Check out Chapter 11 for more details about the testes and the ovaries.

Part II

Understanding the Thorax, Abdomen, and Pelvis

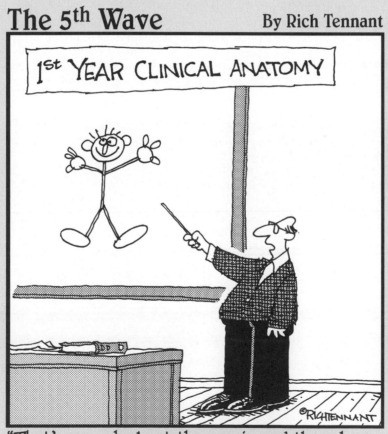

The 5th Wave   By Rich Tennant

"That's enough about the noggin and the schnoz. Let's move on to the tummy-wummy and the keister."

In this part . . .

Part II is a look at the three regions that comprise the body's trunk: the thorax, the abdomen, and the pelvis. Each of these regions has a framework made up of bones, muscles, and other soft tissues. These frameworks give the trunk its shape, and they also protect the delicate organs inside.

The internal organs and structures found in these regions work constantly to provide the rest of the body with oxygen and energy, and then they eliminate waste. In addition to explaining these different organs, this part talks about the anatomical features that make humans male or female.

Chapter 7

Checking Out the Thoracic Cage and Coverings

. . . .

In This Chapter

▶ Getting to know the bones, muscles, and other parts of the thoracic cage

▶ Identifying the thoracic-cage structures on top of the skin

. . . .

*P*hysical examination of the thoracic cage is important because it gives you the first view of the chest and back. You can see the skin, check out how the patient is breathing, and find the surface landmarks (indicated by bones and muscles) that help you locate the thoracic organs.

In this chapter, we look at what's going on under the skin to study the bones, joints, muscles, nerves, and blood vessels. Then we take a look at the surface landmarks for both the posterior and anterior chest walls (with the help of a few imaginary lines).

Getting Under Your Skin: Thoracic Bones, Joints, Muscles, and More

The thoracic cage is made up of bones and cartilage along with joints and an assortment of muscles and other soft tissues. The part that opens into the neck is called the *superior thoracic aperture* (see Figure 7-1), and the bottom of the thoracic cage (the *inferior thoracic aperture*) is closed by a muscle called the *diaphragm*. Its main function is to protect your heart, lungs, and major blood vessels located inside. The following sections explain what you need to know about the main parts of the thoracic cage.

Forming the thoracic cage: The bones

The bones that create the architecture of the thoracic cage include the sternum, the ribs, and the thoracic vertebrae. We talk about the sternum and ribs in the following sections (check them out in Figure 7-1); the thoracic vertebrae are covered in Chapter 15 along with the rest of the back.

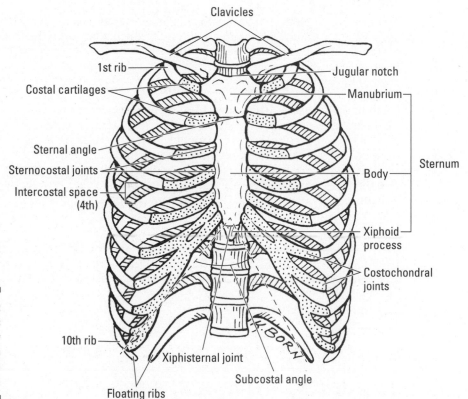

Clavicles
1st rib
Costal cartilages
Jugular notch
Manubrium
Sternal angle
Sternocostal joints
Intercostal space
(4th)
Body
Sternum
Xiphoid
process
Costochondral
joints
10th rib
Xiphisternal joint
Subcostal angle
Floating ribs

Figure 7-1:
The bones
and carti-
lage of the
thoracic
skeleton.

The sternum

The *sternum* is a flat, long bone that forms the medial and anterior part of the thoracic cage (in other words, the middle and front part). It has three parts, which you can see in Figure 7-1: manubrium, body, and xiphoid process.

✔ **Manubrium:** The *manubrium* forms the upper part of the sternum. The superior border (upper edge) has an indentation called the *jugular notch* (or *suprasternal notch*). It articulates (forms a joint) with the clavicles, or collarbones, at the *clavicular notches*. It also attaches to the cartilage of the first two ribs.

✔ ***Body:*** This part of the sternum is longer and more narrow than the manubrium. It articulates with the costal cartilages of the 2nd through 7th ribs on its sides and with the xiphoid process just below.

✔ ***Xiphoid process:*** This small piece of cartilage turns into bone during adulthood. It's located at the inferior (bottom) end of the sternal body at the *xiphisternal joint.*

The ribs

The ribs are 12 pairs (left and right) of flat, curved bones that give the thoracic cage its shape (refer to Figure 7-1). They articulate with the thoracic vertebrae in your back, and most of them are attached directly or indirectly to your sternum by *costal cartilages.* These cartilages help hold the thoracic cage to the sternum and add elasticity to the thoracic cage.

Each rib is separated from neighboring ribs by an *intercostal space* that runs between the ribs along their full lengths. You can see these spaces in Figure 7-1. Each of the 11 intercostal spaces is named for the rib above it. The space below the 12th rib (the last one) is called the *subcostal space.*

The ribs can be grouped in a couple different ways: either by how they're attached to the sternum or by their general anatomy. We start with how they attach to your sternum (refer to Figure 7-1):

✔ ***True ribs:*** The 1st through 7th pairs of ribs have their own costal cartilages that connect directly to the sternum.

✔ ***False ribs:*** The 8th, 9th, and 10th pairs of ribs each have their own costal cartilages, but they attach to the cartilage of the rib just above rather than directly to the sternum.

✔ ***Floating ribs:*** The last two pairs of ribs, the 11th and 12th, have little stumps of cartilage at their tips, but they don't connect with the sternum at all (hence the term *floating*).

Anatomically, all ribs are either *typical* or *atypical.*

✔ **Typical:** The 3rd through 9th ribs are similar anatomically, so they're called the *typical* ribs. The main parts of the typical ribs include the following:

• Each typical rib has a wedge-shaped *head* with two facets. One facet articulates with the vertebra of the same number as the rib, and the other facet joins the vertebra just above the rib.

• The *neck* connects the head to the thin flat *body* (or *shaft*), which curves strongly at the *angle.*

• The *tubercle* is located at the junction of the neck and body; it has a facet that articulates with the transverse process (see Chapter 15 for a description of vertebrae) of the corresponding vertebra.

✔ **Atypical:** The remaining ribs — the 1st, 2nd, 10th, 11th, and 12th — are called *atypical* because they don't look like the 3rd through 9th ribs. They have heads and bodies similar to typical ribs, but they differ from there.

- The 1st rib is an atypical rib that is smaller but wider than typical ribs and mostly horizontal. It has two grooves that allow passage of the subclavian vessels (see Chapter 14 for more info) that are separated by the *scalene tubercle.*

- The 2nd rib is a transitional rib. It is thinner, less curved, and longer than the 1st rib and has two facets on the head that articulate with the 1st and 2nd thoracic vertebrae. It also contains a tubercle (small, rounded point) for muscle attachment.

- The heads of the 10th and 11th ribs have only one facet each, and the 11th and 12th ribs are much shorter than other ribs, with no necks or tubercles.

A patient who comes to you with pain in the thoracic cage that gets worse when he or she bends or twists may have a bruised or cracked rib. A rib fracture isn't always visible on an X-ray, but X-rays can help determine whether the lungs have been damaged by broken ribs. Palpation (medical examination by touch) may identify a rib fracture, but as long as the lungs are undamaged, the treatment is about the same for both a fracture or a bruise: rest and pain relief. Breathing exercises may also be used to prevent pulmonary (lung and airway) complications.

Moving just a little: The joints

The cartilaginous joints in your thoracic cage allow you to breathe, but they don't have a large range of motion compared to a knee joint (see Chapter 20) or elbow joint (see Chapter 17). The 1st ribs don't move at all, but the act of breathing requires the other ribs to move up and down a bit, so the joints formed between the rest of the ribs and thoracic vertebrae allow for some movement. You can see some of these joints in Figure 7-1:

✔ *Manubriosternal joint:* The joint between the manubrium and the body of the sternum; forms the *sternal angle* (angle of Louis)

✔ *Xiphisternal joint:* Formed between the sternal body and xiphoid process

✔ *Costovertebral joints:* Formed between the heads of the ribs and the bodies of the vertebrae and the necks of the ribs and the transverse processes of the vertebrae

✔ *Sternocostal joints:* Join the sternum to the costal cartilages

✔ *Sternoclavicular joints:* Join the sternum and clavicles (which are part of the shoulder girdle covered in Chapter 16)

✔ *Costochondral joints:* Attach the ribs to the costal cartilages

✔ *Interchondral joints:* Join cartilage to cartilage

Helping you breathe: The respiratory muscles

Several muscles of the shoulder are attached to the thoracic cage, so they're discussed with the rest of the shoulder girdle in Chapter 16. The scalene muscles, which elevate the 1st and 2nd ribs and bend the neck to the side, are discussed in detail in Chapter 14, along with other structures in the neck. So what's left? In the following sections, we focus on the muscles of the thoracic cage that help you breathe — namely, the diaphragm and respiratory muscles.

The diaphragm

The main respiratory muscle found in the thorax is called the *diaphragm*. It's a thin muscle that curves up into two dome shapes called *cupulae.* The diaphragm separates the thoracic cavity from the abdominal cavity and has openings that allow structures to pass from one cavity to the other. (Flip to Chapter 10 for details on the abdominal cavity.)

The diaphragm can be divided into three parts:

✔ *Sternal part:* This part of the diaphragm originates (attaches) at the xiphoid process (see the earlier section "The sternum" for more about the xiphoid process).

✔ *Costal part:* This part originates from the lower six ribs and their cartilages.

✔ *Lumbar part:* This part of the diaphragm originates from the vertical columns by two tendinous structures (called *crura*) and by the medial and lateral arcuate ligaments.

The diaphragm is secured to the thoracic cage by the following ligaments and tendons:

✔ *Right crus:* This tendinous structure is attached to the sides of the first three lumbar vertebrae and discs. (Note that *crus* is the singular form of *crura.*) Some of its fibers form a loop around the esophageal orifice *(hiatus)* (see Chapter 10 for details on the esophagus).

- *Left crus:* This structure is attached to the first two lumbar vertebrae and the disc between them.

- *Median arcuate ligament:* This ligament connects the two crura.

- *Medial arcuate ligament:* This ligament attaches to part of the diaphragm as it extends from the 2nd lumbar vertebra to the transverse process of the 1st lumbar vertebra. It passes over the psoas muscles.

- *Lateral arcuate ligament:* This structure also attaches to part of the diaphragm as it runs from the transverse process of the 1st lumbar vertebra to the 12th rib. It lies over the quadratus lumborum muscle.

- *Central tendon:* The diaphragm inserts into this tendon, which is partially fused with the pericardium (see Chapter 8 for more info).

The diaphragm has three openings (hiatuses) that allow passage of various structures. We discuss most of those structures in Chapter 8, along with other thoracic organs, but here's a quick introduction to the openings:

- *Aortic opening:* This opening is just anterior to the 12th thoracic vertebra and allows room for the aorta, thoracic duct, and azygos vein.

- *Esophageal opening:* This opening is at the level of the 10th thoracic vertebra and transmits the esophagus, vagal nerves, esophageal branches of the gastric vessels, and some lymphatic vessels.

- *Caval opening:* At the level of the 8th thoracic vertebra, this opening leaves room for the inferior vena cava and terminal branches of the right phrenic nerve.

A hiccup is an involuntary contraction of the diaphragm. The space between your vocal folds snaps shut to stop the inflow of air caused by the spasm. It can happen after you eat or when the vagus or phrenic nerve is irritated.

The intercostal muscles and other muscles

Three muscles that help your diaphragm during breathing are located in the *intercostal spaces* between each of the ribs: the *external intercostal,* the *internal intercostal,* and the *innermost intercostal* muscles. The innermost intercostals are lined by the *endothoracic fascia* (a sheet of fibrous tissue), which in turn is lined by the parietal pleura (thin serous membrane). When the intercostal muscles contract, they bring the ribs closer together. You can see intercostal muscles in Figure 7-2.

When you breathe in, the 1st rib is held stable by the scalene muscles of the neck, and the rest of the ribs are elevated toward it. When you breathe out, the 12th rib is fixed by the quadratus lumborum and the oblique abdominal muscles (see Chapter 9 for more on abdominal muscles), and the ribs move downward.

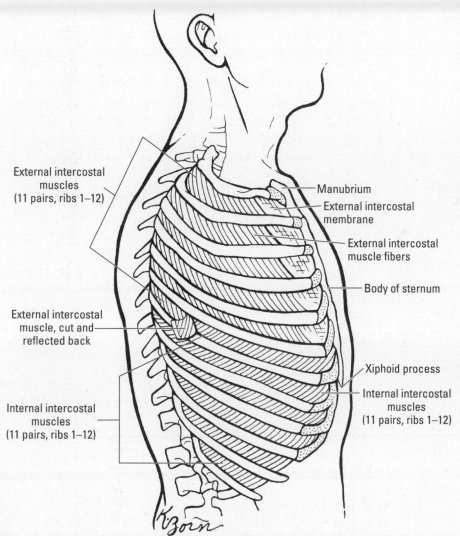

External intercostal
muscles
(11 pairs, ribs 1–12)

External intercostal
muscle, cut and
reflected back

Internal intercostal
muscles
(11 pairs, ribs 1–12)

Manubrium

External intercostal
membrane

External intercostal
muscle fibers

Body of sternum

Xiphoid process

Internal intercostal
muscles
(11 pairs, ribs 1–12)

Figure 7-2:
Intercostal
muscles.

Five additional muscle groups are found on each side of the thoracic cage:

- ✔ *Transversus thoracis muscles:* Run from the posterior (back) part of the sternum to the internal portion of the 2nd through 6th costal cartilages

- ✔ *Subcostal muscles:* Attach to the internal surface of the lower ribs and travel inferiorly to attach to the superior border of the second or third rib below

✔ *Levatores costarum muscles:* Start at the transverse processes of the 7th through 11th thoracic vertebrae and insert into the next rib below

✔ *Serratus posterior superior muscles:* Run from the spinous processes (posterior projections; visible as the bumps down the middle of the back) of the last cervical vertebrae and the first three thoracic vertebrae to the superior borders of the 2nd through 4th ribs

✔ *Serratus posterior inferior muscles:* Start at the spinous processes of the last two thoracic vertebrae and the first two lumbar vertebrae and attach to the inferior borders of the 8th through 12th ribs (near the angles)

Running through the thorax: The nerves and blood vessels

Spinal nerves innervate the muscles of the thoracic cage, and blood is carried through intercostal arteries and veins. You can find the info you need to know about these nerves and blood vessels in the following sections.

The nerves

The thoracic cage is innervated by 12 pairs of spinal nerves. Each spinal nerve leaves the vertebral canal via intervertebral foramina and then branches into an anterior and posterior ramus (see Chapter 15 for more about vertebral and spinal nerve anatomy). The anterior ramus runs along the inferior border of the rib in the intercostal space, becoming the *intercostal nerve.* The 12th anterior ramus is called the *subcostal nerve.* Check out Figure 7-3 to see some nerves as well as some muscles from the preceding section.

The intercostal nerves have many branches:

✔ *Rami communicantes:* These branches connect the intercostal nerves to ganglia of the sympathetic trunk, the string of interconnected sympathetic ganglia along each side of the vertebral column (see Chapter 3 for more info on the sympathetic nervous system).

✔ *Collateral branches:* These branches run just below the main nerve, on the rib below.

✔ *Lateral cutaneous branches:* These nerve branches innervate the skin of the side of the chest.

✔ ***Anterior cutaneous branches:*** These branches are the terminal portions of the anterior rami that innervate the skin of the anterior thorax.

✔ ***Muscular branches:*** These branches innervate the intercostal muscles.

✔ ***Pleural sensory branches:*** These branches innervate the parietal pleura.

✔ ***Peritoneal sensory branches:*** These branches run to the parietal peritoneum (thin serous membrane lining the abdominal wall) on the 7th through 11th intercostal nerves.

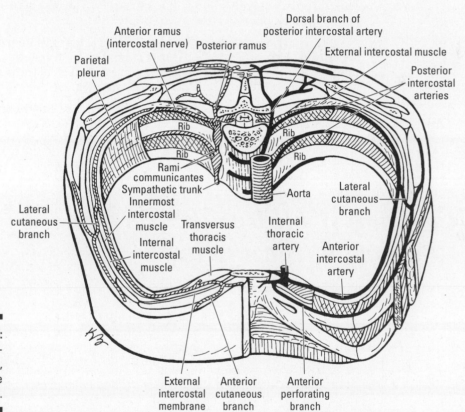

Figure 7-3: An intercostal space, transverse section.

The diaphragm gets its motor-nerve supply from the phrenic nerves (sometimes we say, "C3, 4, 5 keep the diaphragm alive"). The sensory nerve supply comes from the phrenic nerve and the lower six intercostal nerves (see Chapter 3 for more about sensory and motor nerves).

The arteries and veins

The thoracic wall is served by a bunch of arteries and veins (refer to Figure 7-3 to see a few of them).

✔ **Anterior intercostal arteries:** The first six anterior intercostal arteries stem directly from the internal thoracic artery. The rest of them branch off the musculophrenic artery (see Chapter 8).

✔ **Posterior intercostal arteries:** Two of these arteries branch off the superior intercostal artery in the first two intercostal spaces, and the remaining posterior intercostal arteries are branches of the descending thoracic aorta (which we talk about in Chapter 8).

✔ **Anterior intercostal veins:** These veins return blood to the internal thoracic and musculophrenic veins.

✔ **Posterior intercostal veins:** Most of these veins return blood to the azygos and hemiazygos veins (see Chapter 8).

Covering It All Up: The Surface Anatomy of the Thorax

The thoracic cage is covered by skin, which you can assess for color, texture, and visible lesions or disfigurations such as scars, moles, rashes, and/or discolorations (see Chapter 5 for more information on the skin, technically known as the *integumentary system*). As you find out in the following sections, using imaginary lines and bony landmarks on the front and back of the thorax helps you describe locations of the anatomical structures that we describe earlier in this chapter.

Using imaginary lines in your assessment

The easiest way to assess the surface anatomy of the thorax is to use several sets of imaginary lines (you were expecting something more complicated, right?). The lines cover the front, side, and back of the thorax.

Three imaginary vertical lines on the anterior wall give you points of reference:

- *Midsternal (anterior median) line:* Runs down the middle of the sternum (that's easy enough to remember!)

- *Right and left midclavicular lines:* Run parallel with the midsternal line, passing through the midpoint of each clavicle (see Chapter 16 for more about the clavicles)

Three more vertical lines demarcate the lateral portion of the thoracic cage:

- *Anterior axillary line:* Runs along the anterior axial fold (fold of skin where the armpit meets the pectoralis, or chest muscle), close to the front of the thorax

- *Posterior axillary line:* Runs parallel with the anterior axillary line along the posterior axillary fold (where the armpit meets the back muscle), close to the back

- *Midaxillary line:* Runs midway between the anterior and posterior axillary lines, starting at the deepest part of the axilla (armpit)

Finally, three lines help describe surface locations on the back:

- *Midvertebral (posterior median) line:* Runs vertically down the midpoint of the spine

- *Right and left scapular lines:* Run parallel with the midvertebral (posterior median) line but pass through the inferior angles of the scapulae (see Chapter 16)

Looking at the anterior chest wall

The anterior of the chest is a main area for physical examination. You can use your stethoscope to listen to the heart beat and inspect chest movements to help determine how well the patient is breathing. You'll also find the breasts on the anterior chest wall.

Landmarks indicated by bones and muscles

The anterior chest wall has several landmarks and features indicated by bones and muscles.

- *Clavicles:* The *clavicles* are visible and palpable bony structures located just below the neck. They each articulate medially with the manubrium of the sternum. You can palpate the suprasternal (jugular) notch at the top of the manubrium. The superior vena cava (a main vein that enters the heart) passes behind the manubrium.

✔ *Sternal angle:* The sternal angle is located at the level of the 2nd costal cartilages and corresponds to the level of the disc space between the 4th and 5th thoracic vertebrae.

The sternal angle is found at the level of the second ribs, which are easy to locate — just put your fingers on the clavicle near its articulation with the manubrium and slide your fingers inferiorly. You'll feel an indentation (the 1st intercostal space) then the 2nd rib is below that. Don't worry about the 1st rib here, it's hidden behind the clavicle. The primary bronchi (airways to the lungs) split apart from the trachea behind the sternal angle. It's also the location for the beginning of the aortic arch, the large artery that leaves the heart.

✔ *Sternum:* The body of the sternum is palpable in the midline of the chest between the breasts. The right border of the heart lies posterior to it. Near the sternum are four areas that are used for auscultating (listening to with a stethoscope) the heart:

- *Aortic area:* At the 2nd intercostal space to the right of the sternum

- *Pulmonic area:* At the 2nd intercostal space to the left of the sternum

- *Tricuspid area:* Over the lower left sternal border

- *Mitral area:* At the left 5th intercostal space at the midclavicular line

Sternal deformities include *pectus excavatum,* which is a congenital concavity, and *pectus carinatum,* in which the sternum protrudes outwardly. Sternal deformities may have an alarming appearance, but they don't usually cause any functional problems for the patient.

✔ *Subcostal angle:* The *subcostal angle* is at the inferior (lower) portion of the sternum, between the 7th costal cartilages. Imagine drawing lines that follow the *costal margins* (lower borders of the anterior rib cage) and meet at the lower part of the sternum. The angle they form is the subcostal angle. The xiphoid process of the sternum marks the level of the superior portion of the liver, the inferior part of the heart, and the central tendon of the diaphragm.

✔ *Costal margins:* The *costal margins* are formed by the medial portions of the 7th through 10th costal cartilages. They may be visible in a thin patient, and they're easily palpable. (As a matter of fact, all the ribs can be palpated, except for the 1st ribs, and may be visible in thin patients.)

✔ *Apex beat of the heart:* The *apex beat of the heart* is caused by the contractions of the heart as it beats. You can usually feel it at the 5th intercostal space on the left side (the mitral area), about 3.5 inches from the midline. To find the 5th intercostal space, find the 2nd rib (as described earlier in this list) and just slide your fingers inferiorly. Don't forget to keep count as you go.

✔ **Axillary folds:** *Axillary folds* frame the *axillae,* or armpits. The *anterior axillary fold* is formed by the lower border of the pectoralis major muscle, and the *posterior axillary fold* is formed by the latissimus dorsi and teres major muscles. (We talk about everything related to the axillae in Chapter 16.)

The breasts

The *breasts* are prominently displayed on the anterior chest wall, especially in females. The *intermammary cleft* is formed by the cleavage between the breasts. The *nipples* are near the midclavicular line (which we locate in "Using imaginary lines in your assessment") and are surrounded by a raised and pigmented area called the *areola.* In men, the nipples are at the level of the 4th intercostal space, but in women, the level varies greatly.

The *mammary glands* in the breasts of females are normally more developed than in males. They gradually enlarge as a female goes through puberty, partially due to the growth of ducts, but mostly due to fat deposition. These developmental changes are due to various hormonal influences.

The bases of the breasts extend laterally from the edge of the sternum to the midaxillary line. The *axillary tails* of the breasts travel upward and laterally toward the axilla.

Each breast can be divided up into four quadrants to make describing your examination findings easier:

✔ The superolateral quadrant (upper outside)

✔ The inferolateral quadrant (lower outside)

✔ The superomedial quadrant (upper and toward the midline of the body)

✔ The inferomedial quadrant (lower and toward the midline of the body)

The breast consists of 15 to 20 lobes of glandular tissue. Each lobe has a *lactiferous duct* that opens onto the surface of the nipple. Each duct has a dilated portion called the *lactiferous sinus,* or *ampulla,* located in the connective tissue deep to the areola.

The nerves of the breast come from the anterior and lateral cutaneous branches of the 4th to 6th intercostal nerves. They supply sensory fibers to the skin and sympathetic fibers (part of the nervous system that controls autonomic functions like blood flow — see Chapter 3 for more info) to the blood vessels and smooth muscles of the nipple and skin.

The blood supply to the breasts comes from the perforating branches of the internal thoracic artery and the intercostal arteries. The lateral thoracic and thoracoacromial branches of the axillary artery may also supply blood. Venous drainage is mainly through the axillary vein, with some flow through the internal thoracic vein. Check out Figure 7-4 for details.

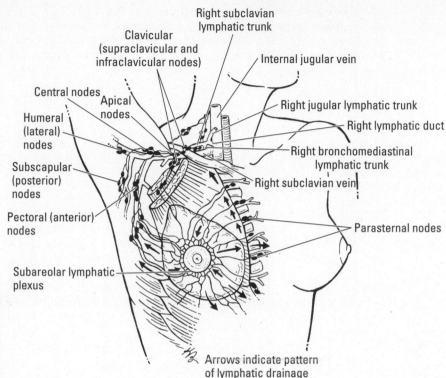

Clavicular
(supraclavicular and
infraclavicular nodes)

Right subclavian
lymphatic trunk

Internal jugular vein

Central nodes

Apical
nodes

Humeral
(lateral)
nodes

Subscapular
(posterior)
nodes

Pectoral (anterior)
nodes

Subareolar lymphatic
plexus

Right jugular lymphatic trunk

Right lymphatic duct

Right bronchomediastinal
lymphatic trunk

Right subclavian vein

Parasternal nodes

Figure 7-4:
The lymph
drainage of
the breast.

Arrows indicate pattern
of lymphatic drainage

Lymph drainage of the breasts is important due to its role in the spread of cancer cells. Lymph flows from the nipple, areola, and lobes to the *subareolar lymphatic plexus.* From there, most lymph drains from the lateral quadrants to the axillary lymph nodes (see Chapter 16). The medial quadrants drain to the *parasternal lymph nodes,* whereas lymph from the inferior quadrants of the breasts passes into the abdominal lymph nodes.

Possible signs of breast cancer include skin dimpling, abnormal contours, edema that causes an orange-peel effect, and nipple retraction and deviation.

Examining the posterior chest wall

When you look at your patient from behind, you see the skin, of course, and depending on the physical condition of the person you may also see the ribs or the outlines of the musculature of the back. Imagine the midvertebral (posterior median) line running down the middle of the back. Some of the spinous processes of the thoracic vertebrae may be visible, or at least palpable. The spinous process for the 7th cervical vertebra (vertebral prominens) is almost always palpable and serves as a good landmark for noting the location of any examination findings of the posterior chest wall. Check out Chapter 15 for detailed information on assessing the surface anatomy of the vertebrae.

The *scapulae,* or shoulder blades, are easy to find on each side of the spine. They're flat, triangular bones located on the upper portion of the posterior chest wall. The superior angles at the top of the scapulae are at the level of the 2nd thoracic vertebrae. The spines of the scapulae are generally easy to palpate as they run obliquely toward the shoulders. You can follow the medial border of each scapula down to the inferior angle, which is at the level of the 7th thoracic vertebra. You can find detailed information on examining the shoulder blades in Chapter 16.

The posterior part of the thoracic cage can be distorted due to certain medical disorders, such as in the following cases:

- *Scoliosis* is a rotation and lateral flexion of the spine that may twist and turn the thoracic cage.

- An arthritic disease of the vertebral joints, *ankylosing spondylitis,* results in hyperkyphosis (an abnormal increase in the thoracic curvature) and may restrict lung expansion if the disease spreads superiorly. It may lead to fusion of intervertebral joints and spinal column rigidity.

Chapter 8

Assessing the Thoracic Organs

. . . .

. . . .

The thoracic cavity is basically the chest, including everything between the neck and the diaphragm. It's home to the thoracic organs and is protected by the thoracic cage described in Chapter 7. The heart and lungs are essential for survival and both are prone to certain diseases, so you need to be able to examine them. This chapter explores the locations and anatomy of the structures in the thoracic cavity, including the heart, lungs, major vessels, and other organs.

Understanding the Mediastinum and Pleural Cavities

The thoracic cavity has three compartments: the mediastinum and two pleural cavities. The mediastinum is home to the heart, trachea, great vessels, and some other structures. The pleural cavities are on either side of the mediastinum and contain the lungs and the pleural linings. We describe all three of these compartments in the following sections.

The mediastinum

The *mediastinum* is the compartment that takes up the middle portion of the thoracic cavity. It's lined by *mediastinal pleura* and extends from the *superior thoracic aperture* (where the thoracic cavity opens into the neck) down to the *diaphragm* (the main muscle for breathing; we discuss the diaphragm in more detail later in this chapter). It has several different regions:

✔ **Superior mediastinum:** This region covers the area from the superior thoracic aperture to a horizontal plane at the level of the intervertebral disc between the 4th and 5th thoracic vertebrae (Chapter 15 has details on vertebrae). It contains the superior vena cava, brachiocephalic veins, arch of the aorta, thoracic duct, trachea, thymus, and vagus and phrenic nerves.

✔ **Inferior mediastinum:** This region of the mediastinum starts where the superior mediastinum leaves off and extends inferiorly (in other words, toward the feet) to the diaphragm. It has three sections:

  • The *anterior mediastinum* contains lymph nodes, fat, connective tissue, and remnants of the thymus (it shrinks after childhood). It's close to the front of the body.

  • The *middle mediastinum* is home to the pericardium, heart, arch of the azygos vein, main bronchi, and roots of the great vessels.

  • The *posterior mediastinum* contains the esophagus, thoracic aorta, azygos and hemiazygos veins, vagus nerve, sympathetic trunks, and splanchnic nerves. It's close to the rear of the thorax.

We cover all the arteries, veins, nerves, and other structures in the preceding list throughout this chapter.

The pleural cavities

Two pleural cavities house the lungs, one on each side of the mediastinum. Each lung is covered by a pleural sac, which is made up of two layers of pleura, which you can see in Figure 8-1:

✔ **Visceral pleura:** This pleura adheres to the lungs.

✔ **Parietal pleura:** Lining the cavities and attached to the thoracic wall, the mediastinum, and the diaphragm, this pleura has four parts:

  • The *costal part* covers the sternum, ribs and cartilage, intercostal muscles (as described in Chapter 7), and sides of the thoracic vertebrae (see Chapter 15).

  • The *mediastinal part* covers the sides of the mediastinum.

  • The *diaphragmatic part* covers the parts of the diaphragm on each side of the mediastinum.

  • The *cervical pleura* runs from the superior thoracic aperture into the root of the neck to form a dome over the lungs.

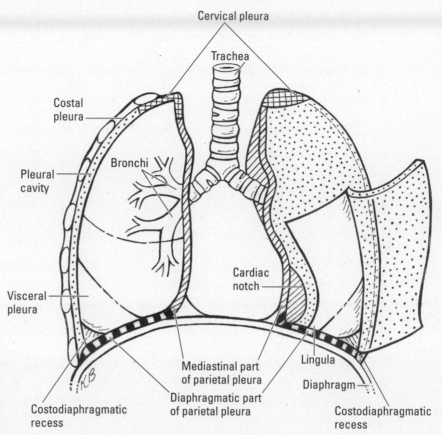

Cervical pleura

Trachea

Costal pleura

Bronchi

Pleural cavity

Visceral pleura

Cardiac notch

Lingula

Mediastinal part of parietal pleura

Diaphragmatic part of parietal pleura

Diaphragm

Costodiaphragmatic recess

Costodiaphragmatic recess

Figure 8-1: Looking at the lungs and pleura.

Each cavity contains recessed spaces called the *costodiaphragmatic* and *costo-mediastinal recesses,* which allow room for full expansion of the lungs during inspiration (breathing in).

Looking at the Lungs

Everyone needs oxygen to live. The *lungs* are pink spongy organs to the left and right of the heart that provide the means to get oxygen from the air into your red blood cells. You can see the lungs in Figure 8-1. In the following sections, we delve into the lungs' surfaces, borders, trachea, bronchi, lobes, nerves, blood vessels, and lymphatics.

Surveying the lungs' surfaces and borders

Each lung has an *apex* at the superior end (in other words, at the end closer to the head) that rises above the level of the 1st rib and into the root of the neck (see Chapter 14 for the scoop on the neck). Each lung also has three surfaces:

- ✔ *Costal surface:* Next to the sternum, ribs, and costal cartilage
- ✔ *Mediastinal surface:* The hilum (see the later section "Branching into the bronchi") and the medial (middle) surfaces of the lung
- ✔ *Diaphragmatic surface:* The underside of the lungs, just above the diaphragm

Each lung has three borders where the surfaces meet:

- ✔ *Anterior border:* Closer to the front of the body; lies between the costal and mediastinal surfaces.

  The anterior border of the left lung is indented by the *cardiac notch* to make room for the heart. You can check out this notch in Figure 8-1. The anteroinferior border of the cardiac notch forms the lingula, a tongue-like projection of the superior lobe.

- ✔ *Inferior border:* Closer to the feet; separates the diaphragmatic surface from the mediastinal and costal surfaces.

- ✔ *Posterior border:* Closer to the rear of the body; lies between the costal and mediastinal surfaces.

Getting air in and out with the trachea

Before the lungs can oxygenate the blood, they need air, which is provided by the airways, starting with the trachea. The *trachea* (which you can see in Figure 8-1), also sometimes called the *windpipe,* is a tube made up of incomplete cartilaginous rings that connects the larynx with the lungs. It terminates in a bifurcation, creating the right and left primary (main) bronchi. The trachea is covered in greater detail in Chapter 14 on the structures of the neck.

Branching into the bronchi

Two primary *bronchi* run from the bifurcation of the trachea to the hila of the lungs. What are hila, you ask? *Hila* is the plural of *hilum,* and the *hilum* is the part of the lung where the bronchus and pulmonary artery enter and the pulmonary vein exits the lungs. The bronchi, arteries, and veins are referred to collectively as the *root of the lung* and reside in the hilar spaces (See the later section "Vital blood vessels" for more about pulmonary arteries and veins.)

The right primary bronchus is wider and shorter than the left primary bronchus. It also runs more vertically. The left primary bronchus passes underneath the arch of the aorta and anterior to the esophagus (we discuss both the aorta and the esophagus later in this chapter).

The primary bronchi enter the hila of the lungs and form the bronchial trees by first dividing into the secondary bronchi (one for each lobe of each lung) and then into tertiary bronchi.

A *bronchopulmonary segment* is a portion of the lung served by a tertiary bronchus, a branch of the pulmonary artery, and is drained by tributaries of the pulmonary veins located in the connective tissue between the adjacent segments (see the later section "Vital blood vessels"). The right lung has ten bronchopulmonary segments, and the left lung has eight.

In each bronchopulmonary segment, the bronchi form more branches that eventually end in *terminal bronchioles*. Each terminal bronchiole divides into many respiratory bronchioles that lead to outpouchings for the exchange of gases. Each respiratory bronchiole has up to 11 *alveolar ducts*. Each duct has up to six outpouchings called *alveolar sacs* surrounded with capillaries. Each alveolar sac contains alveoli where gas exchange between the air and the blood takes place (as we introduce in Chapter 4).

Asthma is a disease of the lungs that causes the walls of the bronchi and bronchioles to swell and become too narrow as a result of inflammatory responses. Asthmatics (people with asthma) also produce extra mucus. Asthma makes breathing difficult and results in coughing, wheezing, and shortness of breath. A pulmonary-function test called *spirometry* confirms the presence of asthma, and it's treated with medication that dilates the bronchi and bronchioles, along with removal of any environmental factors that trigger asthmatic attacks.

Checking out the lobes

The right lung is just a little bit larger than the left lung, and it has three sections, called *lobes*. They're referred to as the *upper, middle,* and *lower lobes*. They're marked by two *fissures,* or deep grooves: the oblique fissure and the horizontal fissure. The horizontal fissure divides the upper and middle lobes, and the oblique fissure divides the middle and lower lobes.

The left lung is a bit smaller, and it has the *cardiac notch,* an indentation that makes room for the heart. The left lung has only two lobes, the *upper lobe* and the *lower lobe,* which are separated by the *oblique fissure*.

Pneumonia is an infection of the lung usually caused by viruses, bacteria, or fungi. Common symptoms include cough, fever, chills, trouble breathing, and possibly headaches, energy loss, and chest pain. Antibiotics may be prescribed if the cause is bacterial. Regardless of the cause, rest, drinking plenty of fluids, and analgesics (painkillers) are the typical courses of action.

Flowing with nerves, blood vessels, and lymphatics

The lungs need nerves to keep you breathing, and they also need blood supply and lymph drainage to perform their vital functions. And don't forget they also need to resupply the blood that comes to the lungs for gas exchange. We discuss the lungs' nerves, blood vessels, and lymphatics in the following sections.

Necessary nerves

The nerves that serve the lungs come from the pulmonary plexuses (networks of nerves) that are located anterior and posterior to the roots. They contain sympathetic fibers from the sympathetic trunks and parasympathetic fibers from the vagus nerve (see Chapter 12).

- **Sympathetic stimulation:** Causes bronchodilation (in other words, it widens the bronchial openings) and constricts the blood vessels

- **Parasympathetic stimulation:** Constricts the bronchi, dilates blood vessels, and increases glandular secretions

Flip to Chapter 3 for more about the sympathetic and parasympathetic nervous systems.

Vital blood vessels

The blood vessels that supply the lungs with blood for gas exchange include the pulmonary arteries that leave the heart with oxygen-poor blood (unlike other arteries in the body) and the pulmonary veins that return oxygen-rich blood to the heart:

- *Pulmonary trunk:* Leaves the right ventricle of the heart and splits into the *right* and *left pulmonary arteries,* each of which go to the respective lung

- *Pulmonary arteries:* Branch off into *lobar* and *segmental arteries* within the lungs

- ✔ *Pulmonary capillaries:* Surround the alveolar sacs

- ✔ *Lobar* and *segmental veins:* Form from the merger of capillaries and drain into four *pulmonary veins* (two for each lung), which empty into the left atrium of the heart

Note: We talk about the ventricles and atria of the heart in the later section "Putting together the four chambers."

Blood supply to the bronchi and connective tissue comes from the bronchial arteries. The left bronchial arteries (usually two) branch off the thoracic aorta. The right bronchial artery may stem from a superior posterior intercostal artery, the thoracic aorta, or a left superior bronchial artery. (See the later section "Circulating blood in the major vessels" for more about these structures.)

Venous blood is returned from the lung structures by bronchial veins and by the pulmonary veins. The right bronchial vein drains into the *azygos vein.* The left bronchial vein drains into the *accessory hemiazygos vein* or the *superior intercostal vein.*

A pulmonary embolism is a blockage in one of the arteries of the lungs. It's usually caused by blood clots that travel up to the lungs from the legs. Blood clots can form after prolonged immobilization in a bed (or even remaining seated during prolonged car trip), after surgery or leg injuries, or due to conditions that increase the clotting of blood cells. Treatment includes giving oxygen, using medications that break up the clots, and using medications to elevate blood pressure if needed.

Lively lymphatics

Two lymphatic plexuses drain lymph from the lungs:

- ✔ *Superficial lymphatic plexus:* Lying under the visceral pleura that we discuss in the earlier section "The pleural cavities," this plexus drains lymph from the lung tissue and the visceral pleura. The plexus drains into the *bronchopulmonary lymph nodes.*

- ✔ *Deep lymphatic plexus:* This plexus is in the mucosal layers and connective tissue of the bronchi. It drains the roots of the lung and passes that lymph into the *pulmonary lymph nodes.*

All lymph from the lungs drains into the *tracheobronchial lymph nodes,* which are located near the bifurcation of the trachea. From there the lymph drains to the *right* and *left bronchomediastinal lymph trunks,* which end near the junction of the subclavian and internal jugular veins (see Chapter 14).

✔ The right bronchomediastinal lymph trunk merges with other trunks to form the right lymphatic duct.

✔ The left bronchomediastinal lymph trunk ends at the thoracic duct.

The right lymphatic duct and thoracic duct return lymph to the blood (more about them later).

Classifying types of lung cancer

Lung cancer is a disease that occurs when abnormal lung cells grow out of control. They don't function like normal cells, so as they grow they impair the function of the lungs. Lung cancers can be classified in one of two groups: small-cell lung cancer or non-small-cell lung cancer.

In small-cell lung cancer, cells multiply quickly and form large tumors that not only grow in the lungs but can spread to other parts of the body. This disease is almost always caused by smoking.

Non-small-cell lung cancers are more common than small-cell cancers; they make up about 80 percent of lung cancers. Following are the different types of non-small-cell cancers:

✔ *Squamous-cell carcinoma* forms in the lining of the bronchi. It's the most common type of non-small-cell cancer and the most common type found in men.

✔ *Adenocarcinoma* occurs in the mucus-producing parts of the lungs. It's the most common form of cancer in women and in nonsmokers.

✔ *Bronchiolavleolar carcinoma* is a rare form of adenocarcinoma that occurs near the alveoli.

✔ *Large-cell undifferentiated carcinoma* forms near the surface of the lungs.

✔ *Mesothelioma* is a type of cancer that occurs in the pleura. It's nearly always caused by exposure to asbestos fibers that were commonly used in building insulation.

Symptoms of lung cancer include chest pain, coughing that won't go away, unexpected weight loss, shortness of breath, wheezing, fatigue, and possibly coughing up blood. Diagnostic procedures include X-rays, CT scans, MRI (see Chapter 23 for more info on ways to look into the body without cutting it open) and taking samples of sputum (spit). Treatment depends on the type of cancer, but may include surgery, chemotherapy medication, radiation, and medications to alleviate pain and improve breathing when necessary.

Having a Heart

The heart is a muscular four-chambered pump that beats constantly to keep blood flowing to the rest of your body, from the top of your head to the tip of your toes. In the following sections, we describe the sac that surrounds the heart, as well as the surfaces, chambers, vessels, and nerves of the heart.

Surrounding the heart with the pericardium

The *pericardium* is a fluid-filled sac that encloses the heart and the proximal part (in other words, the part of the vessel closest to the heart) of the great vessels. It has several parts:

- ✔ *Fibrous pericardium:* This outer covering of the pericardium attaches to the central tendon of the diaphragm.

- ✔ *Serous pericardium:* This internal part has two layers: the parietal layer and the visceral layer.

    • The *parietal layer* lines the fibrous pericardium.

    • The *visceral layer* covers the heart and forms the *epicardium.*

    The pericardial cavity lies between these two layers and contains a small amount of fluid.

Blood is supplied to the pericardium by the *pericardiacophrenic arteries,* which are branches of the internal thoracic arteries. Venous blood is drained by tributaries of the internal thoracic and azygos veins. The pericardium is innervated by the phrenic nerve, the vagus nerve, and branches of the sympathetic trunks (all of which we cover in this chapter).

Examining the surfaces of the heart

The heart is located in the middle of the thorax, with the apex (the more pointed part) facing toward the left and inferiorly, at the level of the 5th intercostal space (between the ribs; see Chapter 7). The base of the heart is the posterior part of the heart (you can see the exterior of the heart in Figure 8-2).

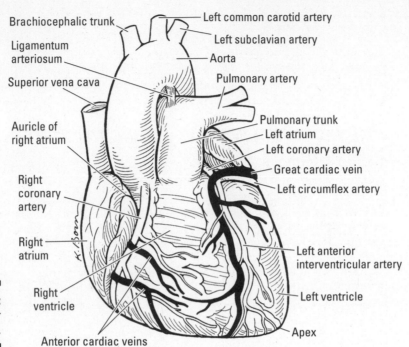

Brachiocephalic trunk — Left common carotid artery
Ligamentum arteriosum — Left subclavian artery
— Aorta
Superior vena cava — Pulmonary artery
Auricle of right atrium
Pulmonary trunk
Left atrium
Left coronary artery
Great cardiac vein
Left circumflex artery
Right coronary artery
Right atrium
Left anterior interventricular artery
Right ventricle
Left ventricle
Apex
Anterior cardiac veins

Figure 8-2: The exterior of the heart.

The heart has four surfaces:

- ✔ *Sternocostal surface:* The anterior portion formed mostly by the right ventricle

- ✔ *Diaphragmatic surface:* The inferior portion formed by the left ventricle and part of the right ventricle

- ✔ *Left pulmonary surface:* Made up of the surface of the left ventricle

- ✔ *Right pulmonary surface:* Made up by the surface of the right atrium

The heart has four *ausculatory areas* (spots on the chest where the sounds produced by the heart's valves closing are strongest). Identifying these areas helps you know where to place the diaphragm of a stethoscope so you can hear the heart:

- ✔ *Aortic area:* This area is located at the 2nd intercostal space to the right of the sternum.

- ✔ *Pulmonic area:* This area is at the 2nd intercostal space, to the left of the sternum.

> ✔ ***Tricuspid area:*** The tricuspid area is over the lower left part of the sternum.
>
> ✔ ***Mitral area:*** This location is at the 5th intercostal space at the midclavicular line on the left side of the chest wall. This area is where the *apex beat* can be heard or palpated. The apex beat is created when the apex of the heart hits the thoracic wall when the ventricles contract.

Putting together the four chambers

As you find out in the following sections, the interior of the heart is divided into four separate chambers: two atria and two ventricles. The divided chambers keep the oxygen-poor blood that needs to go to the lungs away from the blood that's oxygenated and ready to flow to the rest of the body. The walls of the heart consist of three layers: the *epicardium* (external layer formed by the visceral layer of the serous pericardium), the *myocardium* (middle layer of cardiac muscle), and the *endocardium* (internal layer of endothelium).

Atria

The two atria are simply called *the right atrium* and the *left atrium.* The right atrium receives venous blood from the superior vena cava, inferior vena cava, and the coronary sinus (find out more about those blood vessels later in this chapter). The left atrium receives blood from the pulmonary veins. You can see some of these structures in Figure 8-3.

The *right atrium* has a small pouch called the *right auricle,* which provides a little more room for blood. The smooth posterior part of the atrium, called the *sinus venarum,* is where the superior and inferior vena cava and the coronary sinus empty into the chamber. *Pectinate muscles* form a rough wall, and the *interatrial septum* lies between the left and right atria. The *fossa ovalis* is a depression in the wall of the septum. It's the remnant of the *foramen ovale,* which is an opening between the two atria. The foramen ovale allows blood to pass from the right atrium to the left atrium of a developing fetus.

The *left atrium* forms a large part of the base of the heart. Just like the right atrium, it has pectinate muscles and an auricle (the *left auricle,* of course). It has a thicker wall than the right atrium, and it receives oxygenated blood from the four pulmonary veins.

Ventricles

When the atria contract, blood is forced into the left and right ventricles through atrioventricular orifices. The right and left ventricles are visible in Figure 8-3. The right ventricle forms the bulk of the anterior surface, and the left ventricle forms the apex and most of the diaphragmatic and left surfaces of the heart.

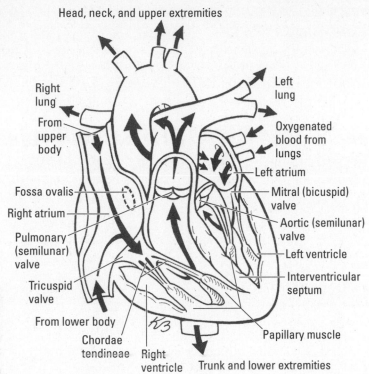

Head, neck, and upper extremities

Right lung

From upper body

Left lung

Oxygenated blood from lungs

Left atrium

Fossa ovalis

Right atrium

Pulmonary (semilunar) valve

Tricuspid valve

Mitral (bicuspid) valve

Aortic (semilunar) valve

Left ventricle

Interventricular septum

Chordae tendineae

Right ventricle

From lower body

Papillary muscle

Trunk and lower extremities

Figure 8-3: The internal parts of the heart.

The *right atrioventricular orifice* is guarded by the *right atrioventricular (tricuspid) valve,* which consists of a fibrous ring and three cusps. Tendinous cords called *chordae tendineae* are attached to the cusps and to the *papillary muscles* of the ventricle. These cords hold the cusps in place during a ventricular contraction, preventing backflow of blood into the right atrium. The left *atrioventricular orifice* is guarded by a similar valve called the *left atrioventricular (bicuspid; mitral) valve,* which has two cusps instead of three.

The interior of the right ventricle is somewhat cone shaped. Its anterior portion, the *conus arteriosus,* is the location of the entrance to the pulmonary trunk (see the earlier section "Vital blood vessels"). It's controlled by the *pulmonary (semilunar) valve,* which consists of three cusps that keep blood from flowing back into the ventricle. The right ventricle has muscular elevations called the *trabeculae carneae* and a muscular ridge called the *supraventricular crest. Papillary muscles* form conical projections.

The interior of the left ventricle has a longer conical cavity, and the walls are much thicker than in the right ventricle. The trabeculae carneae and papillary muscles are larger than those found in the right ventricle. During ventricular contractions, blood is pumped through the *aortic (semilunar) valve* into the aorta. The aortic valve prevents backflow of blood into the left ventricle.

The ventricles are separated by an *interventricular septum*. The *septomarginal trabecula* is a muscular bundle that runs from the interventricular septum to the anterior papillary muscle of the right ventricle.

Feeding the heart: Arteries and veins

The heart needs its own nutrient and oxygen supply so it can keep beating every day, all day long. The right and left coronary arteries supply the heart with oxygenated blood.

The *right coronary artery* starts from the right aortic sinus (see more about the aorta later in this chapter) and travels through the *coronary sulcus* located between the right atrium and ventricle. It has four branches:

- *Sinoatrial nodal artery:* Supplies the sinoatrial node (see the next section)

- *Right marginal artery:* Runs to the inferior part of the heart and apex and serves the right ventricle

- *Posterior interventricular artery:* Runs to the apex via the posterior interventricular groove located on the surface of the heart between the ventricles and supplies blood to both ventricles and the posterior portion of the septum

- *Atrioventricular nodal artery:* Supplies blood to the atrioventricular node (see the next section)

The *left coronary artery* leaves the left aortic sinus and runs through the *atrioventricular groove* that's located between the atria and ventricles on the surface of the heart. Here are three branches:

- *Anterior interventricular artery:* Runs along the anterior interventricular groove to the apex; provides blood to the right and left ventricles and anterior part of the interventricular septum

- *Circumflex artery:* Runs to the posterior part of the heart, and it provides blood to the left atrium and left ventricle

- *Left marginal artery:* Runs on the left side of the heart to provide blood to the left ventricle

Refer to Figure 8-2 to see some of the preceding coronary arteries.

Coronary heart disease is the narrowing of the coronary arteries caused by the buildup of plaque within the walls. This results in decreased blood flow (and decreased oxygen) to the heart muscles. A *myocardial infarction,* or heart attack, can occur when blockage of a coronary artery results in damage to the heart musculature. The symptoms of a myocardial infarction include chest pain that may feel like squeezing or pressure on the chest. Pain may also be present in other parts of the body, including the shoulder and arm (usually on the left), belly, neck, or jaw. Can you prevent a heart attack? Family history is a factor, but the risk can be reduced by lowering elevated blood pressure, addressing high cholesterol levels, losing weight, not smoking, exercising, and eating a healthy diet.

Most of the veins that drain blood from the heart muscles and structures empty into the *coronary sinus,* which is the main vein of the heart. It runs along the backside of the heart. The veins that flow into the coronary sinus include the *great, middle,* and *small cardiac veins,* the *left posterior ventricular vein,* and the *left marginal vein.* You can see some of these veins in Figure 8-2.

Small anterior cardiac veins empty directly into the right atrium, and the *smallest cardiac veins* drain into all four chambers but mostly the atria.

Giving the heart its spark

The constant beating of the heart is controlled by the *conducting system of the heart,* which is a series of specialized nerve tissues that fire through the heart and coordinate the actions of the heart beat (check out Figure 8-4):

- ✔ **Sinoatrial (SA) node:** This pacemaker initiates the impulse. It's located anterolaterally (towards the front and the side) just under the epicardium where the superior vena cava enters the right atrium. The impulse from the sinoatrial node spreads through the myocardium of the right and left atria, and it's also quickly transmitted to the atrioventricular node.

- ✔ **Atrioventricular (AV) node:** This node is located in the posterior and inferior portion of the interatrial septum, close to the opening of the coronary sinus in the right atrium. From there the signal is transmitted to the ventricles by a bundle of nerves called the atrioventricular bundle (also called the *bundle of His*).

- ✔ **Atrioventricular bundle:** This bundle of nerves runs from the atrioventricular node to the ventricles along the interventricular septum. It divides into *left and right bundle branches* that run deep to the endocardium to become the subendocardial branches (also called the *Purkinje fibers*):

- *Subendocardial branches of the right bundle* stimulate the interventricular septum, the papillary muscle, and the wall of the right ventricle.

- *Subendocardial branches of the left bundle* stimulate the interventricular septum, the papillary muscle, and wall of the left ventricle.

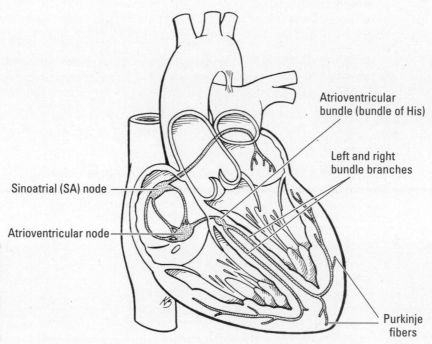

Atrioventricular bundle (bundle of His)

Left and right bundle branches

Sinoatrial (SA) node

Atrioventricular node

Figure 8-4: The conducting system of the heart.

Purkinje fibers

The heart is innervated by the autonomic nerves from *superficial* and *deep cardiac plexuses* (bundles of nerve fibers). The deep cardiac plexus is located on the bifurcation of the trachea, and the superficial cardiac plexus is located on the base of the heart below the arch of the aorta.

The autonomic nervous system is made up of a two-neuron chain (using the presynaptic neuron and the postsynaptic neuron) from the central nervous system to the viscera (in this case, the heart). (See Chapter 3 for a description of the automatic nervous system.) The presynaptic sympathetic fibers branch off the first five or six thoracic segments of the spinal cord. They enter the sympathetic trunks and synapse with postsynaptic neurons located in the cervical and upper thoracic ganglia. Fibers of the postsynaptic neurons join the cardiac plexus and terminate on the SA node, AV node, cardiac muscle fibers, and coronary arteries.

Sympathetic stimulation increases heart rate, force of contraction, and dilation of coronary arteries. Parasympathetic innervation to the heart is provided by the vagus nerve (CN X). The presynaptic parasympathetic fibers of the vagus nerve join the postsynaptic sympathetic fibers in the cardiac plexus. The postsynaptic parasympathetic neurons are located in intrinsic ganglia (within the wall of the heart) and terminate on the SA node, AV node, and coronary arteries. Parasympathetic stimulation has the opposite effect of sympathetic stimulation.

The *cardiac cycle* is the sequence of events of each heart beat:

- ✔ *Diastole:* During this process, the ventricles fill with blood from the atria. The atrioventricular valves are open, and the pulmonary and aortic valves are closed.

- ✔ *Systole:* In this process, the ventricles empty into the aorta and pulmonary arteries. The atrioventricular valves are closed, and the pulmonary and aortic valves are open.

Figure 8-5 demonstrates how blood flows through the heart's chambers to the lungs and back (called pulmonary circulation). It also depicts the pattern of systemic circulation, which includes the arteries and veins of the rest of the body.

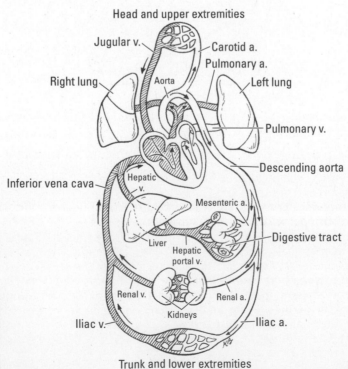

Figure 8-5:
The cardiac cycle.

Exploring Thoracic Circulation

The heart has to pump a large amount of blood to the rest of the body, so the blood vessels closest to it are quite large. The thorax is also home to the *thoracic duct,* the final collecting point of much of the lymphatic fluid in the body. You can discover the details of both processes in the following sections.

Circulating blood in the major vessels

The major blood vessels of the thorax include arteries that branch off the *aorta* and veins that drain into the *vena cava.* You can see some of these vessels in Figure 8-5.

Following are the parts of the aorta and its branches:

✓ **Ascending aorta:** This part of the aorta leaves the left ventricle and ascends up to the sternal angle (see Chapter 7). It has spaces between the walls of the vessel and the cusps of the aortic valve called *aortic sinuses.*

✓ **Arch of the aorta:** Continuing from the ascending aorta, this part arches posteriorly to the left of the trachea and esophagus, above the left primary bronchus. The branches of the aortic arch are covered in Chapter 14:

  • *Brachiocephalic trunk* (only on the right side of the body)

  • *Left common carotid artery*

  • *Left subclavian artery*

✓ **Thoracic aorta:** The thoracic aorta continues from the arch and descends in the posterior mediastinum and left of the vertebral column.

✓ **Posterior intercostal arteries:** These arteries branch off the posterior part of the thoracic aorta and run laterally and anteriorly in the intercostal spaces.

✓ **Bronchial arteries:** These arteries branch off the anterior part of the aorta or a posterior intercostal artery.

✓ **Esophageal arteries:** Starting at the anterior part of the thoracic aorta, these arteries run to the esophagus.

✓ **Superior phrenic arteries:** These arteries start at the anterior part of the thoracic aorta and run to the diaphragm.

Following are the parts of the vena cava and its tributaries:

- *Right and left brachiocephalic veins:* These veins unite to form the *superior vena cava* near the brachiocephalic trunk (at the level of the 1st costal cartilage).

- *Superior vena cava:* This large vein runs inferiorly to enter the right atrium.

   The superior vena cava returns blood to the heart from all the structures above the diaphragm except for the heart and lungs.

- *Inferior vena cava:* This vein is formed by the union of the iliac arteries and is described with the abdominal structures in Chapter 10. It enters the heart at the lowest part of the right atrium.

- *Azygos vein:* This vein arises from the right ascending lumbar vein and passes through the posterior mediastinum to drain into the superior vena cava.

- *Hemiazygos vein:* This vein starts at the left ascending lumbar vein and crosses the vertebral column around the level of the 8th thoracic vertebra to join the azygos vein.

- *Accessory hemiazygos vein:* This vein is formed by the union of the left fourth to the eighth posterior intercostal veins and joins the azygos vein at the level of the 7th thoracic vertebra.

The *ligamentum arterisosum* (refer to Figure 8-2) is a remnant of a fetal vessel called the *ductus arteriosus* that connected the pulmonary artery to the aortic arch in a developing fetus.

Moving lymph through the lymphatic vessels

The lymphatic system moves lymph from all parts of the body to the thorax; lymph from most of the body is returned to the venous system through the *thoracic duct.* It starts at the cisterna chyli (see Chapter 10) and lies along the bodies of the 6th through 12th thoracic vertebrae (see Chapter 15). The thoracic duct has a beaded appearance caused by a large number of valves.

The thoracic duct receives lymph from branches of *collecting trunks* in the intercostal spaces (between the ribs); the jugular, subclavian, and bronchomediastinal lymphatic trunks; and posterior mediastinal structures. The thoracic duct empties into the *left venous angle,* which is the union of the left internal jugular vein and subclavian vein (see Chapter 14).

Lymph from the lower extremities, pelvis, abdomen, left side of the thorax, left upper extremity, and the left side of the head and neck drains into the thoracic duct. Lymph from the rest of the body drains into the right lymphatic duct, which returns lymph to the blood at the right subclavian vein near the right internal jugular vein.

Posterior mediastinal lymph nodes are located behind the pericardium. They receive lymph from the esophagus, posterior portion of the pericardium, diaphragm, and intercostal spaces. The *inferior tracheobronchial lymph nodes* receive lymph from the heart.

Discovering What Else Is in the Thoracic Cavity

Much of the focus is on the heart and lungs, but the following organs also live in the thoracic cavity:

- ✔ **The diaphragm:** The *diaphragm* is a dome-shaped muscle that divides the thorax from the abdomen. Its function is to expand and contract the thoracic cavity during inhalation and exhalation along with the muscles of the thoracic wall (see Chapter 7). The central tendon of the diaphragm is attached to the pericardium. The anatomy of the diaphragm is described in Chapter 7.

- ✔ **The thymus:** The pink-lobed *thymus* is located between the sternum (breastbone) and the pericardium in the anterior portion of the mediastinum. The thymus grows during childhood, but after puberty it shrinks (or involutes). The thymus is the site for the maturation of T cells (see Chapter 5 for more about the immune system and blood cells). The thymus gets its blood supply from the inferior thyroid (see Chapter 14) and internal thoracic arteries.

- ✔ **The esophagus:** The *esophagus* is a tube about 10 inches long that joins the oropharynx (see Chapter 14) to the stomach. It runs downward and to the left through the superior and posterior mediastinum. The esophagus is described fully in Chapter 10 along with the other organs and structures of the digestive system.

- ✔ **The nerves of the thorax:** A number of nerves can be found in the thoracic cavity:

  - • The *right vagus nerve* enters the mediastinum anterior to the right subclavian artery, where it gives off the *right recurrent laryngeal nerve*. The *left vagus nerve* enters the mediastinum between the left common carotid and left subclavian artery. It passes anterior to the arch of the aorta where it gives off the *left recurrent laryngeal nerve*. The left and right vagus nerves join the esophageal plexus and continue into the abdomen.

- On the right side, the *recurrent laryngeal nerve* loops around the subclavian artery (see Chapter 14). On the left, it passes under the arch of the aorta. Both nerves run up to the larynx, one on each side.

- The right and left *phrenic nerves* enter the superior thoracic aperture and travel between the mediastinal pleura and the pericardium to the diaphragm.

- The *cardiac plexus* receives branches from the vagus nerve and the sympathetic trunk and runs to the arch of the aorta and heart.

- The *pulmonary plexus* also receives branches from the vagus nerve and the sympathetic trunk and runs to the bronchial subdivisions in the lungs.

- The *esophageal plexus* receives fibers from the vagus nerve and sympathetic ganglia and form a plexus on the esophagus inferior to the bifurcation of the trachea.

Chapter 9

Bellying Up to the Abdominal Wall

- -

- -

The abdominal wall surrounds the abdominal cavity. It covers the trunk from just below the diaphragm (see Chapter 8) to the pubic symphysis and the pelvis (see Chapter 11). The main function of the abdominal wall is to surround and protect the vital abdominal organs inside as well as assist in posture, bending, twisting, and breathing.

This chapter provides pointers for drawing quadrants and regions so you can easily refer to different abdominal structures. We also describe the nerve and blood supply, the muscles, and the lymph nodes found in the abdominal wall, and we discuss a special area known as the inguinal region. We wrap up with an overview of the wall's surface anatomy. (Turn to Chapter 10 if you're interested in the details of abdominal organs.)

Drawing Quadrants and Regions on the Abdominal Wall

When you examine a patient's abdomen, being able to associate the surface of the abdominal wall with the organs found inside the abdominal cavity is helpful. Well, good news: You can do this with some imaginary lines that divide the abdomen into different areas. You can draw the lines in two ways, as you find out in the following sections: One way uses two imaginary lines to create four quadrants, and the other method uses four lines to create nine regions.

Using two lines: The four quadrants

The abdomen can be divided into four quadrants by drawing two imaginary lines on the abdomen, one vertical and one horizontal, that meet in the middle. These two planes are the following:

- *Transumbilical plane:* Marked by the horizontal line, this plane runs through the umbilicus (navel) and the intervertebral disc between the 3rd and 4th lumbar vertebrae (see Chapter 15 if you need a refresher on these vertebrae).

- *Median (midsagittal) plane:* Marked by the vertical line running through the midline of the body, this plane divides it into the right half and the left half. (Flip to Chapter 2 for more about this plane.)

These lines result in four quadrants: the *right upper, left upper, right lower,* and *left lower.*

Using four lines: The nine regions

In addition to the four quadrants in the preceding section, the abdomen can also be divided into nine regions by two vertical lines and two horizontal lines (imagine a tic-tac-toe board), which provides for a little more accuracy when describing the location of pain or a lesion.

- **Vertical lines:** Two vertical lines are formed by the *midclavicular planes,* which line up with the midpoints of the clavicles.

- **Horizontal lines:** Two horizontal lines are provided by the following planes:

  • The *subcostal plane* is at the level of the bottom of the 10th costal cartilages (see Chapter 7). That's near the bottom of the rib cage.

  • The *transtubercular plane* is at the level of the body of the 5th lumbar vertebra (see Chapter 15) and near the top of the hip bones.

The lines form three rows with three regions each.

- **Top row:** The regions in the superior (top) row consists of the *right hypochondriac, epigastric,* and *left hypochondriac.*

- **Middle row:** The regions in the middle row consists of the *right lumbar (lateral), umbilical,* and *left lumbar (lateral).*

- **Bottom row:** The regions in the inferior (bottom) row consists of the *right inguinal (iliac), hypogastric (pubic),* and *left inguinal (iliac).*

Making Up the Abdominal Wall: Muscles and More

As you find out in the following sections, the abdominal wall is mainly made up of muscles and the tissues that support them. They combine with the spinal column (see Chapter 15) to give the midsection its structure.

Absolutely fabulous abdominal muscles

The abdominal muscles cover the front and sides of the abdomen (known clinically as the *anterolateral* area). They support it, help keep you upright, and assist with breathing. They also allow you to bend and twist the trunk.

The abdominal wall muscles move your middle, but they also have a few other functions:

- ✔ Supporting the abdominal wall while maintaining flexibility
- ✔ Protecting the abdominal organs that we describe in Chapter 10
- ✔ Controlling intra-abdominal pressure, which helps you exhale, cough, yell, and, yes, even belch (on the other end, that intra-abdominal pressure provides force to assist the intestines and bladder for defecating and urinating)

The anterolateral abdominal muscles are divided into four pairs:

- ✔ ***External oblique muscles:*** These abs originate on the 5th through the 12th ribs and insert on the linea alba and pubic tubercle. They flex and rotate the trunk and support the abdominal organs.

    The *linea alba* is a band of fibrous tissue that runs along the midline of the abdominopelvic wall, from the xiphoid process down to the pubic symphysis. Check out Chapter 7 for more about the thoracic wall; Chapter 11 has details about the pubic bone and other structures of the pelvis and perineum.

- ✔ ***Internal oblique muscles:*** These muscles originate on the thoracolumbar fascia (see Chapter 17), iliac crest, and connective tissue under the inguinal ligament that we discuss later in this chapter. They insert onto the 10th through 12th ribs, the linea alba, and the pubic bone. They flex and rotate the trunk and support the abdominal organs along with the external obliques.

✔ *Transversus abdominis muscles:* These abdominal muscles originate on the 7th through 12th costal cartilages, thoracolumbar fascia, iliac crest, and connective tissue under the inguinal ligament. They insert onto the linea alba and pubic bone. The transversus abdominis supports the organs of the abdomen.

✔ *Rectus abdominis muscles:* These muscles originate at the pubic symphysis and pubic crest and insert onto the xiphoid process and the 5th through 7th costal cartilages. They flex the trunk and control the tilt of the pelvis. The rectus abdominis are covered by the *rectus sheath,* which is formed by the aponeuroses (broad tendinous structure) of the abdominal muscles.

Three abdominal muscles are posterior:

✔ *Psoas major muscles:* These muscles originate at the transverse processes (lateral projections), bodies, and intervertebral discs of the 12th thoracic vertebra and the five lumbar vertebrae (see Chapter 15). They insert onto the lesser trochanter (bony protrusion) of the femur (see Chapter 19). The psoas major muscles are innervated by the lumbar plexus (L1–L3), and they flex the thighs.

✔ *Iliacus muscles:* These muscles originate on the iliac fossa (the large indentation — see Chapter 11), sacral ala (sides of the sacrum — see Chapter 15), and the anterior sacroiliac ligaments (see Chapter 19). They insert onto the lesser trochanter and shaft of the femur and to the tendon of the psoas major. They're innervated by the femoral nerve (L2–L4) and work with the psoas major to flex the thighs.

✔ *Quadratus lumborum:* These muscles originate on the medial (toward the midline of the body) parts of the 12th ribs and transverse processes of the lumbar vertebrae. They insert onto the iliolumbar ligament (between the ilium and the L5 vertebra) and the iliac crest (see Chapter 11). The quadratus lumborum muscles are innervated by branches from T12 through L4 nerves, and they extend and laterally flex the vertebral column.

Nerves, blood vessels, and lymphatics for maintaining tissues

The skin, muscles, and other structures of the abdominal wall need nerve supply, blood, and lymphatic drainage. We provide details about these structures in the following sections.

Nerves

A number of nerves run to the muscles and skin of the abdomen. Figure 9-1 shows the abdominal-wall nerves:

- ✔ **Thoracoabdominal nerves:** Five pairs of thoracoabdominal nerves continue from the 7th through 11th intercostal nerves, which are described in Chapter 7. They run between the layers of abdominal muscles to innervate the muscles of the anterolateral abdominal wall. *Anterior* and *lateral* and *cutaneous branches* provide nerve supply to the skin.

- ✔ **Subcostal nerves:** These nerves stem from the anterior rami of the 12th thoracic spinal nerves (see Chapter 15 for details on spinal nerves). They run just inferior to the 12th ribs and down to below the umbilicus (the navel). Subcostal nerves innervate the abdominal wall muscles and the skin (via cutaneous branches) between the iliac crests and the umbilicus.

- ✔ **Iliohypogastric nerves:** The iliohypogastric nerves stem from the anterior rami of the 1st lumbar spinal nerves and form branches that run below the subcostal nerves to the lower part of the abdominal wall. They innervate the skin over the iliac crests, upper iliac (inguinal) regions, and hypogastric (pubic) regions (the area below the navel). They also give nerve supply to the internal oblique and transversus abdominis muscles that we discuss earlier in this chapter.

- ✔ **Ilioinguinal nerves:** These nerves stem from the anterior rami of the 1st lumbar spinal nerves. They run between the layers of abdominal muscle and down to the inguinal canal (which we cover later in this chapter). They innervate the scrotal skin in men and labia majora in women (see Chapter 11), the area over the pubic bone, and the medial portions of the thigh (see Chapter 19). They also innervate the internal oblique and transversus abdominis muscles.

- ✔ **Lateral cutaneous nerves of the thigh:** These nerves run from the 2nd and 3rd lumbar spinal nerves inferiorly on the iliacus muscles to the thighs. They supply the skin on the anterolateral parts of the thighs.

- ✔ **Femoral nerves:** These nerves come from the 2nd through 4th lumbar spinal nerves and run along the lateral part of the psoas major muscles to innervate the iliacus muscle before descending into the thigh to supply extensors of the knee (see Chapter 19).

- ✔ **Obturator nerves:** These nerves come from the 2nd through 4th lumbar spinal nerves and run from the medial part of the psoas major muscle through the pelvis and into the thighs, where they supply the adductor muscles (see Chapter 19).

- ✔ **Lumbosacral trunk:** These nerves come from the 4th and 5th lumbar nerve roots. They pass over the sacrum and descend into the pelvis to help form the sacral plexus (see Chapter 15).

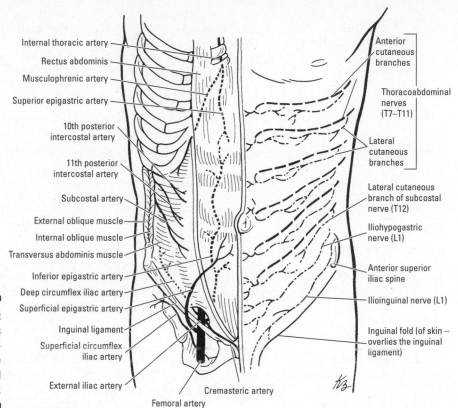

Internal thoracic artery
Rectus abdominis
Musculophrenic artery
Superior epigastric artery
10th posterior intercostal artery
11th posterior intercostal artery
Subcostal artery
External oblique muscle
Internal oblique muscle
Transversus abdominis muscle
Inferior epigastric artery
Deep circumflex iliac artery
Superficial epigastric artery
Inguinal ligament
Superficial circumflex iliac artery
External iliac artery
Cremasteric artery
Femoral artery

Anterior cutaneous branches
Thoracoabdominal nerves (T7–T11)
Lateral cutaneous branches
Lateral cutaneous branch of subcostal nerve (T12)
Iliohypogastric nerve (L1)
Anterior superior iliac spine
Ilioinguinal nerve (L1)
Inguinal fold (of skin – overlies the inguinal ligament)

Figure 9-1: The nerves and arteries of the abdominal wall.

Blood vessels

The abdominal wall has quite a few blood vessels. It includes all the arteries covered here and in Figure 9-1:

- ✔ **Musculophrenic artery:** Branches off the internal thoracic artery and runs along the costal margin to supply the hypochondriac region of the abdominal wall and the anterolateral muscles and the diaphragm (check out Chapter 7 for more on those structures)

- ✔ **Superior epigastric artery:** Stems from the internal thoracic artery and runs down behind the rectus abdominis to supply blood to the rectus abdominis and the superior portion of the anterolateral abdominal wall

- ✔ ***10th and 11th posterior intercostal arteries* and *subcostal arteries:*** Branch off the aorta and run past the ribs to the abdominal wall where they provide blood flow to the lateral part of the abdominal wall

- ✔ ***Common iliac arteries:*** Form the terminal branches of the abdominal aorta; diverge and run inferiorly alongside the psoas muscles to the brim of the pelvis where they divide into the internal and external iliac arteries (see Chapter 11)

- ✔ ***Median sacral artery:*** Rises up from the abdominal aorta at its bifurcation and then descends into the lesser pelvis (see Chapter 11)

- ✔ ***Inferior epigastric artery:*** Branches from the external iliac artery (see Chapter 11) and runs superiorly into the rectus sheath to supply blood to the rectus abdominis and part of the abdominal wall

- ✔ ***Deep circumflex iliac artery:*** Starts at the external iliac artery and runs parallel to the inguinal ligament (which we discuss later in this chapter), supplying blood to the iliacus muscle and inferior part of the anterolateral abdominal wall

- ✔ ***Superficial circumflex iliac artery:*** Branches off the femoral artery (see Chapter 19) and runs along the inguinal ligament to supply blood to the superficial part of the abdominal wall of the inguinal region (the part that's closest to the surface of the skin) and anterior thigh

- ✔ ***Superficial epigastric artery:*** Also branches off the femoral artery, running to the umbilicus in the superficial fascia to supply blood to the skin below the umbilicus and pubic area

Veins are in this area too, of course. They have the same names as the arteries and are located near them.

Lymphatics

Superficial lymphatic vessels (close to the surface of the skin) follow along with the superficial veins. The ones that run above the umbilicus drain into the axillary nodes of the armpits (see Chapter 16), whereas the vessels below the umbilicus drain into the superficial inguinal lymph nodes, which are described in Chapter 11.

Deep lymphatic vessels follow the deep veins and drain into the external iliac, common iliac, and lumbar lymph nodes discussed in Chapter 11.

Lining the abdomen: The peritoneum

A glistening membrane called the *peritoneum* serves as the lining for the innermost part of the abdominal cavity. It has two layers:

- *Parietal peritoneum:* Lines the internal surface of the abdominopelvic wall
- *Visceral peritoneum:* Covers the abdominal organs

Peritonitis is an inflammation of the peritoneum due to bacterial or fungal infection. It's very painful and can be life-threatening if not treated promptly.

Inspecting the Inguinal Region

The *inguinal region* of the abdominal wall includes the area between the anterior superior iliac spine and the pubic tubercle (in other words, the groin or lower lateral parts of the abdomen). This region is particularly important for examination of males because the spermatic cord, the testes (male reproductive organs), and the scrotum are included in this area. In the following sections, we describe these structures and others of the inguinal region (notably, the inguinal ligament, the iliopubic tract, and the inguinal canal); the penis and internal male organs are outlined in Chapter 11, along with the female organs.

The inguinal region is a site for herniations, especially in males where the spermatic cord runs through the inguinal canal.

The inguinal ligament and the iliopubic tract

The *inguinal ligament* (see Figure 9-2) is formed at the inferior end of the external oblique's *aponeurosis* (the broad tendinous structure that attaches a muscle to another muscle). Most of the inguinal ligament fibers insert into the pubic tubercle directly, but some of them form the *lacunar* and *pectineal ligaments* that attach to the superior pubic ramus (discussed in Chapter 11).

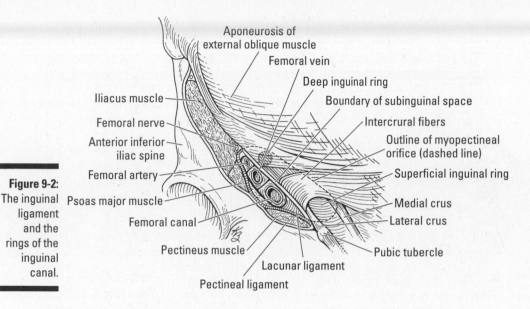

Aponeurosis of
external oblique muscle

Femoral vein

Deep inguinal ring

Boundary of subinguinal space

Iliacus muscle

Intercrural fibers

Femoral nerve

Outline of myopectineal
orifice (dashed line)

Anterior inferior
iliac spine

Superficial inguinal ring

Femoral artery

Medial crus

Psoas major muscle

Lateral crus

Femoral canal

Pubic tubercle

Pectineus muscle

Lacunar ligament

Pectineal ligament

Figure 9-2:
The inguinal
ligament
and the
rings of the
inguinal
canal.

The *iliopubic tract* is a fibrous band that runs just under the inguinal ligament.
It reinforces the posterior wall and the floor of the inguinal canal that we talk
about later in this chapter.

The inguinal canal

Both males and females possess inguinal canals, but the contents vary con-
siderably. For men, the inguinal canal gives passage to the spermatic cord
(see the next section), whereas in women, the inguinal canal houses the
round ligament of the uterus (see Chapter 11). In both men and women, it
also contains blood vessels, lymphatics, and the ilioinguinal nerve mentioned
earlier in this chapter.

The inguinal canal is about four centimeters long in adults. The canal has a
wall, a floor, and a roof that are formed from fascia and the aponeuroses of
the abdominal muscles. It also has a ring at each end (refer to Figure 9-2):

✔ The *deep ring* is the internal entrance to the canal. It's located above the
inguinal ligament and lateral to the inferior epigastric vessels.

✔ The *superficial ring* is where the inguinal canal exits between the fibers
of the aponeurosis of the external oblique near the pubic tubercle. The
edges of the superficial ring are called the *lateral* and *medial crura,* with
intercrural fibers keeping the crura in place so they don't spread apart.

The spermatic cord

The *spermatic cord* contains the structures that go to the testes and back (see the next section), and it also helps hold the testis in the scrotum. The cord starts at the deep inguinal ring (see the preceding section) and ends at the posterior part of the testes. It has three layers of fascia: the *internal spermatic fascia,* the *cremasteric fascia,* and the *external spermatic fascia.*

The cremasteric fascia contains part of the *cremasteric muscle,* which draws each testis superiorly in the scrotum. It's innervated by the *genital branch of the genitofemoral nerve (first and second lumbar spinal nerves).* This effect is more pronounced in a cold environment. When it's warm, the cremasteric muscle tends to relax.

The cremasteric muscle works in conjunction with the *dartos muscle,* the subcutaneous smooth muscle of the scrotum (see Chapter 3 for more information about smooth muscle) to help maintain the testicles at the appropriate temperature for sperm development.

Various vessels, nerves, and other structures that are described in this chapter pass through the spermatic cord:

- ✔ Ductus (vas) deferens
- ✔ Artery to the ductus (vas) deferens
- ✔ Testicular artery
- ✔ Cremasteric artery
- ✔ Pampiniform venous plexus
- ✔ Genital branch of the genitofemoral nerve
- ✔ Lymphatic vessels

The testes

Two oval organs called the *testes* produce spermatozoa and a male hormone called *testosterone.* Spermatozoa are formed in the *seminferous tubules.* They open into a network of channels called the *rete testis.* The rete testis is connected to the epididymis (described later in this section) by *efferent ductules.* Each testis is enclosed by a fibrous capsule called the *tunica albuginea* and covered by the *tunica vaginalis,* which is a double layer of peritoneum that surrounds the testes inside the scrotal sac. (We discuss the peritoneum later in this chapter.)

The testes are served by the *testicular arteries* that come from the abdominal aorta and pass through the spermatic cord (see the preceding section). Venous drainage is provided by the *pampiniform venous plexus* that surrounds the testicular artery and empties into the *left* and *right testicular veins.* The left testicular vein drains into the left renal vein, and the right testicular vein drains into the inferior vena cava. (Turn to Chapter 10 to review the abdominal arteries and veins.)

 The pampiniform venous plexus helps regulate the temperature of the testes, which require a fairly constant temperature to function properly. *Varicoceles* are abnormal enlargements of the veins and can form when these veins remain dilated due to defective valves.

Lymphatic vessels drain the testes and pass through the spermatic cord to empty into the lumbar and preaortic lymph nodes, which are described in Chapter 10.

The coiled and compacted *duct of the epididymis* forms the *epididymis.* Sperm cells are transported from the rete testis to the epididymis through *efferent ductules.* The epididymis has a head at the superior part, a body in the middle, and a tail that becomes the *ductus (vas) deferens,* which is the tube that delivers spermatozoa to the ejaculatory ducts (see Chapter 11 for more info). The ductus deferens receives blood flow from *the artery of the ductus (vas) deferens.*

 A vasectomy is a surgical procedure used as a form of birth control. During a vasectomy the ductus (vas) deferens of each testicle is cut and closed off so spermatozoa can't be transported to the ejaculatory ducts.

The scrotum

The testes are found within the *scrotum,* a sac that's covered with a layer of skin over a layer of fascia called the *dartos fascia,* which contains the *dartos muscle.* Unlike the rest of the abdomen, the scrotum does not have a layer of fat.

 The *dartos muscle* is attached to the skin of the scrotum, and when it contracts, it wrinkles and thickens the skin to reduce the surface area of the scrotum and move the testes closer to the body to conserve heat.

The scrotum is a sensitive area. Following are the several nerves that service the scrotum:

- ✓ *Genital branch of the genitofemoral nerve:* Originates from the 1st and 2nd lumbar spinal nerves and supplies the anterolateral part

- ✓ *Anterior scrotal nerves from the ilioinguinal nerve:* Originate at the 1st lumbar spinal nerves and supply the anterior part

- ✓ *Posterior scrotal nerves from the pudendal nerve:* Originate from the 2nd through 4th sacral spinal nerves and supply the posterior part

- ✓ *Perineal branches of the posterior cutaneous nerve of the thigh:* Originate at the 2nd and 3rd sacral spinal nerves and supply the inferior part

Blood is supplied to the scrotum by the following arteries (and returned by similarly named veins):

- ✓ *Posterior scrotal branches of the perineal artery:* Branches of the internal pudendal artery (see Chapter 11)

- ✓ *Anterior scrotal branches of the deep external pudendal artery:* Stem from the femoral artery (see Chapter 19)

- ✓ *Cremasteric artery:* Branches off the inferior epigastric artery (refer to Figure 9-1)

Seeing the Skin and Surface Anatomy of the Abdominal Wall

One notable structure on the surface of the abdomen is the umbilicus, or navel, which is the spot where the umbilical cord entered the body. The abdominal muscles and linea alba may be visible under the skin in the epigastric, umbilical, and hypogastric (pubic) regions unless they're obscured by adipose tissue (fat).

The iliac crest, anterior superior iliac spine, and pubic symphysis are all easily palpated (medically examined). Find the iliac crest by placing your fingers into the lateral side of the abdominal wall near the transumbilical plane and pressing downward to find the large bone. Follow the crest anteriorly to locate the prominent anterior superior iliac spine (it's the most anterior part of the iliac crest). The pubic symphysis is located at the anterior and midline of the pubic bone that can be palpated above the external genitalia.

The inguinal region features the scrotum in males, lying just behind the penis. The scrotum is often more pigmented than the skin of the abdomen and the thigh, has a wrinkled appearance, and is covered with pubic hair following puberty.

Chapter 10

Probing the Abdominal Organs

Most of the organs and structures of the digestive system are located in the abdomen (including the stomach and lower digestive tract), as are the liver, gallbladder, pancreas, kidneys, ureters, and spleen. Understanding the arrangement of the organs makes physical examination easier to perform. This chapter tells you what you need to know about the organs of the abdomen and the vessels that serve them.

Poking Around the Peritoneum

The *peritoneum* is a membrane made up of two layers. One layer lines the cavity and the other layer lines the organs. The peritoneum helps support the organs in the abdominal cavity and also allows nerves, blood vessels, and lymph vessels to pass through to the organs. As we note in Chapter 9, the *parietal peritoneum* lines the abdominal wall and extends to the organs, whereas the *visceral peritoneum* covers the organs. The *peritoneal cavity* lies between these two peritoneal layers. It contains a thin layer of fluid that lubricates the peritoneal surfaces.

The visceral peritoneum is served by the same blood, lymphatic vessels, and nerves as the organs it covers. The parietal peritoneum, though, shares circulation and nerve supply with the abdominal wall (which we discuss in Chapter 9).

In the following sections, we describe the structures that are formed by the tissues of the peritoneum.

The mesentery and the peritoneal folds and ligaments

The *mesentery* is a double layer of peritoneum with some connective tissue that helps support organs and allows for nerves and blood vessels to travel to those organs. The mesentery anchors the abdominal organs to the posterior abdominal wall, helping keep those organs in place but still allowing for some mobility.

A *peritoneal fold* is a part of the peritoneum that is raised from the abdominal wall by the underlying blood vessels and ducts. Each fold forms a pouch-like *peritoneal recess*. Some peritoneal folds are called *peritoneal ligaments* when they connect an organ to the abdominal wall or to another organ.

The greater and lesser omentums

The omentum is a fatty apron that hangs over the intestines and helps to cushion them. The *greater omentum* and the *lesser omentum* are also composed of double layers of peritoneum (see the preceding section). The greater omentum is actually four layers thick. They both run between the stomach and the first part of the duodenum to other organs (all of which we describe later in this chapter).

The greater omentum is made up of the following ligaments:

- *Gastrophrenic ligament:* This ligament runs from the greater curvature of the stomach to the diaphragm (Chapter 7 has details on the diaphragm).

- *Gastrosplenic ligament:* This ligament runs from the greater curvature of the stomach to the spleen.

- *Gastrocolic ligament:* This quite large ligament runs from the greater curvature of the stomach and first part of the duodenum to the transverse colon. It also forms a fatty apron that overlies the intestines.

The lesser omentum is made up of the following ligaments:

- *Hepatogastric ligament:* This ligament runs from the lesser curvature of the stomach to the liver.

- *Hepatoduodenal ligament:* This ligament runs from the liver to the duodenum.

Digging into the Main Digestive Organs

The *digestive tract* (also called the *alimentary tract*) runs from the mouth to the anus. As you find out in the following sections, the main digestive-tract organs found in the abdomen include part of the esophagus, the stomach, the small intestine, and part of the large intestine. (Flip to Chapter 6 for basics on the digestive system as a whole.)

Entering the esophagus

The *esophagus* is a muscular tube that extends from the pharynx (described in Chapters 13 and 14) to the stomach. It officially enters the abdomen when it passes through the esophageal hiatus (opening) of the diaphragm (see Chapter 7). The esophagus ends at the *esophagogastric junction,* where it joins the stomach (see the next section).

In the abdomen, the esophagus is located just to the left of the midline of the body near the level of the 11th thoracic vertebra (see Chapter 15). It's also located behind the peritoneum, so it's considered to be *retroperitoneal.*

The esophagus has two layers of muscle, a circular layer internally and an external layer that runs from one end to the other longitudinally. In the upper part of the esophagus, the outer layer of muscle is skeletal muscle, whereas the external layer of the lower part of the esophagus is smooth muscle. (See Chapter 3 for more about skeletal and smooth muscle.)

The lining of the esophagus is different than the lining of the stomach, and the area of transition between the two is called the *Z line.* The *inferior esophageal sphincter* (tight ring of muscle) is located just superior to (above) this line.

The esophageal sphincter opens to allow food and liquid to enter the stomach; otherwise it remains shut. Gastroesophageal reflux disease (you may know it as *GERD* or *acid reflux*) results when the sphincter frequently remains open, allowing the acidic stomach juices to flow into the lower part of the esophagus, which is painful and can result in damage to the tissues that line the esophagus. Patients who have GERD complain of heartburn (burning pain in the chest) that's usually worse at night, nausea, and a feeling that food is stuck in the esophagus. Medical treatment includes medications that decrease production or secretion of stomach acid, or antacids that absorb stomach acid. Lifestyle changes can help too, such as avoiding aspirin, ibuprofen, and any foods that appear to trigger the pain. Severe cases may require extra diagnostic tests, such as an upper endoscopy (see Chapter 23) to assess the damage to the lining of the esophagus.

Innervation of the esophagus comes from the anterior and posterior gastric nerves (vagal trunks) and the greater splanchnic nerves (thoracic sympathetic trunks). The esophagus receives blood flow from the esophageal branches of the left gastric artery and from the left inferior phrenic artery. Venous blood is drained by the left gastric vein of the portal system and into the esophageal veins that drain into the azygos vein (described in Chapter 7). Lymph drains into the left gastric lymph nodes, which drain into the celiac lymph nodes. We describe all of these structures later in this chapter.

Churning in the stomach

The *stomach* is a muscular bag that holds food and mixes it with digestive juices. The stomach is covered by peritoneum except for areas where blood vessels run along its exterior and a small area posterior to the cardial orifice. It's located left of the midline of the body in the upper part of the abdominal cavity (see Figure 10-1). The *lesser curvature* forms the right concave (inwardly curving) margin of the stomach. The *greater curvature* forms the left convex (outwardly curving) margin of the stomach.

The stomach has a slightly different shape in each person, but it is divided into the same parts:

- ✔ **Cardia:** The *cardia* surrounds the *cardial orifice,* which is where the esophagus joins the stomach.

- ✔ **Cardial notch:** The *cardial notch* is located between the esophagus and the fundus.

- ✔ **Fundus:** The *fundus* is the superior portion of the stomach. It begins at the top of the stomach (just underneath the left dome of the diaphragm) and ends at a plane at the level of the cardial orifice.

- ✔ **Body:** The *body* is the major part of the stomach between the fundus and the pyloric antrum.

- ✔ **Pyloric portion:** The *pyloric portion* of the stomach forms the rest of the stomach and ends with the *pyloric orifice* that opens into the duodenum (which we discuss later in this chapter). The widest part is called the *pyloric antrum,* and the narrower part of the funnel-shape is the *pyloric canal.* The *pylorus* has a thickened layer of smooth muscle that works like a sphincter to control the release of stomach contents into the small intestine.

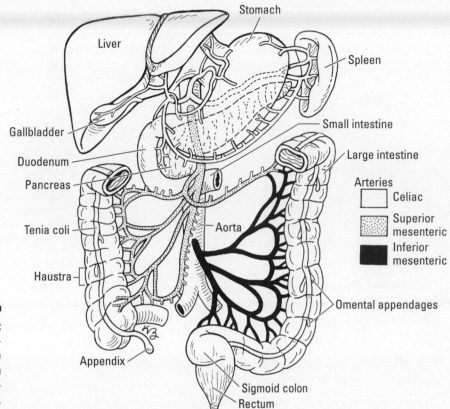

Figure 10-1:
An over-
view of the
organs in
the alimen-
tary tract.

(Labels in figure: Stomach, Liver, Spleen, Gallbladder, Small intestine, Duodenum, Large intestine, Pancreas, Arteries — Celiac, Superior mesenteric, Inferior mesenteric, Tenia coli, Aorta, Haustra, Omental appendages, Appendix, Sigmoid colon, Rectum)

The interior part of the stomach has *gastric folds (rugae)* that appear when the stomach muscle tissue is contracted.

Parasympathetic innervation is provided by the anterior vagal trunk, which is from the left vagus nerve, and by the posterior vagal trunk, which comes from the right vagus nerve. Sympathetic nerve supply comes from the celiac plexus. (Need a refresher on the differences between sympathetic and parasympathetic nerves? Flip to Chapter 3.)

The short gastric arteries supply blood to the fundus, and the right and left gastric arteries (located along the lesser curvature) and the right and left gastro-omental arteries (located along the greater curvature) supply the rest of the stomach. Veins that drain the stomach include the left and right gastric veins, the short gastric veins, the left gastro-omental veins, and the right gastro-omental vein. The veins drain into the hepatic portal circulation.

Lymphatic vessels follow the arteries and drain lymph into the gastric lymph nodes, gastro-omental lymph nodes, pancreaticosplenic lymph nodes, pyloric lymph nodes, and pancreaticoduodenal lymph nodes. Lymph from these nodes passes to the celiac lymph nodes located near the celiac trunk.

We cover all these nerves and vessels later in this chapter.

Winding through the small intestine

The small intestine (refer to Figure 10-1) is the first part of the *intestinal tract,* which includes the large intestine (also called the *colon;* we talk about it later in this chapter). The small intestine starts at the pylorus of the stomach (see the preceding section) and ends at the cecum of the large intestine. The small intestine has three segments: the duodenum, the jejunum, and the ileum. The main function of the small intestine is continued digestion and absorption of nutrients.

The duodenum

The *duodenum* is the first segment of the small intestine and is also the shortest (about 25 centimeters, or roughly 10 inches). It starts at the pylorus and ends at the *duodenojejunal junction.* It has four parts:

- ✔ *Superior part:* This part is horizontal and in front of the 1st lumbar vertebra.

- ✔ *Descending part:* This segment runs inferiorly (toward the bottom) along the right borders of the 2nd and 3rd lumbar vertebrae. It's close to the head of the pancreas, so this part is where the pancreatic and bile ducts are located.

- ✔ *Inferior part:* This part crosses to the left, in front of the inferior vena cava, close to the level of the 3rd lumbar vertebra.

- ✔ *Ascending part:* Starting near the 3rd lumbar vertebra, this part runs upward along the left side of the aorta (refer to Figure 10-1). It joins the jejunum at the *duodenojejunal junction.* It's supported by the *suspensory muscle of the duodenum,* also called the *ligament of Treitz.*

TECHNICAL STUFF

Ailments of the small intestine

Health conditions that can affect the small intestine include ulcers, celiac disease, and Crohn's disease. An *ulcer* is a sore in the lining of the duodenum (and can occur in the stomach too). The most common symptom is burning pain near the stomach. It's usually caused by a bacterium called *Helicobactor pylori* or long-term use of nonsteroidal anti-inflammatory medications. Ulcers can be diagnosed by upper endoscopy (see Chapter 23 for ways to look inside the body without cutting it open). Treatment includes medications that block production or secretion of stomach acid, along with lifestyle changes like smoking cessation and cutting back on alcohol consumption.

Celiac disease is a condition in which the intestinal lining becomes inflamed due to an autoimmune reaction to a protein called *gluten.* Wheat, barley, and rye all contain gluten. The inflammation damages the lining of the intestine, so absorption of nutrients is decreased. Common symptoms include abdominal pain and bloating, diarrhea; pale, foul-smelling stools; and weight loss. It can be diagnosed by a biopsy (taking a sample of tissue through an endoscope) of the small intestine. The only way to treat celiac disease is to remove gluten from the diet.

Crohn's disease is an inflammatory disease that can occur in any part of the digestive system but usually affects the ileum (discussed in the section "The jejunum and the ileum"). The cause isn't known, but it has a connection with the immune system. Symptoms of Crohn's disease include abdominal pain and diarrhea and often rectal bleeding, weight loss, and fever. The disease may be detected by taking an upper GI series, which is a type of X-ray procedure that involves drinking barium, a solution that shows up on X-rays and help to reveal inflammation and damage. Crohn's can't be cured, but it can be treated with medications, nutritional supplements, and surgery in severe cases.

Parasympathetic nerve supply to the duodenum comes from the vagus nerve, and sympathetic nerves in this area include the greater and lesser splanchnic nerves. Blood is supplied to the duodenum by the superior pancreaticoduodenal artery, a branch of the gastroduodenal artery, and the inferior pancreaticoduodenal artery, a branch of the superior mesenteric artery. Blood is drained by the corresponding veins into the hepatic portal system. Lymphatic vessels follow the arteries to the pancreaticoduodenal lymph nodes, pyloric lymph nodes, and the superior mesenteric lymph nodes. Lymph flows from those nodes to the celiac lymph nodes.

We discuss all the nerves and vessels that serve the small intestine in greater detail later in this chapter.

The jejunum and the ileum

The *jejunum* is the middle portion of the small intestine. It starts at the duo-denojejunal junction and changes into the *ileum,* which is the third portion. The jejunum takes up about two-fifths of the length of the small intestine, but no clear line demarcates where it turns into the ileum. The ileum ends at the *ileocecal junction.* The ileum and jejunum are attached to the posterior abdominal wall by the mesentery (which we describe earlier in this chapter).

Sympathetic and parasympathetic (vagus) nerves are brought by the superior mesenteric plexus. Blood is brought to the jejunum and ileum by branches from the superior mesenteric artery. Blood is drained away by the superior mesenteric vein. Lymph nodes that drain this area include the juxtaintestinal lymph nodes, mesenteric lymph nodes, and central nodes that converge on the superior mesenteric lymph nodes. Lacteals are specialized lymphatic vessels found in the small intestine that absorb fat from the foods you eat.

Moving into the large intestine

Most of the large intestine is located in the abdomen; only the final portions (the sigmoid colon and rectum) are located in the pelvic cavity, and they're covered in Chapter 11. As you discover in the following sections, the abdominal portion of the large intestine includes the cecum and the ascending, transverse, and descending colon. The main function of the large intestine is to absorb water from fecal material before it's eliminated from the body. The colon is also home to friendly bacteria that synthesize vitamin K and keep bad microbes in check.

The large intestine has a different appearance than the small intestine (refer to Figure 10-1). It's much larger in diameter and has *omental appendages* (fatty appendages) attached to it. The longitudinal layer of smooth muscle is incomplete and forms three thick bands of smooth muscle called *teniae coli* that run from end to end. Contraction of the tenia coli cause the large intestine to form sacculations (pouches) called *haustra.*

The colon may form *diverticula,* which are small pouches that bulge outside the colon. When these pouches become inflamed, the result is a disease called *diverticulitis.* Symptoms include abdominal pain (usually in the left lower quadrant), fever and chills, bloating, gas, diarrhea or constipation, and nausea. Diverticulitis is diagnosed by X-rays or CT scans. Treatment includes antibiotics (if infection is present), relaxation techniques, heating pads, pain medication, and surgery in severe cases.

The cecum

The *cecum* is the first part of the large intestine. It's basically a pouch of intestine that hangs below the *ileocecal junction* in the right lower quadrant of the abdomen. Folds of mucosal tissue form the *ileocecal valve* that covers the *ileal orifice* (opening between the ileum and the cecum). The *appendix* extends from the posteromedial (back middle) part of the cecum.

Sympathetic and parasympathetic nerves come from the superior mesenteric plexus. Blood supply to the cecum comes via the ileocolic artery, a branch of the superior mesenteric artery. The appendicular artery branches from the ileocolic artery. Lymphatic vessels pass to the ileocolic lymph nodes and the superior mesenteric lymph nodes. (We describe all the nerves and vessels that serve the large intestine later in this chapter.)

The ascending colon

The *ascending colon* travels from the cecum upward on the right side of the abdominal cavity to the *right colic flexure* near the right side of the liver. This part of the colon is retroperitoneal (behind the peritoneum).

Nervous supply is brought to the ascending colon by the superior mesenteric plexus. The arteries that bring blood to the ascending colon include the ileocolic and right colic arteries, branches of the superior mesenteric artery. Blood is drained away by the ileocolic and right colic veins to the superior mesenteric vein. Lymph is drained by the epicolic and paracolic lymph nodes, and then it travels to the ileocolic and right colic lymph nodes. From there, it drains into the superior mesenteric nodes.

The transverse colon

The *transverse colon* crosses from the right side of the abdomen to the left, ending at the *left colic flexure,* which is just in front of the left kidney. The left colic flexure is attached to the diaphragm by the *phrenicocolic ligament.* The *transverse mesocolon* is the mesentery that attaches the transverse colon to the greater omentum (which we cover earlier in this chapter).

The sympathetic nerves that serve the transverse colon come from the superior and inferior mesenteric plexuses; the parasympathetic nerves arise from the vagus nerves and the pelvic splanchnic nerves.

Blood is brought to the transverse colon primarily by the middle colic artery, a branch of the superior mesenteric artery. The distal portion of the transverse colon (farther from its origin) is served by the left colic artery, a branch of the inferior mesenteric artery. Venous blood is removed by the superior mesenteric and inferior mesenteric veins. Lymph is drained into the colic lymph nodes, which drain into the superior mesenteric lymph nodes, and into the colic nodes, which drain to the inferior mesenteric nodes.

The descending colon

The *descending colon* travels behind the peritoneum and downward from the left colic flexure to the left iliac fossa where it continues as the sigmoid colon.

Sympathetic nerve supply comes from the lumbar splanchnic nerves, the inferior mesenteric plexus, and the periarterial plexuses that surround the inferior mesenteric artery. Parasympathetic nerve supply comes from the pelvic splanchnic nerve.

Blood is brought to the descending colon by the left colic and sigmoid arteries, branches of the inferior mesenteric artery. Blood is drained away by the inferior mesenteric vein. Lymph is drained into the epicolic and paracolic lymph nodes, which drain into the intermediate colic lymph nodes. From here the lymph drains into the inferior mesenteric lymph nodes.

Observing Organs that Assist with Digestion

The digestive tract needs a little help when it comes to digesting the food you eat. That help comes from the organs in the following sections:

- ✓ **Liver:** The liver makes bile and works hard to metabolize nutrients.
- ✓ **Gallbladder:** The gallbladder stores bile until you need it.
- ✓ **Pancreas:** The pancreas serves two systems: It makes digestive enzymes for the digestive system and makes the hormone called insulin, so it's also part of the endocrine system (see Chapter 6).

Locating the liver

The *liver* (see Figure 10-2) is the largest organ in the abdomen, and it sits just under the diaphragm in the right upper quadrant. It's a busy organ because just about every substance you eat goes to the liver to be metabolized before going anywhere else in the body. (Fats are the exception — they enter the lymphatic system.) The liver also makes bile, which helps break down fat in the small intestine, and also stores various substances. The following sections cover the parts, nerves, and vessels of the liver.

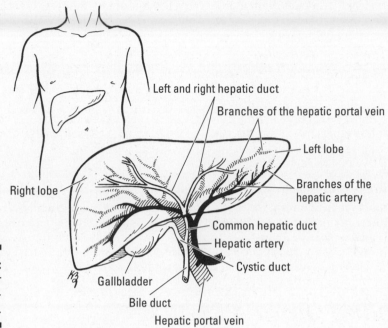

Left and right hepatic duct

Branches of the hepatic portal vein

Left lobe

Branches of the hepatic artery

Common hepatic duct

Hepatic artery

Cystic duct

Right lobe

Gallbladder

Bile duct

Hepatic portal vein

Figure 10-2:
The liver and the gall-bladder.

The surfaces and lobes

The liver has two surfaces: The *diaphragmatic surface* includes the anterior (front), superior (top), and part of the posterior (rear) surface, and the *visceral surface* is located on the posteroinferior (bottom rear) surface.

Most of the liver is covered with peritoneum except for a posterior section that contacts the diaphragm, the bed of the gallbladder, and the *porta hepatis,* which is an opening that allows the passage of the hepatic portal vein, hepatic artery, nerves, ducts, and lymphatic vessels. The visceral surface contacts the following: esophagus, stomach, duodenum, gallbladder, right colic flexure of the colon, right kidney, and suprarenal gland.

The liver is divided into two lobes by the falciform ligament: the larger *right lobe* and the smaller *left lobe.* The *falciform ligament* is a fold of peritoneum that extends from the umbilicus (navel) to the liver. The falciform ligament contains the *round ligament of the liver.*

The presence of *fissures,* or grooves, further divides the liver.

  ✔ ***Right sagittal fissure:*** This groove is formed by the fossa (depression) for the gallbladder and a groove that makes room for the inferior vena cava.

> ✔ **Left sagittal fissure:** This groove is formed by the fissure for the *round ligament of the liver* on the front and the fissure for the *ligamentum venosum* on the back.

The left and right sagittal fissures divide the right lobe to include the *caudate lobe* and *quadrate lobe.*

The round ligament of the liver is leftover from the umbilical vein that carries oxygenated blood to the fetus. The ligamentum venosum is a remnant of the *ductus venosus,* which sends blood from the umbilical vein to the inferior vena cava.

The nerves, blood vessels, and lymphatics

Nerve supply is brought to the liver by the *hepatic plexus,* which has sympathetic fibers from the celiac plexus and parasympathetic fibers from the vagal trunks.

The liver receives blood from the following two sources:

> ✔ **Hepatic artery:** Systemic circulation comes from the *hepatic artery,* which brings oxygenated blood to the liver.

> ✔ **Hepatic portal vein:** This vein carries venous blood from the abdominal part of the digestive tract.

The *hepatic portal system* is made up of the hepatic portal vein and its tributaries: the *superior mesenteric vein,* the *splenic vein,* the *gastric veins,* and the *cystic veins.*

Additional veins of the portal system include:

> ✔ **Gastro-omental veins:** Drain blood from the stomach and greater omentum into the splenic vein (left gastro-omental vein) and superior mesenteric vein (right gastro-omental vein)

> ✔ **Short gastric veins:** Drain blood from the stomach to the splenic vein

> ✔ **Ileocolic vein:** Drains blood from the cecum and appendix into the superior mesenteric vein

> ✔ **Inferior mesenteric vein:** Drains blood from the rectum, sigmoid, and descending colon into the splenic vein

> ✔ **Left colic vein:** Drains blood from the descending colon to the inferior mesenteric vein

> ✔ **Middle colic vein:** Drains blood from the transverse colon into the superior mesenteric vein

> ✔ **Right colic vein:** Drains blood from the ascending colon into the superior mesenteric vein

In the liver, the hepatic portal vein branches out and ends in capillaries called the *venous sinusoids of the liver.* (You can see parts of the hepatic portal venous system in Figure 10-3.) All blood from the liver is drained by the hepatic veins into the inferior vena cava.

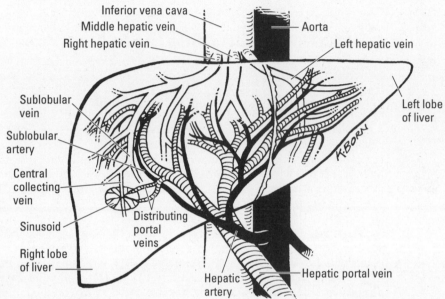

Figure 10-3:
Hepatic
portal
venous
system.

Lymph is drained from the liver by *lymphatic vessels of the liver,* which include superficial and deep lymphatic vessels. Hepatic lymph nodes are found along the hepatic vessels and the lesser omentum. Lymph from these lymphatic vessels drains into the celiac lymph nodes and then into the cisterna chyli. Lymph nodes on the posterior and anterior surfaces of the liver drain into the phrenic lymph nodes (near the diaphragm) and then into the posterior mediastinal lymph nodes (all located in the thorax; see Chapter 8) before draining into the right lymphatic and thoracic ducts (also discussed in Chapter 8).

The bile duct

The liver produces bile and secretes it into *bile canaliculi,* which drain the bile into *interlobular bile ducts.* Those ducts then lead to larger ducts that eventually merge to form the *right* and *left hepatic ducts* (one for each lobe). The two hepatic ducts merge to form the *common hepatic duct.* This duct, along with the *cystic duct,* forms the *bile duct.*

The bile duct runs down to the duodenum to form the *hepatopancreatic ampulla* with the pancreatic duct (the pancreas is discussed later in this chapter). The ampulla opens into the duodenum through the *major duodenal papilla.* The terminal portion of the bile duct is surrounded by the *sphincter of the bile duct.* The hepatopancreatic ampulla has its own sphincter called the *sphincter of Oddi.*

Glancing at the gallbladder

The *gallbladder* (refer to Figure 10-2) is a pouch-shaped organ that stores bile produced by the liver. After you eat a meal, a substance called *cholecystokinin* is secreted by cells in the walls of the duodendum. Cholecystokinin simulates the gallbladder to release the stored bile into the small intestine, where it emulsifies large globules of fats so they're easier to digest. The gallbladder lies in the *gallbladder fossa,* which is on the visceral surface of the liver (see the preceding section). It's surrounded by peritoneum that connects it to the liver. It has three parts: the wide *fundus* (which lies at the midclavicular line at the inferior border of the liver), the *body,* and the tapered *neck* that joins the cystic duct.

Nerve supply is brought by the celiac plexus, the vagus nerve, and the right phrenic nerve. Blood is brought to the gallbladder by the cystic artery, which commonly branches from the right hepatic artery. The gallbladder is drained by the cystic veins into the hepatic portal vein and small veins that drain directly into liver sinusoids. Lymph is drained by the cystic lymph node and the hepatic lymph nodes, which drain into the celiac lymph nodes. (We cover these nerves and vessels later in this chapter.)

Pinpointing the pancreas

The *pancreas* is a multifunctional organ. It synthesizes enzymes that break down carbohydrates, proteins, and fats and secretes them into the duodenum. It also produces bicarbonates that neutralize the acid that passes from the stomach into the duodenum. The pancreas also produces insulin, a hormone that stimulates cells to take up glucose (blood sugar) from the blood. It lies behind the peritoneum and runs transversely along the posterior wall behind the stomach (between the duodenum of the small intestine and the spleen — refer to Figure 10-1). It's divided into four parts:

✔ The *head* is located near the duodenum. It has an *uncinate process* that projects inferiorly and medially to the left.

✔ The *neck* is the short section that connects to the body.

✔ The *body* continues from the neck to the tail.

✔ The *tail* lies near the hilum of the spleen (we talk about the spleen in more detail later in this chapter).

The *main pancreatic duct* starts at the tail and runs to the head. From there it moves inferiorly and meets the bile duct of the liver to form the hepato-pancreatic ampulla. The main pancreatic duct has a sphincter to prevent backflow of bile into the pancreas. The *accessory pancreatic duct* drains the uncinate process and opens up into the duodenum via the *minor duodenal papilla.*

Innervation of the pancreas comes from the celiac and superior mesenteric plexuses. Blood is brought to the pancreas by the superior pancreatico-duodenal arteries, branches of the gastroduodenal artery, the inferior pancreaticoduodenal arteries, branches of the superior mesenteric artery, and branches of the splenic artery. Blood is drained away by tributaries of the splenic, and superior mesenteric veins. Lymph is drained by the pancreatico-splenic nodes and pyloric lymph nodes. These nodes drain into the superior mesenteric lymph nodes or the celiac lymph nodes. (We discuss these nerves and vessels later in this chapter.)

Pancreatitis is an inflammation of the pancreas that begins with pain in the upper abdomen, possibly radiating to the back. A person with pancreatitis is quite sick and may have a fever, a rapid pulse, and possibly nausea that leads to vomiting. Pancreatitis can be diagnosed by blood tests and diagnostic imaging techniques such as CT scans and ultrasound. Patients with pancreatitis usually require hospitalization.

Identifying Renal Anatomy

Renal anatomy refers to anatomy of the kidneys. The two kidneys filter the blood and form urine, which is transported to the urinary bladder (in the pelvis — see Chapter 11) by the ureters. Each kidney is capped by a supra-renal gland, which is a major player in the endocrine system covered in Chapter 6. We describe the kidneys, ureters, and suprarenal glands in the following sections.

Knowing the kidneys

The two kidneys lie behind the peritoneum on the posterior abdominal wall near the 12th thoracic and first three lumbar vertebrae (see Chapter 15 for details about vertebrae). The right kidney is slightly lower than the left kidney. Each kidney and suprarenal gland is encased in a *perinephric fat capsule,* which is covered by a membranous *renal fascia. Paranephric fat* lies outside of the renal fascia.

Each kidney is shaped like a kidney bean (surprised?) with an anterior and posterior surface (see Figure 10-4). The *renal hilum* is located at the medial border and allows the *renal artery* to enter the kidney and the *renal vein* to leave. It also allows the ureter to exit the kidney. The internal part of the kidney includes a section called the *medulla* surrounded by a covering called the *cortex.* The medulla contains *minor calyces* that merge to form *major caly-ces.* The innermost *renal pelvis* is formed by the merger of the major calyces.

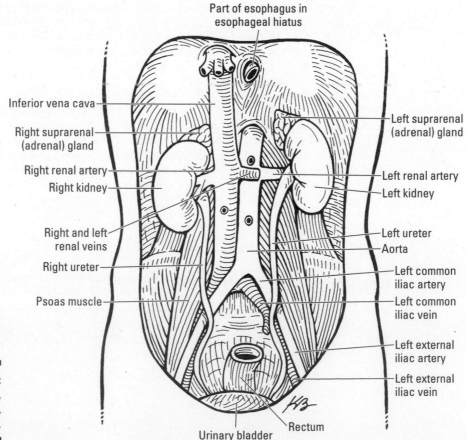

Part of esophagus in esophageal hiatus

Inferior vena cava

Right suprarenal (adrenal) gland

Right renal artery

Right kidney

Right and left renal veins

Right ureter

Psoas muscle

Left suprarenal (adrenal) gland

Left renal artery

Left kidney

Left ureter

Aorta

Left common iliac artery

Left common iliac vein

Left external iliac artery

Left external iliac vein

Rectum

Urinary bladder

Figure 10-4:
The kidneys, ureters, and more.

Nerve supply to the kidneys comes from the renal plexus. The renal arteries leave the abdominal aorta around the level of the 1st or 2nd lumbar vertebrae. Each renal artery travels to the kidney, where it branches into *segmental arteries* that supply the segments of the kidney. Renal veins return from the kidneys to empty into the inferior vena cava. Lymph leaves the kidneys via lymphatic vessels that drain into the *lumbar lymph nodes*. (You find out more about the nerves and vessels that serve all the renal organs later in this chapter.)

Tracing the ureters

The ureters are long, narrow, muscular tubes that leave the renal pelvis and exit the kidney, as shown in Figure 10-4. They run along the posterior abdominal wall next to the transverse processes of the lumbar vertebrae. They cross the external iliac arteries to enter the pelvis and continue to the urinary bladder. We discuss the pelvic portion of the ureters in Chapter 11.

Nerve supply to the ureters comes from the renal nerve plexus. *Arteries to the ureters* branch off the renal, testicular, and/or ovarian arteries and the abdominal aorta. *Veins to the ureters* drain into the renal, testicular, and/or ovarian veins. Lymph drains from the ureters to the *iliac lymph nodes* (discussed in Chapter 11).

Renal calculi, better known as kidney stones, are formed from crystals in the urine. Kidney stones are fairly common and can be quite painful when they move down the ureters. The pain is usually felt in the abdomen or the flank (side of the back) and often moves into the groin area. Additional symptoms may include blood in the urine, chills, fever, nausea, and vomiting. Renal calculi are detected by blood tests, urine tests, and imaging techniques such as ultrasound or X-rays. Treatment depends on the size of the stones. Small stones pass through the urinary tract. Pain medication and extra water can help. Large stones lodged in the kidney may require surgery or lithotripsy, a procedure that uses sound waves to break up the stones.

Spying the suprarenal glands

The *suprarenal glands* (or adrenal glands) are located between the superior part of the kidneys and the diaphragm. They're encased in perinephric fat but are separated from the kidneys by fibrous connective tissue. The right suprarenal gland is more pyramid shaped, whereas the left one is more crescent shaped. You can compare the suprarenal glands by looking at Figure 10-4.

Each suprarenal gland is made up of two portions: the *cortex* and the *medulla.* The cortex produces corticosteroids (which affect immune system response, inflammation, metabolism, and electrolyte levels) and androgen hormones (which are male sex hormones), and the medulla produces epinephrine and norepinephrine (which are hormones that affect heart rate and blood pressure).

Nerve supply comes from the celiac plexus and the abdominopelvic splanchnic nerves. Several suprarenal arteries bring blood to the suprarenal glands:

- *Superior suprarenal arteries:* Six or eight branch off the inferior phrenic artery.

- *Middle suprarenal arteries:* One or more branch off the abdominal aorta.

- *Inferior suprarenal arteries:* One or more branch off the renal artery.

Venous drainage is provided by the *suprarenal veins.* The right suprarenal vein drains into the inferior vena cava, and the left suprarenal vein drains into the left renal vein. Lymph is drained into the lumbar lymph nodes.

Figuring Out What Else Is in the Abdominal Cavity

After all the abdominal organs we talk about earlier in this chapter, we still have one more organ to discuss: the spleen, which doesn't fit into any of the categories in the earlier sections. In addition, all the other organs and structures of the abdomen require nerve supply, blood flow, and lymphatic drainage. The following sections take a look at the spleen along with abdominal nerves, blood vessels, and lymphatics.

The spleen

The *spleen* is an oval-shaped organ that can be found in the left upper quadrant just behind the stomach at the levels of the 9th through the 11th ribs (refer to Figure 10-1). Its job is to destroy old and damaged cells from the blood. It's covered in peritoneum except for the *hilum,* which is the portion of the spleen where the splenic arteries and veins enter and exit. It's connected to the greater curvature of the stomach by the gastrosplenic ligament and to the left kidney by the *splenorenal ligament.*

Nerve supply to the spleen is supplied by the celiac plexus. Blood is brought to the spleen by the splenic artery and drained away by the splenic vein, which unites with the superior mesenteric vein to form the hepatic portal vein. Lymph from the spleen is drained into the pancreaticosplenic lymph nodes located on the pancreas.

Splenomegally, or an enlarged spleen, can occur as the result of diseases such as leukemia (a disease resulting in the overproduction of white blood cells), liver diseases, and viral or bacterial infections. The spleen is also easily injured by traumatic force. A ruptured spleen can cause a large amount of blood loss. It's not easy to repair a spleen, and you can live without it, so if it's badly damaged it can be removed surgically.

Nerves

The organs of the abdomen are under the control of the autonomic nervous system (see Chapter 3). The nerves come from the splanchnic nerves and the vagus nerve (also known as *cranial nerve X* — see Chapter 12). Figure 10-5 depicts the autonomic nervous system of the abdomen. The following sections tell you what you need to know.

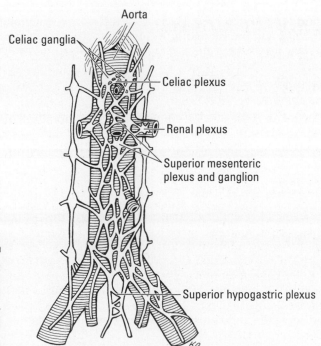

Figure 10-5: Autonomic nerve supply of the abdomen.

Additional abdominal nerves lie along the abdominal wall, and we discuss them in Chapter 9. They include the thoracoabdominal nerves, subcostal nerves, iliohypogastric nerves, and the ilioinguinal nerves.

The sympathetic nerves

The sympathetic (fight-or-flight) nerves include the *abdominopelvic splanchnic nerves,* which carry presynaptic fibers to the abdomen and pelvis. The fibers originate from cell bodies of the intermediolateral cell column (lateral horn) of the 7th thoracic through 2nd lumbar spinal-cord segments (see Chapter 15). The presynaptic fibers pass through anterior roots, anterior rami, and white communicating branches of the spinal nerves on their way to the sympathetic trunks. These presynaptic neurons pass through the paravertebral ganglia without synapsing (a synapse is the junction where nerve impulses pass) and become the abdominopelvic splanchnic nerves. They then enter the prevertebral ganglia and autonomic plexuses located primarily on the abdominal aorta and its branches (see the next section). There they synapse on the cell bodies of postsynaptic neurons. Here are the two main types of abdominopelvic splanchnic nerves:

- ✔ *Lower thoracic splanchnic nerves:* These three nerves *(greater, lesser,* and *least)* contain the most presynaptic sympathetic fibers. They pass through the diaphragm to send fibers to the *celiac, aorticorenal,* and *superior mesenteric* ganglia and plexuses.

- ✔ *Lumbar splanchnic nerves:* These nerves start at the abdominal sympathetic trunk and produce three or four lumbar splanchnic nerves that join the *intermesenteric, inferior mesenteric,* and *superior hypogastric plexuses.*

The parasympathetic nerves

The parasympathetic nerves include *anterior* and *posterior vagal trunks* that are the continuations of the left and right vagus nerves that follow the esophagus into the abdomen. They carry presynaptic parasympathetic and visceral afferent fibers to the aortic and periarterial plexuses.

The *pelvic splanchnic nerves* come from the anterior rami of the 2nd through 4th sacral nerve segments. They carry presynaptic parasympathetic fibers to the pelvic plexus. Parasympathetic ganglia are found in the walls of the abdominal organs.

Abdominal autonomic plexuses

The abdominal autonomic plexuses are networks that contain both sympathetic and parasympathetic fibers. They surround the aorta and its major branches and serve the abdominal and pelvic organs (see Chapter 11 to review the pelvic organs):

✔ *Aortic plexus:* Located around the abdominal aorta and forms periarterial plexuses on the branches of the aorta

✔ *Celiac plexus:* Located around the root of the celiac trunk; has a *parasympathetic root* that contain fibers from the vagus nerves and the *sympathetic roots* are the greater and lesser splanchnic nerves

✔ *Hepatic plexus:* Located around the hepatic artery and comes from the celiac plexus

✔ *Renal plexus:* Surround the renal arteries; formed by fibers from the celiac plexus, aortic plexus, and the least splanchnic nerve

✔ *Superior mesenteric plexus:* Surrounds the superior mesenteric artery; has three branches: the median branch comes from the celiac plexus, and the lateral branches come from the lesser and least splanchnic nerves

✔ *Inferior mesenteric plexus:* Surrounds the inferior mesenteric artery; has a medial root from the intermesenteric plexus and lateral roots from the lumbar ganglia of the sympathetic trunks

✔ *Intermesenteric plexus:* The part of the aortic plexus located between the superior and inferior mesenteric arteries; gives rise to the renal, testicular, ovarian, and uteric plexuses

✔ *Superior hypogastric plexus:* Located anterior to the bifurcation of the aorta; a continuation of the intermesenteric and plexus

✔ *Right* and *left inferior hypogastric plexus:* Located on the sides of the rectum, uterine cervix, and the urinary bladder; formed by hypogastric nerves that come from the superior hypogastric plexus and receives parasympathetic fibers from the pelvic spranchnic nerves

Major abdominal blood vessels

The largest artery is the *abdominal aorta,* which descends from the thoracic cavity, travels through the abdomen, and winds up in the pelvis where it branches into the common iliac arteries (you can see it in Figure 10-1). The abdominal arteries include:

✔ *Anterior* and *posterior inferior pancreaticoduodenal artery:* Branches off the superior mesenteric artery and rises to the head of the pancreas to supply it and the duodenum with blood

✔ *Anterior* and *posterior superior pancreaticoduodenal artery:* Branches off the gastroduodenal artery and runs down to the head of the pancreas; supplies blood to the pancreas and duodenum

- *Appendicular artery:* Branches off the ileocolic artery and supplies the appendix with blood

- *Celiac trunk:* Branches off the abdominal aorta just below the diaphragm; supplies blood to the esophagus, stomach, duodenum, liver, and pancreas

- *Common hepatic artery:* Branches off the celiac trunk and runs between the layers of the hepatoduodenal ligament; divides into the *proper hepatic artery* and the *gastroduodenal artery*

  - *Gastroduodenal artery:* Supplies blood to the stomach, pancreas, and duodenum

  - *Proper hepatic artery:* Branches into the *right* and *left hepatic arteries* and supplies blood to the liver and gallbladder

- *Cystic artery:* Usually branches off the right hepatic artery to supply blood to the gallbladder and cystic duct

- *Gonadal arteries (testicular and ovarian arteries):* Branch off the abdominal aorta and run through the inguinal canal in males or to the ovaries in the female

- *Ileocolic artery:* Branches off the superior mesenteric artery and runs along the mesentery to divide into ileal and colic branches; brings blood to the ileum, cecum, and ascending colon

- *Inferior mesenteric artery:* Branches off the abdominal aorta to supply blood to the descending colon, sigmoid colon, and rectum

- *Inferior phrenic artery:* Branches off the aorta just below the diaphragm; supplies blood to the esophagus, diaphragm, and suprarenal glands

- *Intestinal arteries:* Branch off the superior mesenteric artery and run through the mesentery to supply blood to the jejunum and ileum

- *Left colic artery:* Branches off the inferior mesenteric artery and also supplies blood to the descending colon

- *Left gastric artery:* Branches off the celiac trunk and runs up to the esophagus to supply blood to the esophagus and part of the stomach; anastomoses (connects) with the right gastric artery

- *Left gastro-omental artery:* Branches off the splenic artery and runs through the gastrosplenic ligament to the greater curvature of the stomach to supply it with blood

- *Middle colic artery:* Branches off the superior mesenteric artery and ascends to the transverse mesocolon to supply blood to the transverse colon

✔ *Renal arteries:* Branch off the abdominal aorta and run to the kidneys

✔ *Right colic artery:* Branches off the superior mesenteric artery and runs to the ascending colon to supply it with blood

✔ *Right gastric artery:* Branches off the hepatic artery and supplies the lesser curvature of the stomach

✔ *Right gastro-omental artery:* Branches off the gastroduodenal artery and runs in the greater omentum to supply the greater curvature of the stomach

✔ *Short gastric arteries:* Branch off the splenic artery and run through the gastrosplenic ligament to the fundus of the stomach to supply it with blood

✔ *Sigmoid and superior rectal arteries:* Branch off the inferior mesenteric artery to supply blood to the descending colon, sigmoid colon, and rectum (see Chapter 11)

✔ *Splenic artery:* Branches off the celiac trunk and runs along the superior part of the pancreas and then to the spleen; provides blood flow to the pancreas, spleen, and parts of the stomach

✔ *Superior mesenteric artery:* Branches off the abdominal aorta and runs through the mesentery to the ileocecal junction; provides some branches to the ileum, jejunum, and colon

✔ *Suprarenal arteries:* Branch off the renal arteries and run to the suprarenal glands

The largest vein in the abdomen is the *inferior vena cava,* which is formed by the union of the common iliac veins that carry blood back from the pelvis and lower extremities. It rises up to the thoracic cavity to empty venous blood into the heart (you can see it in Figure 10-4). Following are the tributaries that run to the inferior vena cava:

✔ *Common iliac veins:* Bring blood from the pelvis and lower extremities

✔ *Hepatic veins:* Drain the liver

✔ *Inferior phrenic vein:* Drains blood from the diaphragm

✔ *Left* and *right renal veins:* Receive blood from the kidneys

✔ *Lumbar veins:* Drain the posterior abdominal wall

✔ *Right suprarenal vein:* Receives blood from suprarenal glands

✔ *Right testicular* or *right ovarian vein:* Drain blood from the gonads (the left testicular and ovarian veins drain into the left renal vein)

Lymphatics

A number of nodes and vessels serve the organs and structures of the abdomen. Most of them are located near the abdominal aorta, the inferior vena cava, and the iliac vessel:

- ✔ *Central superior nodes:* Found along the proximal part of the superior mesenteric artery

- ✔ *Colic lymph nodes:* Drain lymph from the colon and include the epicolic, paracolic, and intermediate colic lymph nodes

- ✔ *Cystic lymph nodes:* Found near the gallbladder

- ✔ *Gastric lymph nodes:* Found on the lesser curvature of the stomach

- ✔ *Gastro-omental lymph nodes:* Located on the greater curvature of the stomach

- ✔ *Hepatic lymph nodes:* Located near the liver

- ✔ *Ileocolic lymph nodes:* Lie alongside the ilecolic artery

- ✔ *Juxta-intestinal lymph nodes:* Located alongside the walls of the small intestine

- ✔ *Lateral aortic lymph nodes:* Lie alongside the aorta and drain lymph from the kidneys, suprarenal glands, and pelvic organs

- ✔ *Lymphatic vessels:* The following vessels provide transportation of lymph up to the thoracic duct (see Chapter 8):

  - *Cisterna chyli:* Just below the diaphragm on the right side of the aorta

  - *Intestinal trunk:* Formed from vessels leaving the preaortic lymph nodes

  - *Right* and *left lumbar trunks:* Formed from the vessels leaving the lateral aortic lymph nodes

- ✔ *Pancreaticoduodenal lymph nodes:* Located near the duodenum

- ✔ *Pancreaticosplenic lymph nodes:* Found near the splenic artery

✔ *Preaortic lymph nodes:* Lie near the celiac and mesenteric arteries; drain the lymph from the gastrointestinal tract, spleen, pancreas, gallbladder, and most of the liver. They include:

- *Celiac lymph nodes* are located near the celiac trunk

- *Superior and inferior mesenteric lymph nodes* are found in the mesentery

✔ *Superior* and *inferior pyloric lymph nodes:* Found alongside the pyloric area of the stomach

Chapter 11

Seeing the Pelvis and the Perineum

*T*he pelvis is easy to access during physical examination, so it can tell you a lot if you understand its anatomy. It's especially important to know well when dealing with women's health and pregnancy as well as urinary-tract issues and rectal and prostatic problems.

This chapter goes over the anatomy of the pelvis, including the structures that all people have in common as well as the specific male and female organs. It also includes the perineum, the space between the inner thighs.

Pinpointing the Pelvic Structures

The pelvic organs that we describe later in this chapter are housed in the *pelvic girdle,* which is made up of the bones, joints, and muscles just inferior and posterior to the abdomen and above the lower extremities. (In other words, the pelvic girdle is below and behind the abdomen.) It includes the perineal region between the thighs that we talk about later in this chapter.

The *pelvic cavity* is the interior portion of the pelvis. It's bounded superiorly (at the top) by the *pelvic inlet,* which is the opening to the abdomen. Inferiorly, it's bounded by an opening called the *pelvic outlet.* It's bounded anteriorly (to the front) by a pelvic joint called the pubic symphysis and posteriorly by the coccyx (which we discuss in Chapter 15).

The pelvic inlet is formed by the following structures:

- ✔ Superior part of the pubic symphysis

- ✔ Posterior border of the pubic crest (between the pubic tubercle and the pubic symphysis joint)

- ✔ Superior ramus of the pubic bone

- ✔ Arcuate line of the ilium (a line that resembles a ridge on the internal surface of the ilium)

- ✔ Anterior portion of the sacral ala (large triangular portions on either side of the sacral base)

- ✔ Sacral promontory (most superior and anterior part of the sacrum)

The pelvic outlet is formed by these structures:

- ✔ Inferior portion of the pubic symphysis

- ✔ Inferior rami of the pubic bones and ischial tuberosities of the ischial bones

- ✔ Sacrotuberous ligaments (running from the sacrum to the ischial tuberosities)

- ✔ Tip of the coccyx (tailbone)

In the following sections, we survey the structures that form the pelvis: the bones, joints, muscles, fascia, peritoneum, nerves, blood vessels, and lymphatics. (See the later section "Comparing Pelvic Organs" for details on the items that fill the pelvic cavity.)

Did you know you have two pelvises? The *false pelvis* is bound by the abdominal wall and the upper part of the hip bones, so really it's just part of your lower abdomen, and it contains parts of the intestinal tract covered in Chapter 10. What we discuss here is the *true pelvis,* the portion of the pelvis located below the pelvic inlet.

Forming the pelvic girdle: Bones and joints

The pelvic girdle is formed by the strong bones of the hips and sacrum and the joints that hold them together; we describe these bones and joints in the following sections. (**Note:** The pelvic bones are described here, but the sacrum, which is part of the back, is described in Chapter 15.)

Bones

The left and right pelvic bones (called the *ossa coxae*) create a basin shape and form the *pelvic walls,* which include the posterior wall, an anterior wall, and two lateral pelvic walls. They *articulate* (form joints) with the sacrum and the femurs of the thighs (see Chapter 19).

The pelvic bones are the ilium, the ischium, and the pubis. These three bones are joined together at the *acetabulum,* which forms the socket for the hip joint.

- ✔ **Ilium:** The *ilium* is the flat upper part of the pelvic bone. The large fan-shaped portion is called the *ala,* and the *body* is at the bottom of the fan. It has an *iliac crest* running between the *anterior* and *posterior superior iliac spines.* The *iliac fossa* is the interior concave (bowl-shaped) part formed by the ala.

  The iliac crest is generally easy to *palpate* (medically examine by touch). Press your fingers into the patient's side near the waist and move your fingers inferiorly until you feel the large bony crest — that's the iliac crest.

- ✔ **Ischium:** This bone has two portions: the *body* and the *ramus.* The body forms part of the acetabulum, and the ramus forms the posterior portion of the *obturator foramen,* which is a large opening. The ischium also has a projection near the area where the body and ramus merge. This projection is called the *ischial spine.* The *ischial tuberosity* is a large protuberance on the posteroinferior aspect of the ischium.

- ✔ **Pubis:** The *pubis* is the most anterior portion of the pelvic bone. Its *superior pubic ramus* forms part of the acetabulum (the socket where the head of the femur forms a joint with the pelvic bone), and its *inferior pubic ramus* completes the obturator foramen (the opening created by the ischium and pubis through which nerves and blood vessels travel). The *body* of the pubis has a *pubic crest,* which turns into the *pubic tubercle.*

The inferior ramus of the pubis and the ischial ramus meet to form the ischiopubic ramus. The *pubic arch* is formed where the right and left ischiopubic rami meet at the pubic symphysis. The angle formed by the joining of the rami is called the *subpubic angle.*

The subpubic angle is wider in females than in males. The male pelvis, however, is thicker and heavier than the female pelvis, with a smaller pelvic outlet and a heart-shaped pelvic inlet.

Joints

The joints of the pelvis include the *pubic symphysis;* the *sacroiliac joints,* which are covered with the hip and thigh in Chapter 19; and the *sacrococcygeal joint* that's covered in Chapter 15.

The *pubic symphysis* is a cartilaginous joint formed between the two hip bones (see Chapter 3 for more information on types of joints). It's located at the front of the pelvis where the left and right pubic bones meet. This joint has a fibrocartilaginous disc between the bones and is surrounded by ligaments. It's a very sturdy joint that has almost no movement; however, hormones that circulate through a pregnant woman's body soften the ligaments to allow some movement so that the baby is able to move through the pelvic outlet during delivery.

Making note of muscles and fascia

The pelvis may not move as much as other parts of the body, but it does have several muscles. The *pelvic diaphragm* (also known as the pelvic floor) is the combination of the following two muscles and their fascial coverings (see Figure 11-1):

- *Coccygeus muscles:* These muscles originate at the ischial spines (see the earlier section "Bones") and insert at the bottom of the sacrum and coccyx. They help support the pelvic organs.

- *Levator ani muscle:* This muscle is attached to the pubic bones, the ischial spines, and the *tendinous arch of levator ani.* The levator ani has three parts: *puborectalis, pubococcygeus,* and *iliococcygeus.* Together these three parts support pelvic organs and resist any increase in abdominal pressure (like when you sneeze or cough) to maintain fecal and urinary continence.

The *pelvic fascia* is fibrous connective tissue that lies between the pelvic walls and the peritoneum (see the next section). The fascia has two layers: the parietal pelvic fascia and the visceral layer of pelvic fascia.

- *Parietal layer:* Lining the pelvic walls, this layer is a continuation of the abdominal fascia discussed in Chapter 9. The parietal pelvic fascia covers muscles of the pelvis.

- *Visceral layer:* This layer covers and helps support the pelvic organs that we talk about later in this chapter.

Note: The obturator internus and the piriformis muscles also are near the pelvis; we cover those muscles with the rest of the hip in Chapter 19. A few pelvic muscles also work with specific organs such as the urethra and vagina; we discuss them later in this chapter.

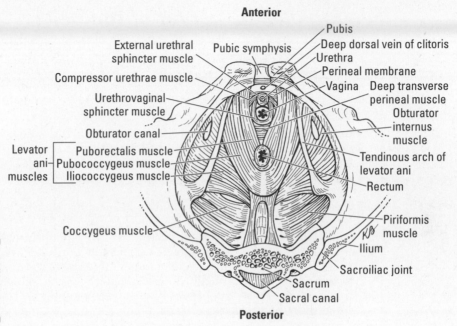

Anterior

External urethral
sphincter muscle

Pubic symphysis

Pubis

Deep dorsal vein of clitoris

Urethra

Compressor urethrae muscle

Perineal membrane

Urethrovaginal
sphincter muscle

Vagina   Deep transverse
          perineal muscle

Obturator
internus
muscle

Obturator canal

Levator   Puborectalis muscle
ani   Pubococcygeus muscle
muscles   Iliococcygeus muscle

Tendinous arch of
levator ani

Rectum

Coccygeus muscle

Piriformis
muscle

Ilium

Sacroiliac joint

Sacrum

Sacral canal

Posterior

Figure 11-1:
Muscles of
the pelvic
diaphragm.

Personal space: The peritoneum

The *peritoneum* that lines the abdominal cavity (see Chapter 9) continues into the pelvis where it forms a number of folds and fossae (depressions) as it covers the superior and lateral surfaces of the pelvic organs:

- ✔ *Supravesical fossa:* On the superior surface of the bladder

- ✔ *Paravesical fossae:* Located on each side of the bladder

- ✔ *Vesico-uterine pouch:* Formed between the bladder and uterus in females

- ✔ *The broad ligament:* A portion of the peritoneum that covers the uterus and vagina in females; surrounds the uterine tubes and round ligaments and suspends the ovaries

- ✔ *The ureteric fold:* Covers the ureters, ductus deferentes, and superior portion of seminal vesicles in males

- ✔ *Recto-uterine pouch:* Located between the uterus and rectum in females

- ✔ *Rectovesical pouch:* Located between the bladder, seminal vesicles and rectum in males

- ✔ *Pararectal fossae:* Run along each side of the rectum

Feeling out the nerves of the pelvis

The pelvic girdle is *innervated* (provided with nervous supply) by nerves that come from the sacral plexus, coccygeal plexus, and pelvic autonomic nerves. You find out more about these groups of nerves in the following sections.

The sacral plexus

The 4th and 5th lumbar spinal nerves (see Chapter 15) form the *lumbosacral trunk*. The lumbosacral trunk goes on to join the 1st through 4th sacral nerves as they exit the sacrum to form the *sacral plexus*. The sacral plexus runs down on the posterior pelvic wall anterior to the piriformis muscle.

The nerves that stem from the sacral plexus include the following:

- *Sciatic nerve:* This nerve is formed by the 4th lumbar through 3rd sacral spinal nerves. It's the largest nerve in the body. It leaves the pelvis through the greater sciatic foramen (opening in the posterior portion of the pelvis formed by the sciatic notch of the ischium and the sacrospinous and sacrotuberous ligament; see Chapter 13) to enter the gluteal area (buttocks; see Chapter 19).

- *Pudendal nerve:* This nerve is formed from the 2nd through 4th spinal sacral nerves. It exits the pelvis through the greater sciatic foramen and enters the perineum through the lesser sciatic foramen to innervate the muscles and skin of the perineum (which we discuss later in this chapter).

- *Superior gluteal nerve:* Formed by the 4th lumbar through the 1st sacral spinal nerves, this nerve leaves the greater sciatic foramen to innervate gluteal muscles.

- *Inferior gluteal nerve:* This nerve's formed by the 5th lumbar through 2nd sacral spinal nerves. Like the superior gluteal nerve, it runs through the greater sciatic foramen to innervate gluteal muscles.

- *Nerve to the quadratus femoris muscle:* This nerve is formed from the 4th lumbar through the 1st sacral spinal nerves. It leaves the greater sciatic foramen to innervate hip muscles.

- *Nerve to the obturator internus muscle:* This nerve is formed by fibers from the 5th lumbar through the 2nd sacral spinal nerves. It also leaves the greater sciatic foramen to innervate hip muscles.

- *Nerve to the piriformis muscle:* Stemming from the 1st and 2nd sacral spinal nerves, this nerve innervates the piriformis muscle.

- *Perforating cutaneous nerve:* This nerve is formed from the 2nd and 3rd sacral spinal nerves and innervates the skin over the lower and medial portion of the buttock.

 ✔ *Posterior femoral cutaneous nerve:* This nerve's formed from the 2nd and 3rd sacral spinal nerves and innervates the skin of the perineum and the back surface of the thigh and leg.

 ✔ *Pelvic splanchnic nerves:* Stemming from the 2nd through 4th sacral spinal nerves, these nerves provide the parasympathtetic innervation to the pelvic organs (which we talk about later in this chapter).

The coccygeal plexus

The *coccygeal plexus* of nerve fibers is formed by the 4th and 5th sacral spinal nerves and the *coccygeal nerves.* It supplies the coccygeus and levator ani muscles and the sacrococcygeal joint. *Anococcygeal nerves* innervate the skin between the coccyx and anus.

Obturator nerve

The *obturator nerve* arises from the from the lumbar plexus and doesn't innervate anything in the pelvis, but it runs through the pelvis to the medial thigh. Its function is discussed in Chapter 19.

Pelvic autonomic nerves

Pelvic autonomic nerves innervate the pelvic cavity; in general, autonomic nerves control things like blood flow, hormone levels, and body functions that you don't consciously think about (see Chapter 3 for details). Pelvic autonomic nerves include the following:

 ✔ *Sacral sympathetic trunks:* These nerves are a continuation of the *lumbar sympathetic trunks.* They run in front of the sacrum and behind the rectum. The sacral sympathetic trunks each have four ganglia (collection of neuron cell bodies; see Chapter 3). The right and left sacral sympathetic trunks unite at the *ganglion impar* anterior to (in front of) the coccyx. These trunks provide *postganglionic sympathetic fibers* to the sacral plexus that innervate the lower extremities (we discuss the sacral plexus earlier in this chapter). In addition, they provide fibers to the hypogastric plexus discussed later on.

 ✔ *Superior hypogastric plexus:* This nerve sits in front of the sacral promontory (most superior portion of the anterior surface of the sacrum). It contains sympathetic fibers from the aortic plexus (see Chapter 10). It descends into the pelvis and divides into the *left* and *right hypogastric nerves.*

 ✔ *Inferior hypogastric plexuses:* These plexuses are formed when the right and left hypogastric nerves are joined by preganglionic parasympathetic fibers from the *pelvic splanchnic nerves.* The plexuses are located on each side of the rectum and the base of the bladder. They contain both sympathetic and parasympathetic fibers (see Chapter 3 for more about nerve fibers).

Pelvic splanchnic nerves (S2–S4): These nerves are preganglionic parasympathetic fibers that originate from the 2nd, 3rd, and 4th sacral spinal segments. They join the hypogastric nerves to form the inferior hypogastric plexuses.

Parasympathetic stimulation increases peristalsis and contraction of the bladder and rectum for urination and defecation. Parasympathetic stimulation of the genital erectile tissue stimulates erection. Sympathetic stimulation inhibits peristalsis and stimulates muscle contraction of genital organs during orgasm.

Viewing blood vessels

The abdominal aorta branches into the *right* and *left common iliac arteries* at the level of the 4th lumbar vertebra. The common iliac arteries descend to the pelvic brim, where they divide into the *external* and *internal iliac arteries.*

The external iliac arteries leave the abdominal cavity to supply the lower extremities. They have two branches, the *inferior epigastric* and *deep circumflex iliac arteries.*

The *internal iliac artery* enters the pelvis to supply blood to pelvic organs, gluteal muscles, and the perineum. It has many branches that stem from its two divisions (anterior and posterior). You can see some branches of the anterior division in Figure 11-2:

- ✔ *Umbilical artery* and *superior vesical artery:* Supply the upper part of the bladder

- ✔ *Obturator artery:* Runs along the lateral pelvic wall and supplies pelvic muscles, ilium, and head of the femur (see Chapter 19)

- ✔ *Inferior vesical artery:* In males only; supplies blood to the base of the bladder and gives rise to the prostatic artery that supplies blood to the prostate, seminal glands, and the *artery of the vas deferens,* which supplies blood to the vas deferens (see the later section "Male internal organs")

- ✔ *Middle rectal artery:* Supplies blood to the rectum

- ✔ *Internal pudendal artery:* Enters the perineum through the lesser sciatic foramen (see Chapter 13); supplies blood to the anal muscles, the skin and muscles of the perineum, and *dorsal artery* to the penis and clitoris; also gives rise to the inferior rectal artery

✔ *Inferior gluteal artery:* Also runs through the greater sciatic foramen and supplies blood to the piriformis, coccygeus, levator ani, and gluteal muscles

✔ *Uterine artery:* Runs medially on the floor of the female pelvis and then crosses the ureter to reach the broad ligament; supplies blood to the ureter, uterus, uterine tube, ovary, and vagina; has a branch called the *vaginal artery* that replaces the male *inferior vesical artery*

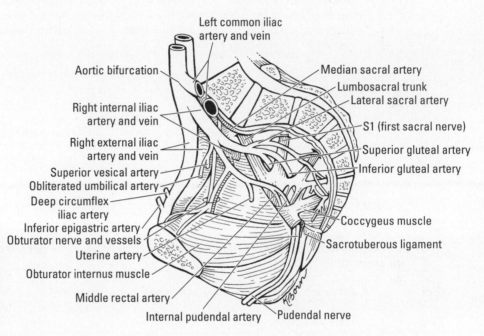

Left common iliac artery and vein

Aortic bifurcation

Median sacral artery
Lumbosacral trunk
Lateral sacral artery

Right internal iliac artery and vein

S1 (first sacral nerve)

Right external iliac artery and vein

Superior gluteal artery
Inferior gluteal artery

Superior vesical artery
Obliterated umbilical artery
Deep circumflex iliac artery
Inferior epigastric artery
Obturator nerve and vessels
Uterine artery
Obturator internus muscle
Middle rectal artery
Internal pudendal artery

Coccygeus muscle

Sacrotuberous ligament

Pudendal nerve

Figure 11-2: Some arteries and veins of the pelvis.

The posterior division of the internal iliac artery supplies blood to the pelvic wall and the gluteal region (refer to Figure 11-2 to see some of these arteries):

✔ *Iliolumbar artery:* Ascends in front of the sacroiliac joint to supply blood to the iliacus and psoas major (covered in Chapter 19), quadratus lumborum muscles, and the cauda equina (see Chapter 15)

✔ *Lateral sacral arteries:* Descend in front of the sacral plexus and provide blood to the piriformis and vertebral canal (see Chapter 15)

✔ *Superior gluteal artery:* Leaves the pelvis through the greater sciatic foramen and supplies blood to the gluteal muscles and tensor fascia latae (find more info about them in Chapters 19 and 20)

The remaining arteries also supply blood to various organs of the pelvis:

- ✔ *Superior rectal artery:* A continuation of the inferior mesenteric artery in the abdomen (described in Chapter 10); supplies blood to the rectum and anal canal

- ✔ *Median sacral artery:* Starts at the bifurcation of the aorta (see Chapter 9) and runs down to the front of the sacrum and coccyx

- ✔ *Ovarian arteries:* In females only; start at the abdominal aorta around the level of the 1st lumbar vertebra and run down behind the peritoneum and enter the suspensory ligaments of the ovaries (we talk more about the ovaries later in this chapter)

The masculine counterpart of the ovarian arteries are the *testicular arteries,* but they go through the inguinal canals and do not enter the pelvis.

The principal veins that return blood from the pelvis include the *external* and *internal iliac veins* and the *median sacral veins.* They accompany the arteries of the same names.

Looking at lymphatics

Several groups of lymph nodes facilitate lymphatic drainage from the pelvis (see more about the lymphatic system in Chapter 5). The nodes are located along the vessels in the pelvic region.

- ✔ *External iliac lymph nodes:* Receive lymph from the *inguinal lymph nodes,* which are located along the femoral vein in the anterior thigh, and from pelvic organs

- ✔ *Internal iliac lymph nodes:* Receive lymph from the pelvic organs, perineum, and gluteal region

- ✔ *Sacral lymph nodes:* Receive lymph from the pelvic organs and drain into the internal or common iliac nodes

- ✔ *Common iliac lymph nodes:* Receive lymph from the other pelvic nodes

- ✔ *Pararectal nodes:* Lie in the connective tissue next to branches of the internal iliac lymphatic vessels

- ✔ *Superficial inguinal* and *deep inguinal nodes:* Drain lymph from the inferolateral part of the trunk and perineum

- ✔ *Lumbar nodes:* Associated with the aorta and inferior vena cava; receive lymph from the previously listed nodes

The lymph nodes of the pelvis are interconnected quite extensively, which means some of the nodes can be removed without disturbing lymphatic drainage. However, it also means cancerous cells can easily spread to any pelvic or abdominal organs.

Comparing Pelvic Organs

The pelvis is home to the reproductive organs, which, of course, vary greatly from males to females. All people have some pelvic organs in common, though, including some of the urinary organs and the rectum. We give you the info you need about all these organs in the following sections.

Locating pelvic organs that everyone has

Males and females have similar ureters and urinary bladders, and the rectum is about the same as well. We discuss all these organs in the following sections.

Urinary organs

The kidneys (organs that filter the blood and produce urine) are located retroperitoneally (behind the peritoneum) in the abdominal cavity (see Chapter 10 for details), but the urine has to get down into the pelvis where it is stored until urination. The pelvic organs involved in that function are the ureters and the urinary bladder.

- ✔ **Ureters:** These muscular tubes start at the kidneys and travel down into the pelvis near the bifurcation of the common iliac arteries that we talk about earlier in this chapter. From there, they continue down the lateral walls of the pelvis before entering the posterior surface of the urinary bladder.

  Ureters are innervated by the autonomic plexuses. Blood is supplied to the pelvic portion of the ureters by the uterine arteries in females and inferior vesical arteries in males. Lymph drains into the lumbar, common iliac, external iliac, and internal iliac nodes.

- ✔ **Urinary bladder:** This hollow organ is shaped somewhat like a pyramid when empty. Its job is to store urine. The *apex* of the bladder points toward the front of the body and lies behind the pubic symphysis. The *fundus* is the back of the bladder. The *body* is between the apex and the fundus. In males, the fundus is adjacent to the rectum, whereas in females it lies against the vagina. The urinary bladder nestles in a *bladder bed,* which is formed by the pubic bones, fascia, and either the rectum or vagina.

The walls of the bladder are made up by three layers of involuntary muscle called the *detrusor muscle.* In males, this muscle forms an *internal urethral sphincter.* On the inside of the bladder, the walls are covered in a mucous membrane. The membrane-covered area at the base of the bladder is called the *trigone.* The openings of the ureters and urethra demarcate this area.

The urinary bladder receives blood flow from branches of the internal iliac arteries (that is, the superior and inferior vesical arteries in males, and the superior vesical and vaginal arteries in females). Blood is drained via the *vesical venous plexus.* The internal and external iliac lymph nodes provide lymph drainage, and the inferior hypogastric plexuses innervate the urinary bladder.

Although the muscles of the urinary bladder and internal urethra sphincter are smooth muscle and under autonomic (involuntary) control, after a person is toilet trained the cerebral cortex can override the urge to urinate, voluntary inhibiting the act of *micturtion* (urination). Injuries to the spinal cord can disrupt the brain's control of micturition.

Understanding the anatomy of the urinary organs is important because kidney stones can cause flank pain as they pass through the ureters (the urine tubes). The pain is often described as radiating from "loin to groin." Cystitis or bladder infections are common, too, especially in women.

The rectum

The *rectum* is the final portion of the colon (see Chapter 10). It starts where the sigmoid colon ends, at the *rectosigmoid junction.* The rectum follows the curve of the anterior part of the sacrum and ends in front of the coccyx. The lower end dilates to form the *rectal ampulla.* From there, it takes a sharp posterior turn and turns into the *anal canal.* That angle is called the *anorectal flexure.*

The rectal ampulla holds fecal matter until defecation, but the sharp angle of the anorectal flexure helps keep it in place until you make it to the restroom.

The rectum has a mucous membrane that's covered in a *muscular coat* that consists of two layers of muscle arranged in circular and longitudinal layers. In three places, the membrane and muscles form folds that jut into the interior of the rectum. They're called the *transverse rectal folds.*

The rectum is innervated by the inferior hypogastric plexuses (see the earlier section "Pelvic autonomic nerves" for more info). The rectum receives blood flow from the superior, middle, and inferior rectal arteries and returns blood through the superior, middle, and inferior rectal veins. (The superior rectal vein drains into the portal venous system. You can find out more about portal blood flow in Chapter 10). Lymph from the rectum drains into the pararectal nodes and the internal iliac nodes.

Finding Mars: The male pelvic organs

The male organs include the penis and various glands and ducts, as you find out in the following sections. Figure 11-3 features an overview of the male pelvis. The testicles and scrotum are also important male structures, and we cover them in the Chapter 9 discussion of the abdominal wall.

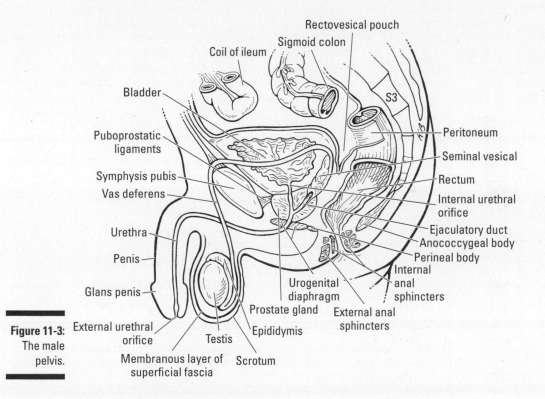

Figure 11-3:
The male pelvis.

The male urethra and the penis

The *male urethra* (refer to Figure 11-3) is a muscular tube that runs through the prostate, perineal membrane and muscles, and the penis from the *internal urethral orifice* of the urinary bladder to the *external urethral orifice* located at the tip of the *glans penis* (the bulbous structure at the distal end). It conveys urine, as well as semen, out of the body.

The urethra is divided into the following four parts:

- ✔ *Preprostatic part:* Surrounded by the *internal urethral sphincter,* which prevents semen from entering the bladder during *ejaculation* (the release of semen through the urethra)

- ✔ *Prostatic part:* Surrounded by the prostate gland (we get to that organ in the next section)

- ✔ *Intermediate (membranous) part:* Surrounded by another sphincter called the *external urethral sphincter*

- ✔ *Penile (spongy) part:* Runs through the penis

The *prostatic nerve plexus* provides innervation to the first three parts of the urethra. The penile (spongy) urethra is innervated by the dorsal nerve of the penis. The first two parts of the urethra get their blood supply from the inferior vesical and middle rectal arteries, while the rest of the urethra gets its blood flow from the internal pudendal artery. Blood is returned through their accompanying veins. Lymph drainage is mostly through the internal iliac lymph nodes, but some also goes to the external iliac lymph nodes and the deep inguinal lymph nodes. (We discuss pelvic nerves, blood vessels, and lymphatics earlier in this chapter.)

The penis consists of three parts, a *root, body,* and *glans penis:*

- ✔ **Root:** The *root* contains three groups of erectile tissue called the *bulb* and the *left* and *right crura.* The bulb surrounds the urethra and is covered by *bulbospongiosus muscles.* Each crus is covered by *ischiocavernosus muscle,* which is attached to the pubic arch.

- ✔ **Body:** The *body* contains the *corpus spongiosum,* which is a cylindrical continuation of the bulb, and the *corpora cavernosa,* which are formed by continuations of the two crura. All three cylinders of erectile tissue are surrounded by Buck's fascia.

- ✔ **Glans:** The *corpus spongiosum* expands distally to form the *glans penis.* The glans forms the *corona of the glans,* which is separated from the body by the *neck of the glans.* The external urethral orifice is the slit-like opening at the tip.

  The glans penis is covered by a double layer of skin called the *prepuce,* or foreskin. The *frenulum* is a fold of skin that runs from the prepuce to the urethral surface of the glans.

The pudendal nerve via the dorsal nerve of the penis innervates the skin and glans. Parasympathetic innervation from the inferior hypogastric plexus supplies the vasculature of the erectile tissue. Blood is supplied to the penis by the branches of the internal pudendal arteries called the *deep arteries of the penis,* the *arteries of the bulb,* and the *dorsal arteries of the penis.* Blood returns via the pudendal veins. Lymph drains into the superficial inguinal nodes and internal iliac nodes.

Internal male organs

The internal male organs, or genital organs, include the testes, epididymides, vasa deferentia (ductus deferentia), seminal vesicles, ejaculatory ducts, prostate gland, and the bulbourethral glands. (The testes and epididymides are covered in Chapter 9 along with the abdominal wall.)

The *vas deferens* is a long tube that carries sperm from the epididymis to the ejaculatory duct. It starts from the epididymis, goes through the inguinal canal, crosses the external iliac vessels, and enters the pelvis. It runs along the lateral wall of the pelvis and ends its course with a dilation called the *ampulla of the vas deferens,* and joins the duct of the seminal gland on the medial side of the *seminal vesicle* to form the *ejaculatory duct* (refer to Figure 11-3). Each seminal vesicle lies on the posterior surface of the urinary bladder. They secrete thick fluid into the ejaculatory duct, which mixes with the sperm.

Blood supply to the vasa deferentia is from the superior vesicle arteries, and blood supply to the seminal vesicles comes from the inferior vesicle and middle rectal arteries and returns via the internal iliac veins. Lymph drains into the internal iliac nodes.

The *prostate gland* (refer to Figure 11-3) surrounds the prostatic part of the urethra. It's about the size of a walnut. Its *base* sits near the neck of the urinary bladder, and its *apex* is next to the *urogenital diaphragm.* It's covered in a thick fibrous capsule, which houses the prostatic plexuses of nerves and veins. The prostate has five lobes, the anterior, middle, posterior, and two lateral lobes. The prostate secretes a milky fluid that's added to the seminal fluid at the time of ejaculation. Blood is supplied to the prostate by the inferior vesical, internal pudendal, and middle rectal arteries. Blood is returned via the *prostatic venous plexuses,* which is located around the base and sides of the prostate.

The fluids produced by the glands are alkaline in pH, which helps to neutralize the acidity of the female vagina.

The *bulbourethral glands* are two small glands located within the external urethral sphincter. They secrete a mucus-like fluid into the urethra during sexual arousal.

Finding Venus: The female pelvic organs

The female pelvic organs include the egg-producing ovaries and the uterine tubes that carry the eggs into the uterus for potential fertilization by male sperm. They also include the vagina, which is the entryway to the uterus. We cover these parts, along with the female urethra, in the following sections. Figure 11-4 provides an overview of the female pelvis.

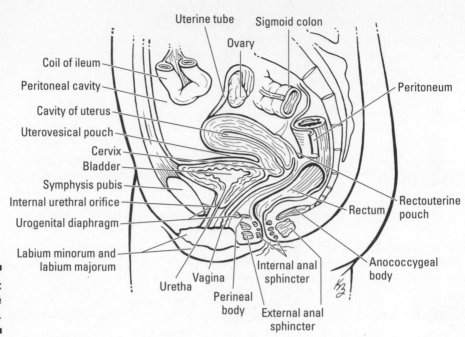

Uterine tube

Sigmoid colon

Ovary

Coil of ileum

Peritoneal cavity

Cavity of uterus

Uterovesical pouch

Cervix

Bladder

Symphysis pubis

Internal urethral orifice

Urogenital diaphragm

Labium minorum and labium majorum

Peritoneum

Rectouterine pouch

Rectum

Anococcygeal body

Internal anal sphincter

Vagina

Uretha

Perineal body

External anal sphincter

Figure 11-4: The female pelvis.

The female urethra

The *female urethra* (refer to Figure 11-4) runs from the *internal urethral orifice* of the urinary bladder, anterior to the vagina, to the *external urethral orifice* in the *vulva.* Two *paraurethral glands* open into the urethra near the external urethral orifice.

The urethra is innervated by the *vesical plexus* as well as the pudendal nerve (refer to the earlier section "Feeling out the nerves of the pelvis" for a reminder of those). The urethra receives blood from the internal pudendal and vaginal arteries and returns blood through their accompanying veins. Lymph drains into the internal iliac and sacral nodes. (We describe these structures earlier in this chapter.)

The uterus and the vagina

The *uterus* is a pear-shaped hollow organ with muscular walls. Its function is to nourish a fertilized ovum. In a nonpregnant female, it lies on the urinary bladder (refer to Figure 11-4). The *fundus* lies above the entrance of the uterine tube; the *body* is the part below. The *cervix* is the narrow part that protrudes into the vagina. It has a *cervical canal,* which opens into the vagina through the *external os,* which is the opening of the uterus (see Figure 11-5).

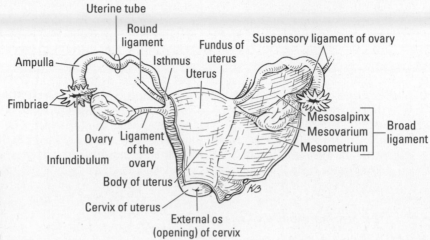

Uterine tube

Round ligament

Fundus of uterus

Suspensory ligament of ovary

Ampulla

Isthmus

Uterus

Fimbriae

Mesosalpinx

Mesovarium

Mesometrium

Broad ligament

Ovary

Ligament of the ovary

Infundibulum

Body of uterus

Cervix of uterus

External os (opening) of cervix

Figure 11-5: The parts of the uterus.

The external os is circular in a woman who hasn't given birth, but after childbirth, the external os becomes a transverse slit.

The walls of the uterus consist of three layers.

- ✓ *Perimetrium:* A fascial layer
- ✓ *Myometrium:* A thick layer made up of smooth muscle and connective tissue
- ✓ *Endometrium:* Lines the body of the uterus and is the part of the uterus that's involved with the menstrual cycle

Uterine fibroids are benign (noncancerous) tumors that grow in the lining of the uterus. The cause isn't known, but it appears to be linked with the female hormone, *estrogen*. If they're small, there's no problem, but if they grow into larger masses, they can cause longer and heavier menstrual periods, pain, and a feeling of fullness in the pelvis. Treatment may include birth-control pills to regulate the hormones, intrauterine devices to reduce bleeding, iron supplements to prevent anemia, nonsteroidal anti-inflammatory medications for pain relief, and surgery if necessary for large and troublesome fibroids.

The uterus is supported by several ligaments, including the *round ligament* (attaches to the uterus near the junction of the uterine tube and runs through the inguinal canal to the labia majora), the *ligament of the ovary* (attaches to the uterus just posterior and inferior to the uterine tube), the *broad ligament* (extends from the sides of the uterus to the lateral walls and floor of the pelvis), the *cardinal ligament* (runs from the cervix to the lateral wall), and the *suspensory ligament* (attaches to the ovary). You can find these ligaments in Figure 11-5.

Nerve supply comes from the inferior hypogastric plexuses. The uterus receives blood flow from the uterine artery and returns blood via the uterine vein. Lymph drains into the para-aortic, internal iliac, external iliac, and superficial inguinal nodes. (We discuss these items earlier in this chapter.)

The *vagina* is a mostly muscular tube that extends from the uterus to an external opening surrounded by the labia and vulva. The part of the vagina that surrounds the cervix is divided into four *fornices:* anterior, posterior, and left and right lateral. The vagina is also known as the birth canal, because the baby passes through the vagina during birth. It also allows excretion of menstrual flow. Nerve supply comes from the inferior hypogastric plexus. Blood flow comes from the vaginal artery and vaginal veins. Lymph drains into the external and internal iliac nodes and the superficial inguinal nodes.

The uterine tubes and the ovaries

The *uterine tubes* lie between the ovaries and uterus, in the *broad ligament.* Each tube starts with the funnel-shaped *infundibulum,* which has *fimbriae,* finger-like projections that lie over the ovary. The *ampulla* is the widest part of the tube, which narrows to form the *isthmus.* The *intramural part* opens into the uterine wall. (Refer to Figure 11-5.)

An ectopic pregnancy occurs when the fertilized ovum implants outside of the uterus, usually within the walls of the uterine tubes. Symptoms include abnormal vaginal bleeding, amenorrhea, breast tenderness, lower back pain, and pain or pelvic cramps. The pregnancy cannot continue, and the implanted cells must be removed to save the woman's life.

The *ovaries* are two oval-shaped organs attached to the broad ligament. The *suspensory ligament of the ovary* conveys blood vessels and nerves to the ovaries, while the *round ligament* runs between the uterus and the ovaries.

The nerve supply for the uterine tubes comes from the inferior hypogastric plexuses. The nerve supply to the ovaries comes from the aortic plexus. The uterine tubes and ovaries receive blood flow from the uterine and ovarian arteries, and they return blood via veins of the same names. Lymph drains into the internal iliac and para-aortic nodes.

Exit Strategy: The Perineum

The *perineum* is the region between the thighs inferior to the pelvic diaphragm. The boundaries of this region are the same as that for the pelvic outlet, namely the pubic symphysis, ischiopubic rami, sacrotuberous ligaments, and coccyx. The perineum has a roof formed by the pelvic diaphragm and a floor of fascia and skin. It also contains the muscles and neurovasculature associated with urogenital structures and the anus (described later in this chapter).

When the legs are abducted (spread apart), the perineum forms a diamond shape that can be divided into two triangles by drawing a line connecting the ischial tuberosities: the urogenital triangle and the anal triangle.

- *Urogenital triangle:* The urogenital triangle makes up the anterior portion of the perineum. The female urogenital triangle is home to the opening of the vagina, the urethra, and the clitoris. Figure 11-6 shows the muscles of the perineum, and you can also see the differences by gender.

  The *perineal fascia* of the urogenital triangle includes superficial and deep layers. The *superficial perineal fascia* has a fatty layer and a deeper membranous layer (*Colles fascia*). The fatty layer makes up the thickened areas of the *labia majora* and *mons pubis.* In males, the fatty layer is much thinner and is absent in the penis and scrotum.

- *Anal triangle:* The anal triangle contains the *anus* and the *ischioanal fossae,* which are two wedge-shaped spaces between the skin around the anal canal and the pelvic diaphragm. They contain fat and loose connective tissue, which helps support the anal canal but is pliable enough to allow for expansion during bowel movements.

The anal canal becomes the anus after it passes the pelvic diaphragm. The *internal anal sphincter* is an involuntary muscle surrounding the superior portion of the anal canal. The *external anal sphincter* is a large voluntary muscle that forms a band on each side of the inferior portion of the canal. The *pectinate line* is the landmark that divides the upper half of the anal canal from the lower half. The external anal sphincter has three parts:

- The *subcutaneous part* circles the lower end of the anal canal.

- The *superficial part* is attached to the coccyx and the perineal body.

- The *deep part* circles the upper end of the canal.

Hemorrhoids are painful, swollen veins in the anal canal or anus. Internal hemorrhoids occur in the anal canal, but they may not be painful because the rectum doesn't have many nerves that sense pain. External hemorrhoids affect the anus and are easy to see and palpate by inspecting the anus. More sensory nerves are located around the anus, so external hemorrhoids may be quite painful. They may also result in itching and bleeding. Topical medications may help shrink hemorrhoids, and dietary changes may prevent their occurrence; however, surgery may be indicated when reoccurrences are frequent.

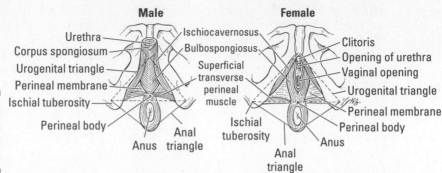

Figure 11-6:
The muscles
of the
perineum.

The anal region is innervated by the inferior hypogastric plexuses and the *inferior rectal nerve.* The blood supply to the anal area is provided by the superior and inferior rectal arteries. Blood is retuned by their accompanying veins. Lymph drains into the pararectal nodes and superficial inguinal nodes. (We describe these items earlier in this chapter.)

The *pudendal canal* lines the lateral wall of the ischioanal fossa. It's a passageway for the pudendal arteries, veins, and nerves that serve the perineum with their branches.

Wait — you're not finished with the perineum yet! The preceding text describes the perineum parts that everyone has in common, but males and females do have some differences, as you find out in the following sections.

The male perineum

The male perineum includes the penis, scrotum, and the perineal muscles in the urogenital triangle, along with the anal triangle. (We talk about the penis and perineal muscles earlier in the chapter.)

The *scrotum* is the fibromuscular sac that houses the testes (refer to Figure 11-3). It's located behind and below the penis. On the surface, you can see the *scrotal raphe,* which is a ridge that runs along the midline of the scrotum. It continues on the penis as the *penile raphe.* Internally, the scrotum is divided by a *septum of the scrotum.*

The female perineum

The female perineum includes the external genitalia, orifices of the urethra and vagina, and the perineal muscles (we describe the orifices and the perineal muscles earlier in this chapter). Pelvic examinations begin with the inspection of these areas.

The external genitalia are collectively referred to as the *vulva*. They include the mons pubis, the labia majora, the labia minora, and the clitoris. The vestibule, the region between the labia minora that the urethra and vagina open into, is also located here. Following are decriptions of these parts:

- *Mons pubis:* This rounded, fatty eminence is anterior to the pubic symphysis.

- *Labia majora:* These prominent folds of fat and skin help to protect the orifices of the urethra and vagina. The labia majora are separated by the *pudendal cleft.*

- *Labia minora:* Inside the pudendal cleft you find these two folds of skin, but they don't contain fat. The anterior portions of the labia minora unite to form laminae that become the *frenulum* and *prepuce* of the clitoris.

- *Clitoris:* This small erectile organ corresponds with the male penis. (Refer to Figure 11-6.) It's located where the labia minor meet at the front of the vulva. The *root* of the clitoris is made up of the *bulb of the vestibule* and the *left* and *right crura of the clitoris.* The *body* of the clitoris contains two *corpora cavernosa* and *ischiocavernosus muscles.* The *glans* of the clitoris is a mass of erectile tissue that has many nerve endings. The blood supply is provided by the branches of the internal pudendal arteries and veins.

- *Vestibule:* This feature is a space between the labia minora. You can find the external urethral orifice there, along with the vaginal orifice. *Greater vestibular glands* and *lesser vestibular glands* lie on either side of the vestibule posterior to the vaginal orifice. The vestibular glands secrete slippery fluids during sexual arousal.

The anterior vulva is innervated by *anterior labial nerves* (branches of the ilioguinal and genital branch of the genitofemoral nerves). *Posterior (labial) nerves* supply the labia minora, vagina, and clitoris (via a branch called *the dorsal nerve of the clitoris*). Blood flow to the vulva is provided by external and internal pudendal arteries. Blood is returned by the labial and internal pudendal veins. Lymph drains into the superficial inguinal lymph nodes, deep inguinal nodes, and internal iliac nodes.

Part III
Looking at the Head, Neck, and Back

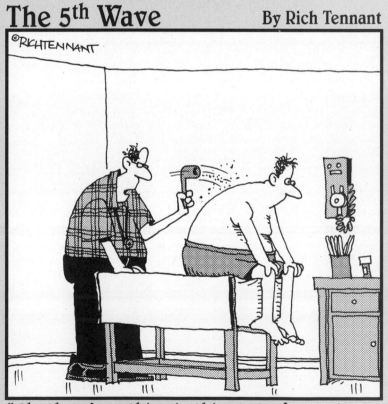

"Oh, there's nothing in this part of your back. I'm just cleaning my pipe."

In this part . . .

Part III includes everything from the neck up, but the
chapters start from the top down. First up is the
head, which includes the brain, the facial features, and the
organs that feed your senses of sight, sound, smell, and
taste. We then discuss the neck, which connects the head
to the rest of the body and is filled with an impressive
array of organs and structures. Finally, we cover the back,
including the bones and the spinal cord.

Chapter 12

Head of the Class

The head doesn't take up a large amount of space compared to the rest of the body, but it contains a number of complicated organs and structures, including the brain, which is in control of the nervous system and lets you think about things and make various decisions throughout each day.

Don't forget about your face, either. Not only is it the placeholder for your eyes, nose, and mouth, but it also presents the world with an array of emotions.

This chapter explains the anatomy of the head, including the skull, the brain, the facial muscles, and various nerves and blood vessels. We look at the eyes, ears, nose, and mouth in Chapter 13.

Sticking to the Skull Bones

The skull, or more officially, the *cranium,* has bones that protect your brain and form your face. The bones that protect the brain are strong and have very little movement at the joints. Their main purpose is to protect the delicate tissues of the brain and its coverings.

The cranium also has some delicate bones that form your beautiful face. The facial bones don't move much, either, except for the jawbone (which moves a lot).

In the following sections, we tell you all about the bones of the skull that protect the brain and form the face.

Need help with keeping all these cranial and facial bones straight? Check out Chapter 22 for some handy mnemonic devices.

Cradling the brain in the cranial cavity

The part of the cranium that holds your brain is called the *neurocranium,* which contains the cranial cavity. It has a rounded dome shape *(calvaria)* on the top and *cranial base* at the bottom. The neurocranium is formed by the following bones (which you can see in Figure 12-1).

- **Frontal bone:** The *frontal bone* is best seen from the front of the skull. It forms the forehead and top portions of the orbits (what most people call the eye sockets). It has two *supercilliary arches* above the eyes and two *supraorbital foramina* (notches) on the medial (middle) part of the arches. The frontal bone also has two hollow spaces called the *frontal sinuses* that are lined with mucous membranes.

- **Parietal bones:** A pair of *parietal bones* form much of the sides and top of the cranium. They meet in the midline at the *sagittal suture,* which is a jagged immobile joint. They join the frontal bone at the *coronal suture.* The meeting point of the sagittal and coronal sutures is the *bregma.* Each parietal bone has two arched lines called the *inferior* and *superior temporal lines.* The area inferior to (below) the inferior temporal line is part of the *temporal fossa,* which is a shallow depression on the side of the skull.

- **Occipital bone:** The *occipital bone* forms the posterior (rear) portion of the skull. It features a large bump, the *external occipital protuberance,* that you can palpate (medically examine) in the midline just above the neck. *Superior* and *inferior nuchal lines* extend laterally from the protuberance. The occipital bone joins the parietal bones at the *lambdoid suture.* The point where the three bones meet is called the *lambda,* and sometimes it can be felt as a slight depression at the top and back of your head. The occipital bone has a large opening called the *foramen magnum,* which transmits the spinal cord. It also has two *occipital condyles,* which are two rounded bony prominences that articulate with the first cervical vertebra (see Chapter 15).

- **Temporal bones:** Two *temporal bones* form the lower parts of the sides of the cranial vault (the space occupied by the brain). Each one meets a parietal bone at the *squamous suture* and forms part of the temporal fossa. Two processes (bony projections) extend from the inferior portion of each bone: the *styloid process* and *mastoid process.* Another process, called the *zygomatic process,* joins the zygomatic bone (coming up in the next section — it's a facial bone). The temporal bones also join the sphenoid bone.

- **Sphenoid bone:** The *sphenoid bone* is a butterfly-shaped bone situated anterior to (in front of) the temporal bones. The *body* has hollow spaces called the *sphenoid air sinuses.* It also has two larger and two smaller wings and two processes called the *pterygoid plates* that project inferiorly. Three pairs of openings, the *foramen rotundum, foramen ovale,* and *foramen spinosum,* are situated on the greater wings near the body. A depression called the *sella turcica* houses the pituitary gland. It's bound by the two *middle clinoid processes* anteriorly and a portion of bone called the *dorsum sella* posteriorly. It also forms the posterior walls of the orbits.

The *pterion* is the meeting point of the sphenoid, frontal, parietal, and temporal bones. You can find it in the anterior part of the temporal fossa, superior to the middle of the zygomatic arch. Immediately deep to the pterion, inside the cranial cavity, is the middle meningeal artery. Trauma to this region may result in damage to the artery and an epidural hematoma.

✔ **Ethmoid bone:** The *ethmoid bone* is spongy and cube shaped. It sits between the orbits at the top of the nasal cavity and has two bony plates called the *superior* and *middle concha*. The *crista galli* is a ridge that projects upward. The perpendicular plate of the ethmoid bone projects inferiorly into the nasal cavity to form the nasal septum.

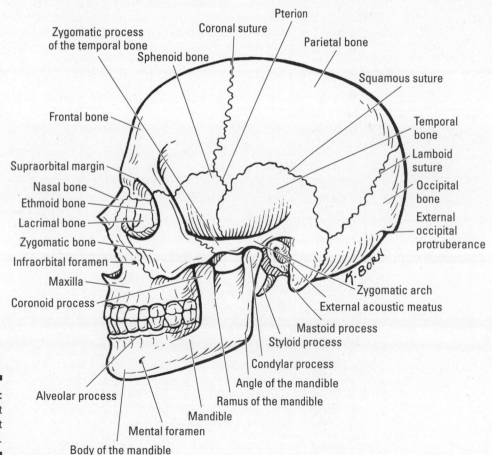

Figure 12-1:
A look at the adult cranium.

Facing forward with the facial bones

The rest of the cranial bones (the ones we don't discuss in the preceding section) form the face by completing the orbits, leaving room for the nose and creating the jaw and mouth. The first two bones appear as single bones, but the rest occur in pairs, with one on each side of the face. You can see some of these bones in Figure 12-1 (see Chapter 13 for more details on structures related to the teeth, nose, and eyes):

✔ **Mandible:** The *mandible* is a U-shaped bone that forms the lower jaw, and it's easily palpated. The horizontal part of the jaw is called the *body,* which contains *alveolar processes* that form sockets for the teeth. The *mental protuberance* is the part of the lower anterior body that juts forward. The body has two small openings called the *mental foramina.*

The vertical portions are called the *rami.* The *angle* of the mandible marks the transition between the body and ramus on each side. Each ramus has two parts that project upwards: the *coronoid process* is anterior and the *condylar process* is posterior. The condylar process forms the inferior portion of the *temporomandibular joint* where it articulates (forms a joint) with the mandibular fossa of the temporal bone.

✔ **Vomer:** The thin *vomer* joins the perpendicular plate of the ethmoid bone to form part of the *nasal septum.* It's located in the midline of the skull, with the *choanae,* or posterior nasal openings, on either side.

✔ **Maxillae:** Two *maxillae* form the upper jaw. *Alveolar processes* form sockets for the teeth, and the *palatine processes* form the roof of the mouth. The tops of the maxillae form the inferior parts of the orbits, and they each have an opening just below the orbit called the *infra-orbital foramen.* Medially, they surround the *piriform aperture,* which is the pear-shaped anterior portion of the nasal opening. They meet each other at the *intermaxillary suture* and join the zygomatic bones below the eyes at the cheeks.

✔ **Zygomatic bones:** The *zygomatic bones* form the lateral sides of the orbits and the cheekbones. Each one has a small *zygomaticofacial foramen* just inferior and lateral to the orbit. The *temporal process* meets the zygomatic process of the temporal bone. This union forms the *zygomatic arch.*

✔ **Nasal bones:** The two small *nasal bones* form the bridge of the nose. They meet the frontal bone at the *nasion* and join the maxillary bones laterally.

✔ **Lacrimal bones:** The thin, small *lacrimal bones* are located on the medial aspect of the orbit between the ethmoid and maxilla bones. A small groove called the *lacrimal fossa* houses the lacrimal sac. The *lacrimal sac* is the dilated portion of the nasolacrimal duct that conveys tears from the eyes to the nasal cavity.

✔ **Inferior concha bones:** The *inferior conchae* are two bony plates that extend along the lateral wall of the nasal cavity. The inferior conchae, along with the middle and superior conchae of the ethmoid bone form the *nasal turbinates.*

✔ **Palatine bones:** The *palatine bones* form the posterior portion of the roof of the mouth, part of the orbits, and part of the inferior wall of the nasal cavity.

Encasing the Brain: The Meninges

The *meninges* are the coverings of the brain. They protect the brain by housing a fluid-filled space, and they function as a framework for blood vessels. The meninges have three layers: the *dura mater,* the *arachnoid mater,* and the *pia mater.* The arachnoid mater is attached to the pia mater by *arachnoid trabeculae,* which is a weblike matrix of connective tissue. The space between the two layers, the *subarachnoid space,* is filled with *cerebrospinal fluid (CSF).* The subarachnoid space includes several *cisterns,* areas where the space between the pia and arachnoid mater is widened due to an accumulation of CSF, that function as reservoirs.

Pressure from the cerebrospinal fluid presses the arachnoid mater against the dura mater. The pia mater adheres to the surface of the brain.

The dura mater is the most superficial layer of the meninges and contains folds and sinuses, as you find out in the following sections. The dura mater contacts the endosteum (see Chapter 3) that lines bones of the cranial cavity. The dura mater is a strong fibrous membrane that surrounds the brain and is continuous with the dura that covers the spinal cord (see Chapter 15).

Meningitis is an infection of the meninges caused by viruses or bacteria. Generally, the bacterial forms are much more serious. Patients with meningitis usually are sensitive to light and have a fever, severe headache, stiff neck, mental disturbances, nausea, and vomiting. Meningitis can be diagnosed by blood tests and by performing a *lumbar puncture,* in which cerebrospinal fluid is collected and analyzed for cell counts, glucose, and protein. Treatment requires antibiotics and may require hospitalization.

The dural infoldings

The meningeal layer folds up to form *dural infoldings* that divide the cranial cavity into different compartments. You can see these four infoldings in Figure 12-2:

✔ *Falx cerebri:* The largest infolding, the falx cerebri is found in the *longitudinal cerebral fissure,* which divides the two hemispheres of the cerebrum (find out more about the areas of the brain in the next section).

✔ *Tentorium cerebelli:* This infolding separates the occipital lobes of the cerebrum from the cerebellum. The falx cerebri (see the next bullet) connects to the tentorium cerebelli at the midline and helps to hold it in place, except for the anterior part, which is left free, making a gap called the *tentorial notch.*

✔ ***Falx cerebelli:*** This vertical infolding is below the tentorium cerebelli. It helps to separate the cerebellar hemispheres.

✔ ***Diaphragma sellae:*** This smaller infolding forms a roof over the pituitary gland.

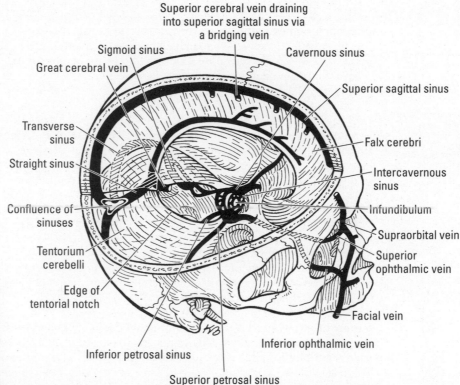

Superior cerebral vein draining into superior sagittal sinus via a bridging vein

Sigmoid sinus

Great cerebral vein

Cavernous sinus

Superior sagittal sinus

Transverse sinus

Straight sinus

Falx cerebri

Intercavernous sinus

Confluence of sinuses

Infundibulum

Supraorbital vein

Tentorium cerebelli

Superior ophthalmic vein

Edge of tentorial notch

Facial vein

Figure 12-2: The meninges and dural infoldings.

Inferior petrosal sinus

Inferior ophthalmic vein

Superior petrosal sinus

The dural venous sinuses

The dural infoldings form spaces between the two layers of the dura mater. These spaces are called *dural venous sinuses,* and they collect blood from veins on the surface of the brain. Blood from the sinuses empties into the internal jugular veins (see Chapter 14). The sinuses include the following:

✔ ***Superior sagittal sinus:*** Formed in the superior part of the falx cerebri, this sinus runs from the crista galli of the ethmoid bone that we describe earlier in this chapter to the *confluence of sinuses* near the occipital bone.

✔ *Inferior sagittal sinus:* This sinus runs along the bottom of the falx cerebri to the straight sinus.

✔ *Straight sinus:* This dural venous sinus is formed where the inferior sagittal sinus merges with the *great cerebral vein.* It follows the place where the tentorium cerebelli attaches to the falx cerebri and joins the confluence of sinuses.

✔ *Transverse sinuses:* The transverse sinuses run laterally from the confluence of sinuses where the tentorium cerebelli attaches to the occipital bones. Where they reach the temporal bone they become the sigmoid sinuses.

✔ *Sigmoid sinuses:* These sinuses run along an S-shaped course and pass through the *jugular foramen,* which is located at the base of the occipital and temporal bones. From there, they become the internal jugular veins.

✔ *Occipital sinus:* The occipital sinus runs along the falx cerebelli up to the confluence of sinuses.

✔ *Cavernous sinuses:* Found on each side of the sella turcica of the sphenoid bone, the cavernous sinuses drain into the superior and inferior petrosal sinuses.

✔ *Superior petrosal sinuses:* These sinuses continue from the cavernous sinuses to the transverse sinuses.

✔ *Inferior petrosal sinuses:* Running from the posterior part of the cavernous sinuses, these sinuses empty into the internal jugular veins.

Arachnoid granulations protrude from the arachnoid mater into the dural venous sinuses. They move cerebrospinal fluid from the subarachnoid space to the venous system. *Emissary veins* connect the dural venous sinuses with veins that run outside of the cranium.

The dura mater receives arterial blood from the *middle meningeal artery.* The *frontal* (anterior) *branch* runs deep to the pterion and then moves posteriorly toward the top of the cranium. The *parietal* (posterior) *branch* runs posteriorly and superiorly along the cranium. The meningeal arteries are accompanied by veins of the same name. The dura mater is innervated by the cranial nerves (coming up later in this chapter).

Locating the Areas and Structures of the Brain

The brain is composed of several parts that control what you think; how you feel; where you move; what you see, hear, and taste; and many other functions. The brain also has a system of ventricles that drain cerebrospinal fluid, along with a number of nerves and blood vessels. You can see some of these structures in Figure 12-3, and we give you the details on these parts in the following sections.

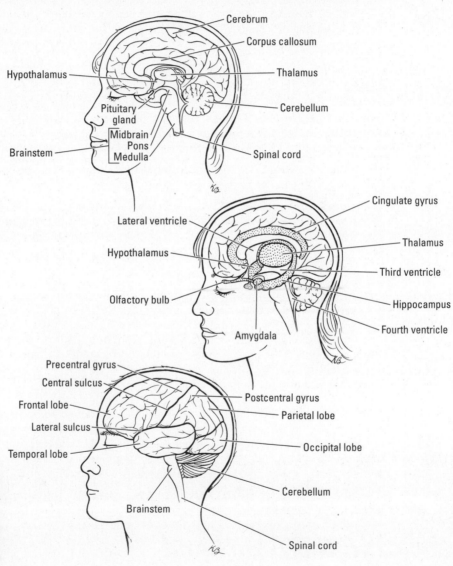

Figure 12-3:
The structures of the brain.

Thinking about the cerebrum

The *cerebrum* is the largest part of the brain, and it's made up of the left and right *cerebral hemispheres,* separated by the falx cerebri. Each hemisphere has five lobes: the *frontal lobe* in the front (of course!), the *temporal* and *parietal lobes* on the sides, the *occipital lobe* in the back, and the *insular lobe* located between the temporal lobe and the frontal lobe. The *cerebral cortex* is the outer layer of the cerebrum. The surface of the cerebral cortex isn't smooth; it has folds, grooves, and clefts. The folds are called *gyri,* the grooves are *sulci* (singular: *sulcus*), and the clefts are called *fissures.* These features increase the surface area of the brain while still allowing into to fit into its bony vault.

The cerebral hemispheres are connected by the *corpus callosum,* a band of nerve fibers that allows each side to communicate with the other. The *cingulate gyrus* is located superior to the corpus callosum. It helps coordinate emotions. The *hippocampus* and the *amygdala* are located in the temporal lobe and are important for memory.

The cerebrum has many different higher functions. It's involved in controlling cognitive functions; shaping your personality, feelings, and perceptions; and handling motor functions and sensory interpretation.

Going inside the diencephalon

The *diencephalon* takes up the central part of the brain, underneath the cerebrum. It includes the *epithalamus* (the posterior part), *thalamus* (the middle part), and *hypothalamus* (the most inferior part). The diencephalon serves as a relay station, interconnecting different parts of the nervous system, and controls many autonomic nervous functions (see Chapter 3 for more on the autonomic nervous system).

Balancing the cerebellum

The *cerebellum* is the portion of the brain lying beneath the tentorium cerebelli in the posterior part of the cranium. It's made up of two hemispheres connected by the narrow wormlike part of the cerebellum called the *vermis.* The cerebellum controls balance, coordinates movement, and maintains muscle tone.

Surveying the brainstem

The *brainstem* connects the cerebrum with the spinal cord (see Chapter 15). It includes three parts: the *midbrain* is the most superior part, the *pons* is in the middle, and the *medulla oblongata* (medulla) is the most inferior portion and connects to the spinal cord. The brainstem controls your levels of alertness, arousal, respiratory rate, blood pressure, digestion, heart rate, and other autonomic functions.

Draining the brain with the ventricles

Cerebrospinal fluid protects the brain from damage by cushioning it during a blow to the head and by helping hold up the brain, which takes the pressure off the base of brain. The fluid is produced by the *choroid plexus,* which is located in four ventricles in the brain.

Two *lateral ventricles* extend into the cerebral hemispheres. They open into the third ventricle through the *interventricular foramina* (also called the *foramina of Monro*). That *third ventricle* is located in the midline of the brain. The *fourth ventricle* is located in the brain stem and is connected to the third ventricle by *cerebral aqueduct,* or *aqueduct of Sylvius.* The fourth ventricle is connected to the *central canal.* The *median aperture* (also called the *aperture of Magendie*) and the two *lateral apertures* (or *apertures of Luschka*) connect the fourth ventricle to the subarachnoid space.

Getting the glands

The cranial cavity contains two glands: the pituitary gland and the pineal gland. They're tiny little things, but they're so important, especially the pituitary gland. It's so significant that it's referred to as the *master gland.*

- ✔ *Pituitary gland:* This small gland is about the size of a pea. It's located in the sella turcica of the sphenoid bone that we talk about earlier in this chapter. It is connected to the hypothalamus by a stalk called the *infundibulum.* It's called the master gland because it secretes several hormones that influence the activity of many other endocrine glands that regulate a variety of body functions, including blood pressure, childhood growth, urine production, testosterone production in males, and estrogen production in females. It has two parts: the anterior portion, the *adenohypophysis,* and the posterior portion, called the *neurohypophysis.*

- ✔ *Pineal gland:* Also called the *epiphysis,* this gland is a small pine-cone-shaped body located at the posterior end of the roof of the third ventricle. It synthesizes melatonin, a hormone that regulates sleep and circadian rhythm based on the body's exposure to light. A problem with the pineal gland can lead to a lot of sleepless nights.

Counting the cranial nerves

The 12 pairs of cranial nerves branch off the brain or brainstem and innervate many different places in the body. Some of them have motor functions, some have sensory functions, and a few have both. (Look at Chapter 3 for more about motor and sensory nerves.) Here are the cranial nerves in numerical order (you can see them in Figure 12-4):

- ✔ **CN I:** *Olfactory nerve:* Located in the olfactory epithelium (see Chapter 13), this nerve leaves the cranium at the foramina in the cribiform plate of the ethmoid bone (see Chapter 13) and enters the olfactory bulb (refer to Figure 12-3). Fibers in the olfactory tract convey sensory impulses to the cerebral cortex. It's a sensory nerve responsible for the sense of smell.

- ✔ **CN II:** *Optic nerve:* This nerve starts at the retina and passes through the optic canal and forms the optic chiasm (see Chapter 13). In the optic chiasm, the fibers from the medial part of the retina cross to the optic tract of the opposite side. The fibers from the lateral portion of the retina travel to the optic tract of the same side. This crossing is necessary for binocular vision (seeing with both eyes). The majority of fibers in the optic tract synapse (communicate) with neurons in the lateral geniculate nucleus of the thalamus. The axons of cells from the lateral geniculate nucleus travel to the visual cortex of the cerebral hemispheres. CN II is a sensory nerve necessary for vision.

- ✔ **CN III:** *Oculomotor nerve:* Starting in the midbrain and leaving the cranium at the superior orbital fissure, this motor nerve innervates the levator palpebrae superioris, the muscle that raises the eyelid. It also innervates the superior rectus, medial rectus, inferior rectus, and inferior oblique, the muscles that turn the eyeball superiorly, medially, and inferiorly. This nerve also provides the parasympathetic input that constricts the pupil and affects the lens (see Chapter 13).

- ✔ **CN IV:** *Trochlear nerve:* This motor nerve leaves the posterior side of the midbrain and exits with the oculomotor nerve at the superior orbital fissure. It innervates a muscle, the superior oblique muscle, that turns the eyeball inferiorly and laterally.

- ✔ **CN V:** *Trigeminal nerve:* This large nerve emerges from the pons and contains both a sensory and motor root. The cell bodies of the sensory neurons are located in the large trigeminal ganglion (grouping of nerve cells). The sensory fibers from the trigeminal ganglion form three nerves that provide the primary sensory innervation of the head. The motor fibers are distributed with the mandibular nerve (CN V_3 — see the following list):

  - **CN V_1:** The *ophthalmic nerve* is a sensory nerve that emerges from the trigeminal ganglion and leaves the cranium at the superior orbital fissure. It transmits sensory impulses from the cornea, skin of the forehead, and scalp, eyelids, nose, nasal cavity, and paranasal sinuses.

- **CN V₂:** The *maxillary nerve* is a sensory nerve that also emerges from the trigeminal ganglion and exits the cranium at the foramen rotundum. It receives sensory input from the skin over the maxilla, upper lip, maxillary teeth, nasal mucosa, maxillary sinuses, and palate.

- **CN V₃:** The *mandibular nerve* has both sensory and motor fibers. The sensory fibers exit the trigeminal ganglion, and the motor fibers branch off the pons. All fibers leave the cranium through the foramen ovale. It receives sensory input from the skin over the chin, lower lip, side of the head, mandibular teeth, temporomandibular joint, inside of the mouth, and the anterior two-thirds of the tongue. Its motor fibers innervate muscles of mastication, mylohyoid, anterior belly of the digastric, tensor veli palatini, and the tensor tympani (check out Chapter 13 to learn more about these muscles).

✔ **CN VI: *Abducent nerve:*** This motor nerve starts in the pons and leaves the cranium through the superior orbital fissure. It innervates the lateral rectus muscle that moves the eyeball laterally.

✔ **CN VII: *Facial nerve:*** This nerve has both sensory and motor fibers. The sensory fibers start at the geniculate ganglion and exit the cranium at the internal acoustic meatus. The facial nerve transmits sensory impulses from the skin of the external acoustic meatus of the ear (which you can see in Figure 12-1). It also carries the sense of taste from the anterior two-thirds of the tongue. The motor fibers of CN VII start at the pons and leave the cranium at the internal acoustic meatus. They innervate muscles of facial expression, the stapedius muscle of the inner ear, and the stylohyoid and digastric muscles (see Chapters 13 and 14).

The facial nerve is also the source of presynaptic parasympathetic fibers that stimulate the lacrimal glands, glands of the nose and palate, and the submandibular and sublingual salivary glands (these structures are described in Chapter 13).

✔ **CN VIII: *Vestibulocochlear nerve:*** This sensory nerve has two divisions:

- The *vestibular nerve* starts in the vestibular ganglion and leaves the cranium via the internal acoustic meatus. It's needed for equilibrium.

- The *cochlear nerve* starts at the *spiral ganglion* and leaves the cranium via the internal acoustic meatus. It's needed for hearing.

✔ **CN IX: *Glossopharyngeal nerve:*** This nerve branches from the medulla oblongata and has both sensory and motor fibers. It leaves the cranium via the jugular foramen. It provides parasympathetic input to the parotid salivary gland and somatic motor fibers that innervate the stylopharyngeus muscle for swallowing. The sensory nerves serve the pharynx, external and middle parts of the ear, the carotid body and sinus, and general sense and taste from the posterior part of the tongue (see Chapters 13 and 14).

✔ **CN X:** *Vagus nerve:* This nerve originates from the medulla oblongata. It has both motor and sensory fibers and exits the cranium through the jugular foramen. The vagus nerve provides motor innervation to the muscles of the palate, pharynx, larynx, and esophagus for swallowing. It's the source of presynaptic parasympathetic fibers that innervate the trachea, bronchi, digestive tract, and heart. It also transmits taste sensations from the palate and epiglottis and somatic sensation from the external acoustic meatus and auricle (external portion of the ear).

✔ **CN XI:** *Spinal accessory nerve:* This motor nerve starts on the spinal cord and leaves the cranium through the jugular foramen. It innervates the sternocleidomastoid and trapezius muscles (see Chapters 14 and 15).

✔ **CN XII:** *Hypoglossal nerve:* This motor nerve starts on the medulla and exits the cranium at the *hypoglossal canal.* It innervates the tongue.

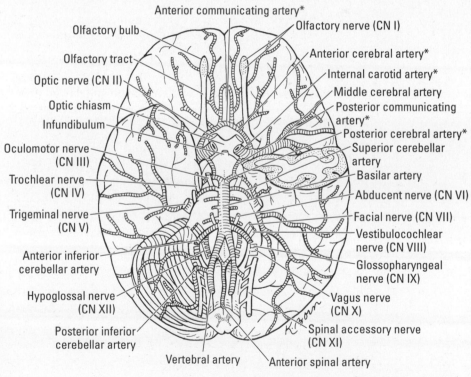

Figure 12-4: The brain's nerves and blood supply.

Anterior communicating artery*
Olfactory bulb
Olfactory tract
Optic nerve (CN II)
Optic chiasm
Infundibulum
Oculomotor nerve (CN III)
Trochlear nerve (CN IV)
Trigeminal nerve (CN V)
Anterior inferior cerebellar artery
Hypoglossal nerve (CN XII)
Posterior inferior cerebellar artery
Vertebral artery

Olfactory nerve (CN I)
Anterior cerebral artery*
Internal carotid artery*
Middle cerebral artery
Posterior communicating artery*
Posterior cerebral artery*
Superior cerebellar artery
Basilar artery
Abducent nerve (CN VI)
Facial nerve (CN VII)
Vestibulocochlear nerve (CN VIII)
Glossopharyngeal nerve (CN IX)
Vagus nerve (CN X)
Spinal accessory nerve (CN XI)
Anterior spinal artery

* Components of cerebral arterial circle of Willis

Turn to Chapter 22 to discover our mnemonic to help you remember the cranial nerves.

Serving the brain: The blood supply

The brain receives a substantial amount of blood and oxygen. That blood comes from the following arteries, which are shown in Figure 12-4:

- ✔ **Internal carotid artery:** This artery branches from the common carotid artery (see Chapter 14) in the neck. It passes through the carotid canal in the temporal bone to enter the cavernous sinus where it serves the pituitary gland and trigeminal ganglion. It supplies most of the blood to the anterior part of the brain and participates in the *circle of Willis*, which is a circle of communicating arteries (anastomosis) at the base of the brain.

- ✔ **Anterior cerebral artery:** Coming from the internal carotid artery, this artery brings blood to most of the cerebral hemispheres (but not the occipital lobes). It also forms part of the circle of Willis.

- ✔ **Middle cerebral artery:** This artery comes from the internal carotid artery and serves the lateral surfaces of the cerebral hemispheres.

- ✔ **Anterior communicating artery:** Connecting the two anterior cerebral arteries, this artery also forms part of the circle of Willis.

- ✔ **Vertebral artery:** This artery starts at the subclavian artery (see Chapter 14) and travels up along the cervical vertebrae to bring blood to the meninges and cerebellum.

- ✔ **Posterior inferior cerebellar artery:** This artery branches off the vertebral artery and serves the inferior part of the cerebellum.

- ✔ **Anterior spinal artery:** The right and left arteries stem from the vertebral artery and anastomose (join together) and run to the spinal cord.

- ✔ **Basilar artery:** This artery is created by the union of the left and right vertebral arteries.

- ✔ **Anterior inferior cerebellar artery:** This artery starts at the basilar artery and runs backward to the anterior part of the cerebellum.

- ✔ **Superior cerebellar artery:** This artery branches off the basilar artery and supplies blood to the superior surface of the cerebellum.

- ✔ **Posterior cerebral artery:** Stemming from the basilar artery, this artery serves the inferior parts of the cerebral hemispheres and the occipital lobes. It's part of the circle of Willis.

- ✔ **Posterior communicating artery:** This artery connects the posterior cerebral artery with the internal carotid artery. It also forms part of the circle of Willis.

Blood from the brain is drained by *cerebral veins,* dural venous sinuses (which we describe earlier in this chapter), and the *great cerebral vein* (called the *vein of Galen*).

An *ischemic stroke* happens when blood flow is cut off to part of the brain. It may cause neurological deficits and even death. This type of stroke is commonly caused by blood clots in the arteries that supply the brain. *Hemorrhagic strokes* occur when a blood vessel ruptures due to an *aneurysm,* which is a weakened dilatation of the blood vessel wall, or cerebral or subarachnoid hemorrhages. High blood pressure increases the risk that an aneurysm may burst.

Putting on a Face

The facial bones are covered with muscles and skin, and although everyone has the same basic facial parts, we all look different in appearance due to slight differences in the shapes of the bones. In the following sections, we take a look at some of the facial muscles underneath the skin (but we save the muscles that move the eye and tongue for Chapter 13). Lots of nerves and arteries serve the face, so we list them, too.

Expressing yourself with facial muscles

The face is so expressive. You can show how happy you are with a smile, frown when you're displeased, and show your flirtatious side with a wink. You can show the world you're angry or sad or maybe even bored. You can do other things with your face too, like kiss your baby goodbye, play a French horn, and keep your food in your mouth when you eat. All these movements are accomplished with the facial muscles.

The muscles of facial expression are located in the subcutaneous layer on the scalp, face, and neck:

- ✔ *Occipitofrontalis:* This muscle has two bellies (the thickest part of the muscle):

    - The *frontal belly* originates from the *epicranial aponeurosis* (fibrous tendon) and inserts into the skin and subcutaneous tissues of the eyebrows and forehead. It elevates the eyebrows and wrinkles the skin of the forehead.

    - The *occipital belly* originates at the superior nuchal line of the occipital bone and inserts at the epicranial aponeurosis. It retracts the scalp.

✔ *Orbicularis oculi:* Originating on the medial part of the orbit and lacrimal bone, this muscle inserts into the skin around the orbit. It closes the eyelid.

✔ *Orbicularis oris:* This muscle originates on the medial mandible and maxilla and the skin around the mouth. It inserts into the lips. It closes the mouth and protrudes the lips. (You can see this facial muscle and a few others in Figure 12-5.)

✔ *Buccinator:* This muscle originates on the mandible and the alveolar processes of both the mandible and maxilla. It inserts at the angle of the mouth and the orbicularis oris. It presses the cheek against the molars and helps keep food between the teeth when chewing.

✔ *Platysma:* Originating in the subcutaneous tissue of the areas above and below the clavicles, or collarbones, this muscle inserts into the mandible, the skin of the cheek, the lower lip, the angle of the mouth, and the orbicularis oris. It depresses the mandible and tenses up the skin of the neck and lower part of the face.

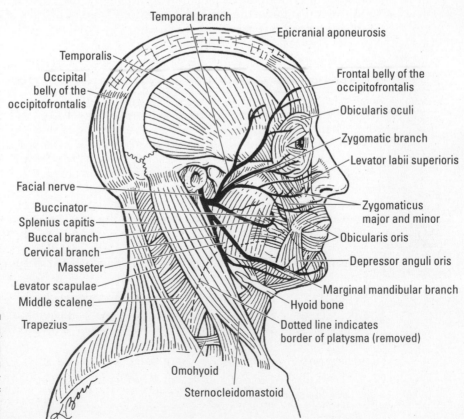

Figure 12-5: Selected muscles and motor nerves of the face.

Temporal branch
Epicranial aponeurosis
Temporalis
Occipital belly of the occipitofrontalis
Frontal belly of the occipitofrontalis
Obicularis oculi
Zygomatic branch
Levator labii superioris
Facial nerve
Buccinator
Splenius capitis
Buccal branch
Cervical branch
Masseter
Levator scapulae
Middle scalene
Trapezius
Zygomaticus major and minor
Obicularis oris
Depressor anguli oris
Marginal mandibular branch
Hyoid bone
Dotted line indicates border of platysma (removed)
Omohyoid
Sternocleidomastoid

Moving with motor nerves

The face has so many movements, so how do you control them? With nerves — lots of nerves. The motor nerves for the muscles of facial expression come from the facial nerve (CN VII). The muscles of mastication (the ones that move your mouth and jaw when you eat) are innervated by the mandibular nerve (motor fibers of CN V). Check out the earlier section "Counting the cranial nerves" for an introduction to the facial and mandibular nerves.

The branches of the facial nerve include the following (some of which you can see in Figure 12-5):

- ✔ **Buccal branch:** Innervates the muscles in the cheek and above the mouth

- ✔ **Cervical branch:** Innervates the platysma (see the preceding section for more about this and other facial muscles)

- ✔ **Marginal mandibular branch:** Innervates the muscles of the lower lip and chin (branches of this nerve are covered in Chapter 13)

- ✔ **Posterior auricular branch:** Has branches that innervate the muscles around the ear and the occipitofrontal muscle

- ✔ **Temporal branch:** Innervates the muscles that wrinkle the forehead, close the eyelids, and wiggle the ear

- ✔ **Zygomatic branches of the facial nerve:** Innervate muscles that close the eye and raise the corners of the mouth

Feeling out sensory nerves

The cutaneous nerves of the face and forehead come from the branches of the trigeminal nerve (CN V). Sensory nerves to the skin covering the neck and posterior scalp come from the cervical nerves (see Chapter 15 to learn more about spinal nerves). In the following sections, we break down the sensory nerves of the face by the major nerves from which they originate.

Sensory nerves originating from the ophthalmic nerve

The following sensory, cutaneous nerves originate from the ophthalmic nerve (CN V_1) (some of the tissues and organs are covered in Chapter 13):

- ✔ **Supraorbital nerve:** This nerve branches from the frontal nerve (largest branch of the ophthalmic nerve) and runs along the roof of the orbit, emerging from the supraorbital notch to the forehead. It innervates the frontal sinus, upper eyelid, and anterolateral part of the forehead and scalp.

- *Supratrochlear nerve:* Branching from the frontal nerve, this nerve runs anteriorly and medially along the roof of the orbit to the forehead. It innervates the medial superior eyelid and anteromedial forehead.

- *Lacrimal nerve:* This nerve branches from the ophthalmic nerve and runs through the orbit. It innervates the lacrimal gland and lateral part of the superior eyelid.

- *Infratrochlear nerve:* Branching off the nasocillary nerve and running along the medial wall of the orbit, this nerve innervates the skin just lateral to the nose, the medial-most parts of the eyelids, the lacrimal sac, and the lacrimal caruncle (the red, fleshy part in the medial corner of the eye, covered in Chapter 13).

- *External nasal nerve:* This nerve branches from the anterior ethmoidal nerve (which supplies the nasal cavity; see Chapter 13) and runs between the nasal bone and lateral nasal cartilage. It innervates the skin of the nose.

Sensory nerves originating from the maxillary nerve

The following three sensory, cutaneous nerves come from the maxillary nerve (CN V_2):

- *Infraorbital nerve:* This nerve comes from the maxillary nerve and runs through the orbital floor, emerging from the infraorbital foramen. It innervates the maxillary sinus, maxillary teeth, inferior eyelid, skin of the cheek, lateral nose, nasal septum, and upper lip.

- *Zygomaticofacial nerve:* Branching from the zygomatic nerve and running along the zygomatic bone at the inferiolateral part of the orbit, this nerve exits the zygomaticofacial foramen of the zygomatic bone and innervates skin on the cheek.

- *Zygomaticotemporal nerve:* This nerve branches off the zygomatic nerve. It exits via the zygomaticotemporal foramen of the zygomatic bone and innervates the skin over the temple.

Sensory nerves originating from the mandibular nerve

Three more cutaneous nerves stem from the mandibular nerve (CN V_3):

- *Auriculotemporal nerve:* Branching off the mandibular nerve near the middle meningeal artery, this nerve runs posteriorly deep to the mandibular ramus and parotid gland. It innervates the skin in the posterior part of the temporal region, the skin of the auricle of the ear, the external acoustic meateus, and the external surface of the tympanic membrane.

✔ *Buccal nerve:* This nerve is different from the buccal branch of the facial nerve. It branches from the mandibular nerve, runs between the pterygoid muscle, and emerges near the mandibular ramus. It innervates the skin and mucosa of the cheek and part of the gums.

✔ *Mental nerve:* This nerve branches from the inferior alveolar nerve (which supplies the teeth — see Chapter 13) and emerges from the mandible through the mental foramen. It innervates the skin of the chin and the inside of the lower lip.

Sensory nerves originating from cervical spinal nerves

The following four sensory, cutaneous nerves are branches of the upper cervical spinal nerves:

✔ *Great auricular nerve:* This nerve branches from the anterior rami of the 2nd and 3rd cervical spinal nerves and runs upward across the sternocleidomastoid posterior to the external jugular vein (see Chapter 14). It innervates the skin over the angle of the mandible, the parotid gland, and the earlobe.

✔ *Lesser occipital nerve:* Also branching from the anterior rami of the 2nd and 3rd cervical spinal nerves, this nerve runs along the posterior border of the sternocleidomastoid and goes up to the ear. It innervates the scalp behind the ear.

✔ *Greater occipital nerve:* Branching off the posterior ramus of the 2nd cervical spinal nerve and passing through the trapezius (see Chapter 15), this nerve innervates the scalp of the occipital area.

✔ *3rd occipital nerve:* This nerve branches off the posterior ramus of the 3rd cervical nerve and pierces the trapezius. It innervates the scalp in the occipital and suboccipital areas.

Viewing blood vessels

A lot of arteries and veins provide circulation of blood to the various tissues of the face. You see some of the following arteries in Figure 12-6.

✔ *Facial artery:* This artery stems from the external carotid artery (see Chapter 14), follows the inferior border of the mandible, and enters the face. It provides blood to the muscles of the face.

✔ *Submental artery:* This artery starts from the facial artery and supplies blood to the tissues under the chin.

- ✔ *Inferior labial artery:* Starting from the facial artery at the angle of the mouth, this artery runs medially to the lower lip, where it provides blood flow.

- ✔ *Superior labial artery:* This artery starts with the inferior labial artery, but it runs medially to the upper lip and provides blood flow there.

- ✔ *Lateral nasal artery:* Starting at the facial artery alongside the nose and running out to the ala of the nose (part of the nose that flares out around the nostril), this artery provides blood to the skin of the nose.

- ✔ *Angular artery:* This last branch of the facial artery passes to the medial angle of the eye. It provides blood to the inferior eyelid and the cheek just below.

- ✔ *Occipital artery:* This artery branches from the external carotid artery and passes to the occipital region. It provides blood flow to the scalp on the back of the head.

- ✔ *Posterior auricular artery:* This artery also branches from the external carotid artery and runs to the areas around the mastoid process and the ear. It provides blood to the ear and scalp behind the ear.

- ✔ *Maxillary artery:* This artery also starts from the external carotid artery. It runs deep to the neck of the mandible to supply blood to deeper structures of the face and meninges.

- ✔ *Inferior alveolar artery:* This artery branches off the maxillary artery (see Chapter 14) and enters the mandible to supply the teeth.

- ✔ *Infraorbital artery:* This artery branches from the maxillary artery and supplies blood to the maxilla, teeth, lower eyelid, cheek, and nose.

- ✔ *Superficial temporal artery:* Starting at the termination of the external carotid artery and ascending in front of the ear to the temporal region, this artery supplies blood to the facial muscles and skin in the frontal and temporal areas.

- ✔ *Zygomaticoorbital artery:* This artery branches off the superficial temporal artery and runs to the orbit (eye socket).

- ✔ *Transverse facial artery:* This artery stems from the superficial temporal artery and crosses the face to just below the zygomatic arch. It supplies blood to the parotid gland and muscles and skin of the face.

- ✔ *Mental artery:* The terminal branch of the inferior alveolar artery, this artery emerges from the mental foramen, where it supplies blood to the facial muscles and skin of the chin.

- ✔ *Supraorbital artery:* This artery branches from the ophthalmic artery (see Chapter 13) and runs upwards to supply blood to the muscles and skin of the forehead and scalp.

- ✔ *Supratrochlear artery:* Also a branch of the ophthalmic artery, this artery passes from the supratrochlear notch to supply blood to the muscles and skin of the scalp.

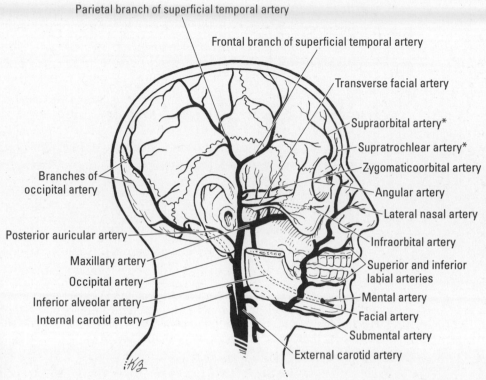

Parietal branch of superficial temporal artery

Frontal branch of superficial temporal artery

Transverse facial artery

Supraorbital artery*

Supratrochlear artery*

Zygomaticoorbital artery

Branches of occipital artery

Angular artery

Lateral nasal artery

Infraorbital artery

Posterior auricular artery

Superior and inferior labial arteries

Maxillary artery

Occipital artery

Mental artery

Inferior alveolar artery

Facial artery

Internal carotid artery

Submental artery

External carotid artery

Figure 12-6: Selected arteries of the face and scalp.

* Branches off the internal carotid artery

Important veins in the face include the following:

- *Angular vein:* This vein runs obliquely (at an angle) down the side of the nose.

- *Facial vein:* The facial vein drains most of the blood from the face. It begins at the *angular vein* in the medial angle of the eye. The *deep facial vein* joins the facial vein, which goes on to drain into the internal jugular vein (see Chapter 14).

- *Maxillary vein:* This vein accompanies the maxillary artery and drains blood from the face.

- *Superficial temporal vein:* This vein drains the forehead and scalp.

- *Retromandibular vein:* This vein is formed by the superficial temporal vein and the maxillary vein. It receives blood from the region of the temple and the face.

✔ *Posterior auricular vein:* This vein is joined by a branch of the retro-mandibular vein to form the external jugular vein (see Chapter 14).

✔ *Supraorbital* **and** *supratrochlear veins:* These veins descend from the scalp to form the angular vein.

Getting a handle on lymphatics

Of course, the face also includes some lymphatic tissues. The nodes are categorized into several groups:

✔ *Parotid lymph nodes:* Receive lymph from the side of the face and scalp

✔ *Submandibular lymph nodes:* Get lymph from the upper lip and part of the lower lip as well as most of the oral cavity

✔ *Submental lymph nodes:* Get lymph from the chin and center of the lower lip

Lymph from these nodes eventually drains into the deep cervical lymph nodes. The deep cervical lymph nodes drain into the jugular lymphatic trunk, which joins the internal jugular vein or brachiocephalic vein on the right side and thoracic duct on the left side (see Chapter 14).

Enveloping the Head: Facial Surface Anatomy and the Scalp

The skull is covered with epidermis (see Chapter 3 for more information on the layers of skin). When examining the face, you can palpate (medically examine by touch) the following features:

✔ **Mandible:** The mandible (the mental protuberance and the angle) can be felt as the lower bone of the jaw.

✔ **Zygomatic arch:** The zygomatic arch can be palpated by feeling for the bony arch just above the temporomandibular joint (joint between the jaw and the temporal bone; it's described in Chapter 13).

✔ **Maxillary bones:** These bones can be palpated as the upper part of the jaw (below the nose).

✔ **Nasal bones:** The nasal bones can be palpated on the sides of nose (behind the wiggly cartilage).

✔ **Frontal bone:** This bone can be palpated by touching the forehead.

Of course, you'll also see eyes, ears, a mouth, and a nose, but we've got those items covered in Chapter 13.

Males may have thick facial hair growth, whereas females generally have little to no hair on the face with the exception of eyebrows, a feature shared by both genders.

The *scalp* covers your head. Some scalps are covered in long, luxurious hair, and others are shiny and bald. The scalp is made up of skin and connective tissue that covers the neurocranium from the top of the frontal bone to the occipital region. It has five layers:

- *Skin:* Contains sweat and sebaceous glands and hair follicles

- *Connective tissue:* Forms a thick subcutaneous layer

- *Aponeurosis:* A strong tendinous sheet that serves as the attachment for the occipitofrontalis and superior auricular muscles

- *Loose connective tissue:* A spongy layer that allows for free movement of the upper layers of scalp over the cranium

- *Pericranium:* A dense layer of connective tissue (periosteum) firmly attached to the cranium

You can remember the layers of the scalp starting from the most superficial to the deepest layer by using the letters S-C-A-L-P. If you like memory devices, you can turn to Chapter 22 for ten more.

Chapter 13

Seeing, Smelling, Tasting, and Hearing

Although the brain takes up much of the cranium, the head is also home to the organs that allow you to see, smell, taste, and hear. Examination of these organs allows you to understand the health of those individual organs as well as the nervous, cardiovascular, and other systems.

In this chapter, we delve into the details of the eyes, nose, mouth, and ears. For the full scoop on the rest of the head (including the brain and the face), flip to Chapter 12.

Seeing into the Eyes

The eyes are housed in the bony orbits that are formed by eight different bones and covered in *periorbita* (a type of *periosteum,* which is a covering of fibrous connective tissue). The orbits protect the eyeballs and the structures they need to function. A bit of orbital fat takes up any space not occupied by other parts. The walls of the orbit are made up of bones, which are covered in Chapter 12 in detail:

> ✔ The superior (top) wall of the orbit is formed in large part by the orbital part of the frontal bone and a small amount from the lesser wing of the sphenoid bone. The *fossa* (indentation) *for the lacrimal gland* is found in this orbital part of the frontal bone.

✔ The medial (middle) wall is formed mostly by the ethmoid bone and parts of the frontal, lacrimal, and sphenoid bones. The medial wall contains the *lacrimal groove* and the *fossa for the lacrimal sac.*

✔ The lateral (side) wall is made up of the frontal processes (bony projections) of the zygomatic bone and the greater wing of the sphenoid bone.

✔ The inferior (bottom) wall is formed mostly by the maxilla with parts of the zygomatic and palatine bones. It's separated from the lateral wall by the *inferior orbital fissure.*

In the following sections, we describe the eyelid and the eyeball, and we talk about the muscles, nerves, and blood vessels of the eye area.

Taking cover with eyelids

The eyes are covered with *eyelids* that open and close — sometimes for long periods, to sleep or avoid seeing something you don't like, and sometimes just to blink to keep your eyes moist.

Externally, the eyelids are covered with skin and lined internally with a mucous membrane called the *palpebral conjunctiva.* This membrane continues onto the surface of the eyeball, where it's known as the *bulbar conjunctiva.* The fold of conjunctiva from the eyelid onto the eyeball creates two recessed areas between the eyeball and the eyelid, one superior (above) and one inferior (below) to the eyeball. They're called the *superior* and *inferior fornices.* The area inside the fornices is called the *conjunctival sac.*

Dense bands of connective tissue called *superior* and *inferior tarsi* strengthen the eyelids. The tarsi (singular: *tarsis*) are connected to the medial and lateral margins of the orbit by *medial* and *lateral palpebral ligaments.* The *orbital septum* is a weak membrane running between the tarsi and the edges of the orbit. *Tarsal glands* secrete fluids that prevent the edges of your eyelids from sticking together when they're closed.

Eyelashes grow at the edges of the eyelids near modified sweat glands called *ciliary glands.* The superior and inferior eyelids meet at the corners of your eyes. These junctions are called the *medial* and *lateral palpebral commissures.* The medial palpebral commissure is located at the medial angle of the eye, and the lateral palpebral commissure is the at the lateral angle of the eye.

Located at the *medial angle of the eye* is a pinkish red mound of tissue called the *lacrimal caruncle.* Tears collect in this area, forming the *lacrimal lake.* The *lacrimal apparatus* generates and acts as a conduit for the tears.

The lacrimal apparatus is made up of several structures. The *lacrimal gland* is located in the fossa for the lacrimal gland. It secretes tears that are conveyed to the conjunctival sac by the *lacrimal ducts.* Tears cover the eyeball to keep it moist and to flush away bacteria and foreign materials. The tears drain into the lacrimal lake, where they enter openings (called *lacrimal punta*) into tiny canals (called the *lacrimal caniculi*) on their way to the *lacrimal sac.* From there, the tears drain through *nasolacrimal duct* into the nasal cavity.

Having a ball — an eyeball, that is

The eyeball holds the structures that allow you to see things. Its posterior portion is covered by a layer of connective tissue that connects the eyeball to the orbit called the *fascial sheath of the eyeball.* The *episcleral space* lies between the fascial sheath and the rest of the eyeball. This little space allows your eyeball to move around.

The eyeball has three layers surrounding its inner chambers (you can see a lot of these parts in Figure 13-1):

✔ *Fibrous layer:* This external layer gives shape to the eyeball. It includes the *sclera,* or the white of the eye, which is a tough coat that covers most of the eyeball. The *cornea* is the transparent part of the fibrous layer covering the anterior portion of the eyeball. A *corneoscleral junction* is formed at the intersection of the cornea and sclera.

✔ *Vascular layer:* This middle layer is called the *uvea.* It includes the *choroid,* which is a dark reddish-brown layer that lines the sclera and contains a dense vascular bed. This layer has several important structures:

  • The *ciliary body* is a thickened muscular part of the uvea found behind the corneoscleral junction. It serves as the attachment point for the lens. It also controls the thickness of the lens by contraction and relaxation of the ciliary muscle contained within.

  • *Ciliary processes* lie on the internal surface of the ciliary body. They secrete *aqueous humor,* a fluid that fills the anterior segment of the eyeball.

  • The *iris* is the colored portion of the eye that surrounds the *pupil,* an opening through which light is transmitted.

  • The muscles that control the iris include the *sphincter pupillae* (parasympathetically innervated), which decreases the diameter of the pupil, and the *dilator pupillae* (sympathetically innervated), which increases the size of the pupil.

✔ *Retina:* This innermost layer has an optic part that's sensitive to light and a nonvisual part that extends over the ciliary body and the posterior part of the iris. The optic part contains photoreceptors called *rods* and *cones* that are sensitive to light. The *ora serrata* is the border between the optic part and the nonvisual part. The posterior part of the retina is what you see when you view the eye through an ophthalmoscope. The *fundus* (the part of the retina you see) includes the following parts:

- *Optic disc:* This blind spot is the location where the sensory fibers that form the optic nerve (cranial nerve II; see Chapter 12) exit the eyeball. It has no photoreceptors.

- *Macula:* This small oval area is equipped with cells specialized for visual acuity.

- *Fovea centralis:* This small depression is in the middle of the macula.

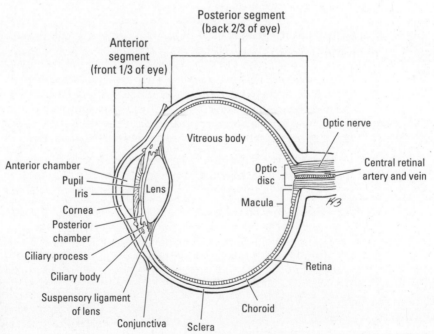

Figure 13-1:
Looking at
the eyeball.

The interior of the eyeball has two segments, anterior and posterior. The anterior segment contains aqueous humor and is divided into an *anterior chamber* and a *posterior chamber,* as shown in Figure 13-1. The anterior chamber is the space between the cornea and the iris. The posterior chamber is the space between the iris and the lens.

Aqueous humor provides nutrients for the lens and the cornea because they aren't served by any blood vessels. It's produced in the posterior chamber and passes through the pupil to the anterior chamber. From there it drains through the *iridocorneal angle* into the *scleral venous sinus* (canal of Schlemm). It's removed by the *limbal plexus* of veins.

Glaucoma is a condition in which the outflow of aqueous humor is blocked, causing intraocular pressure to build up in the eye. Blindness can result from the compression of the retina. People with glaucoma may not have any symptoms, so glaucoma screening is important for early detection. Tonometry is a test that checks the pressure in the eye. Treatment includes laser therapy, medications, and possibly eye surgery.

The *lens* lies between the posterior chamber and the *vitreous body*. The lens is transparent and biconvex (bends outward) on both front and back. The *suspensory ligaments* (refer to Figure 13-1) anchor the lens and its elastic capsule.

The ciliary muscle changes the shape of the lens to allow you to focus on near or far objects. The process of this shape changing for near-vision is called *accommodation.* As people age, their eyes have more difficulty accommodating, so they have to rely on reading glasses.

The *vitreous body* is a jellylike substance that contains a fluid called *vitreous humor.* It fills the posterior segment of the eyeball. It transmits light from the lens to the retina and helps hold the retina in place.

Rolling your eyes with extraocular muscles

You need to be able to move your eyes around so you can look in all different directions and even use them to display emotion. Six muscles, collectively called the *extraocular muscles,* move the eyeball. A seventh muscle moves the eyelid and is also found in the orbit. (Figure 13-2 shows most of these muscles):

- ✔ *Levator palpebrae superioris:* This muscle originates on the sphenoid bone above the optic canal (opening for the optic nerve, CN II). It inserts into the superior tarsis and skin of the eyelid. It's innervated by the oculomotor nerve (CN III — see Chapter 12 for details on all the cranial nerves) and elevates the superior eyelid.

- ✔ *Superior oblique:* This muscle originates on the sphenoid bone and inserts into the sclera deep to (underneath) the superior rectus muscle. It's innervated by the trochlear nerve (CN IV) and abducts (moves away from the midline of the body), depresses, and medially rotates the eyeball.

✔ *Inferior oblique:* Originating on the anterior part of the orbital floor (bottom part of the orbit), this muscle inserts onto the sclera deep to the lateral rectus muscle. It's innervated by the oculomotor nerve and abducts, elevates, and laterally rotates the eyeball.

✔ *Superior rectus:* This muscle originates on the common tendinous ring and inserts into the sclera behind the corneoscleral junction. It's innervated by the oculomotor nerve, and it elevates, adducts (moves toward the midline of the body), and medially rotates the eyeball.

✔ *Inferior rectus:* This muscle originates on the common tendinous ring and inserts into the sclera behind the corneoscleral junction. It's innervated by the oculomotor nerve and depresses, adducts, and laterally rotates the eyeball.

✔ *Medial rectus:* Originating on the common tendinous ring and inserting into the sclera behind the corneoscleral junction, this muscle is innervated by the oculomotor nerve and adducts the eyeball.

✔ *Lateral rectus:* This muscle originates on the common tendinous ring and inserts into the sclera behind the corneoscleral junction. It's innervated by the abducent nerve (CN VI) and abducts the eyeball.

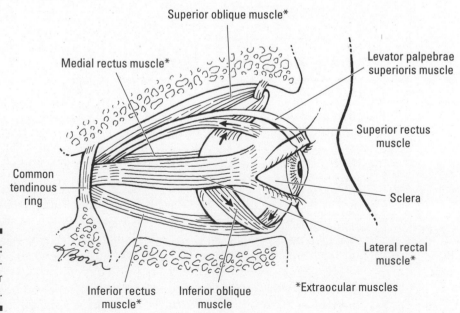

Superior oblique muscle*

Medial rectus muscle*

Levator palpebrae superioris muscle

Superior rectus muscle

Common tendinous ring

Sclera

Lateral rectal muscle*

Inferior rectus muscle*

Inferior oblique muscle

*Extraocular muscles

Figure 13-2:
The extra-ocular muscles.

Serving the eyes: The nerves

The eyes are served by the following cranial nerves and their branches:

- *Optic nerve* (CN II): The large optic nerve is a sensory nerve that transmits impulses from the retina to the brain (refer to Figure 13-1 for an illustration and see Chapter 12 for details on all the cranial nerves).

- *Oculomotor nerve* (CN III), *trochlear nerve* (CN IV), and *abducent nerve* (CN VI): These nerves enter the orbital space through the superior orbital fissure to innervate the extraocular muscles described in the previous section.

- *Ophthalmic nerve* (part of the trigeminal nerve, CN V): This nerve has three branches:

  - The *lacrimal nerve* runs to the lacrimal gland and gives off branches to the conjunctiva and skin of the superior eyelid.

  - The *frontal nerve* enters through the superior orbital fissure and provides sensory innervation to the superior eyelid, scalp, and forehead.

  - The *nasociliary nerve* is the sensory nerve to the eyeball. It also has branches that serve the orbit and other parts of the face. One of its branches, the infratrochlear nerve, supplies the eyelids, conjunctiva, and lacrimal sac.

- *Ciliary ganglion:* This group of postsynaptic parasympathetic nerve cell bodies is associated with the oculomotor nerve and ophthalmic nerve (CN V_1). Presynaptic parasympathetic fibers from the oculomotor nerve synapse on the cell bodies of postsynaptic parasympathetic neurons in the ciliary ganglion.

Short ciliary nerves emerge from the ciliary ganglion and enter the eye. The short ciliary nerves contain postsynaptic parasympathetic fibers from the ciliary ganglion, afferent fibers of the nasociliary nerve, and postsynaptic sympathetic fibers from the internal carotid plexus. Postsynaptic parasympathetic fibers innervate the ciliary muscle and sphincter pupillae muscle. Afferent fibers convey sensory impulses from the iris and cornea. Postsynaptic sympathetic fibers innervate the dilator pupillae muscle.

The *long ciliary nerves* contain afferent and postsynaptic sympathetic fibers from the nasociliary nerve. Long ciliary nerves bypass the ciliary ganglion and run to the iris, cornea, and dilator pupillae muscle. (Flip to Chapter 3 for an introduction to the autonomic nervous system, which contains these types of cell bodies and fibers.)

Providing blood flow to and from the eyes

Blood flow to the orbit (and beyond) comes from branches of the internal carotid artery (see Chapter 14), chiefly via the ophthalmic artery and its branches:

- ✔ *Ophthalmic artery:* Branches from the internal carotid artery and passes through the optic canal into the orbital cavity

- ✔ *Central artery of the retina:* Runs from the ophthalmic artery to the eyeball alongside the optic nerve; it branches at the optic disc and supplies the retina (refer to Figure 13-1)

- ✔ *Supraorbital artery:* Starts at the ophthalmic artery and exits the orbit at the supraorbital notch to supply the forehead and scalp

- ✔ *Supratrochlear artery:* Runs from the ophthalmic artery to the forehead and scalp

- ✔ *Lacrimal artery:* Runs from the ophthalmic artery along the lateral rectus muscle to supply the lacrimal gland, conjunctiva, and the eyelids

- ✔ *Dorsal nasal artery:* Branches from the ophthalmic artery and runs along the nose to supply it with blood

- ✔ *Short posterior ciliary arteries:* Branch from the ophthalmic artery and pierce the sclera at the edge of the optic nerve; they supply the choroid and the rods and cones of the retina

- ✔ *Long posterior ciliary arteries:* Branch from the ophthalmic artery and pierce the sclera to supply the ciliary body and iris

- ✔ *Posterior ethmoidal artery:* Leaves the ophthalmic artery to supply blood to ethmoidal cells (coming up later in this chapter)

- ✔ *Anterior ethmoidal artery:* Runs from the ophthalmic artery to supply ethmoidal cells, frontal sinus, nasal cavity, and skin over the nose

- ✔ *Anterior ciliary artery:* Runs from the *muscular branches of the ophthalmic artery* through the sclera near the rectus muscles and forms an arterial network in the iris and ciliary body

- ✔ *Infraorbital artery:* Runs from the maxillary artery along the infraorbital groove and out to the face

Blood is returned from the orbits via the *superior* and *inferior ophthalmic veins,* which pass through the superior orbital fissure into the *cavernous sinus*. The *central vein of the retina* may join an ophthalmic vein or enter the cavernous sinus directly. *Vorticose veins* drain the vascular layer of the eyeball, and the *scleral venous sinus* encircles the anterior chamber of the eyeball.

Knowing the Nose

The nose is the part of the respiratory tract that sits front and center on your face (flip to Chapter 4 for an introduction to the respiratory system). You use it to breathe air in and to stop and smell the roses. Smell is a powerful sense: Just the smell of your favorite food starts you salivating. In the following sections, we check out the nose's exterior, nasal cavity, paranasal sinuses, nerves, blood supply, and lymphatics.

Sniffing out the exterior of the nose

The external part of the nose includes the *root* (between the eyes), the *dorsum* that runs down the middle, and the *apex* at the tip of the nose. Two openings called *nostrils* (nares) allow air in. They're divided by the *nasal septum* (dividing wall of cartilage and bone), and the parts that surround the nostrils are called the *alae (ala singular)*.

The nose has a bony part that's formed by the bony nasal septum, the nasal bones, and parts of the maxillae, palatine, and frontal bones (see Chapter 12 for more about these bones). The cartilaginous part of the nose is formed by two *lateral cartilages,* two *alar cartilages,* and a *septal cartilage*.

Scoping out the nasal cavity

The nares serve as the entryway to the *nasal cavities,* which open posteriorly into the nasopharynx (described in Chapter 14) via the choanae. The walls of the nasal cavity include the following features:

- ✔ **Roof:** The roof is divided into three parts: frontonasal, ethmoidal, and sphenoidal. Each part corresponds to the underlying bone of the same name (see Chapter 12 for the details on facial bones).

- ✔ **Floor:** The floor consists of the palatine process of the maxilla and the horizontal plate of the palatine bone.

- ✔ **Medial wall:** This wall is the nasal septum, which is formed by the per-pendicular plate of the ethmoid bone, the vomer, cartilage, and the nasal crests of the maxillary and palatine bones.

- ✔ **Lateral wall:** This wall is hallmarked by three *nasal conchae* (superior, middle, and inferior; see Chapter 12) that project inferiorly from the wall (see Figure 13-3). They divide the nasal cavity into four passages that have openings to the paranasal sinuses that we talk about in the next section:

- The *sphenoethmoid recess* lies posterior to the superior concha and has the opening for the *sphenoidal sinus.*

- The *superior nasal meatus* (recess) lies between the superior and middle conchae and has openings to the *posterior ethmoidal sinuses.*

- The *middle nasal meatus* is longer and deeper than the superior nasal meatus. The frontal sinus communicates with the middle nasal meatus via the *infundibulum,* a passageway that opens into the *semilunar hiatus* (groove in the ethmoid bone). The maxillary sinus opens into the semilunar hiatus. An *ethmoidal bulla* (a round swelling formed by the middle ethmoidal cells, or air-filled cavities) is formed just above the semilunar hiatus. The middle and anterior ethmoidal sinuses drain into the middle nasal meatus.

- The *inferior nasal meatus* is found below the inferior nasal concha. The nasolacrimal duct opens into this meatus.

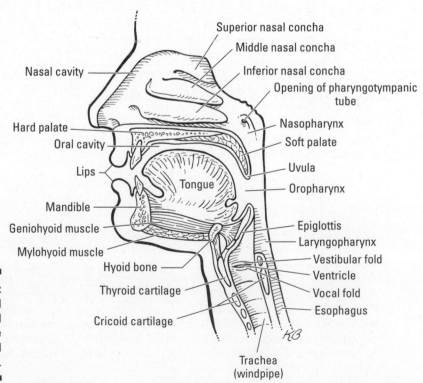

Figure 13-3: The nasal and oral cavities, the palate, and the pharynx.

Superior nasal concha

Middle nasal concha

Nasal cavity

Inferior nasal concha

Opening of pharyngotympanic tube

Hard palate

Nasopharynx

Oral cavity

Soft palate

Lips

Uvula

Tongue

Oropharynx

Mandible

Geniohyoid muscle

Epiglottis

Laryngopharynx

Mylohyoid muscle

Vestibular fold

Hyoid bone

Ventricle

Thyroid cartilage

Vocal fold

Esophagus

Cricoid cartilage

Trachea (windpipe)

The nasal cavity is lined with nasal mucosa (membranous lining that secretes mucus), except for the *nasal vestibule* (just inside the nostrils), which is lined with skin. The mucosa over the superior one-third of the nasal cavity is the *olfactory area,* which is the area where olfaction (sense of smell) begins. Air is drawn past the specialized mucosal cells called the *olfactory epithelium* as air is sniffed though the nose. The olfactory epithelium contains receptors of olfactory neurons that detect smells. Olfactory neurons (from CN I) join together to form nerve bundles that run up through the cribiform plate of the ethmoid bone to the olfactory bulb. The olfactory tract transmits the sensory information about smell from the olfactory bulb to the cerebral cortex.

Insinuating your way into the paranasal sinuses

The *paranasal sinuses* are air-filled cavities in the frontal, ethmoid, maxilla, and sphenoid bones (covered in Chapter 12). They're lined with a mucosal membrane and have small openings into the nasal cavity:

- ✔ *Maxillary sinus:* This sinus is located in the body of the maxilla behind the cheek just above the roots of the premolar and molar teeth. It's shaped like a pyramid. It opens into the nasal cavity in the preceding section via the semilunar hiatus.

- ✔ *Frontal sinuses:* Found within the frontal bone, each of these sinuses is triangular in shape and runs above the medial end of the eyebrow and backward to the orbit. They open into the nasal cavity via the semilunar hiatus.

- ✔ *Sphenoid sinuses:* These sinuses are found in the sphenoid bone. Each opens into the sphenoethmoid recess.

- ✔ *Ethmoid sinuses:* The anterior, middle, and posterior ethmoid sinuses are located in the ethmoid bone between the nose and the eye. The anterior sinus opens into the nasal cavity by the infundibulum, the middle sinus opens into the ethmoidal bulla, and the posterior sinus opens into the superior meatus.

Infection can spread from the nasal cavity into the sinuses, causing sinusitis with inflammation and pain of the mucosal lining. Symptoms of sinusitis include headaches, nasal congestion, bad breath, cough, fatigue, fever, and sore throat or postnasal drip. Sinusitis can be detected by applying pressure to the skin over the sinuses, which will be painful. Treatment includes warm compresses, inhaling steam, nasal saline sprays, and pain medications, and antibiotics may be used if bacterial infection is indicated by a high fever or blood tests.

Sensing the nerves, blood vessels, and lymphatics

Nerve supply to the external nose is provided by the *infratrochlear* and *external nasal branches* of the *ophthalmic nerve* and *the infraorbital branch of the maxillary nerve,* both of which are part of the trigeminal nerve (CN V) (see Chapter 12). The olfactory nerves (CN I) pass through the cribiform plate of the ethmoid bone (for the sense of smell). General sensory innervation (touch, pain, temperature) of the nasal cavity and the paranasal sinuses is from the ophthalmic nerve (CN V_1) and maxillary nerve (CN V_2).

Blood is supplied to the external part of the nose by branches of the ophthalmic and maxillary arteries. The skin of the ala and septum are supplied by the facial artery (see Chapter 12). Blood is brought to the walls of the nasal cavity and sinuses by branches of the maxillary artery. The most important is the sphenopalatine artery, which anastomoses (connects) with a branch of the superior labial artery. Venous blood is returned from the nasal cavity by veins that accompany the arteries.

Lymph from the nasal cavity drains into the submandibular lymph nodes and vessels that drain into the upper deep cervical lymph nodes (see Chapter 14).

Investigating the Mouth

The mouth, or *oral cavity,* and its structures allows you to eat and drink as well as breathe when your nose is plugged. Your mouth also works with the larynx (see Chapter 14) to help you speak. The following sections cover the oral cavity and its structures.

Open wide: The oral cavity

The *oral cavity* (refer to Figure 13-3) is home to your teeth, gums, palate, tongue, tonsils, and salivary glands. Anteriorly, it begins behind the opening of the lips, called the *oral fissure,* and posteriorly it opens into the oropharynx (see Chapter 14).

The oral cavity is divided into the oral cavity proper and the vestibule.

> ✔ **Oral cavity proper:** This space includes everything behind the teeth. The *roof of the mouth* is formed by the hard palate that we discuss later in this chapter, and the *floor* is formed by the anterior two-thirds of the tongue and the mucous membrane that covers the sides of the tongue and attaches it to the mandible.

✔ *Vestibule:* This space is between the cheeks and lips externally and the teeth and gums internally. Two muscular fleshy folds (the lips) surround the oral fissure (opening). Skin covers the lips externally, and the interior is lined with a mucous membrane. Median folds of the mucous membrane called the *labial frenulae* connect the lips to the gums. The lips contain the orbicularis oris, which puckers the lips and is sometimes referred to as the kissing muscle. The little groove that runs from the upper lip toward the nose is called the *philtrum*.

The walls of the vestibule are formed by the internal surface of the cheeks, which contain the buccinator muscles (see Chapter 12), and are also covered internally with mucous membrane.

Chew on this: The teeth and gums

The *teeth* are firmly affixed to the upper and lower jaws in sockets called *dental alveoli.* Teeth are used for biting, chewing, and assisting with speaking. Children have 20 primary teeth (baby teeth), and adults have 32. Sixteen teeth are in each jaw (maxillary and mandible): Moving from the back of the mouth to the front, adults have three molars, two premolars, one canine tooth, and two incisors on each side of the upper and lower jaw. Most of these teeth erupt (break through the skin) by the middle of the teenage years, but the third molars (wisdom teeth) may not erupt until the 20s.

Each tooth has a *crown, neck,* and *root.* The crown varies in size and shape for the different types of teeth. The neck is simply the part between the crown and the root. The root is fixed in the dental alveolus by the *periodontal ligament.* Most of the tooth is made up of a substance called *dentin,* which surrounds the *pulp cavity.* The surface of the crown is covered in a whitish *enamel,* and the root is covered with *cement.* An *apical foramen* located at the bottom of each root opens to a *root canal* that allows nerves and vessels to travel up to the tooth.

The *gingivae,* also known as the gums, are made of fibrous connective tissue and covered with a mucous membrane. The gingivae are attached to the alveolar processes of the mandible and maxilla and the necks of the teeth.

Picking on the palate

The palate forms the roof of the mouth and the floor of the nasal cavities. It has two parts: a *hard palate* and a *soft palate* (both of which you can see in Figure 13-3).

The hard palate

The hard palate forms the anterior part of the palate. It's formed by the palatine process of the maxilla and the horizontal plates of the palatine bones (see Chapter 12). The hard palate is covered by a mucous membrane and has the following three foramina (openings):

- ✔ *Incisive fossa:* This opening is posterior to the central (incisor) teeth. It allows passage of the nasopalatine nerves. (We talk about different nerves and vessels in the mouth later in this chapter.)

- ✔ *Greater palatine foramen:* This opening is located on the lateral portion of the palate. It allows passage of the greater palatine vessels and nerve.

- ✔ *Lesser palatine foramen:* Posterior to the greater palatine foramen, this opening allows the lesser palatine nerves and vessels to pass through to the soft palate.

The soft palate

The soft palate extends posteriorly and inferiorly from the hard palate and is strengthened by the *palatine aponeurosis,* which is a tendinous sheet. A conical, fleshy process called the *uvula* hangs from the back of the soft palate and is visible when the mouth is open wide. Laterally, the soft palate connects to the wall of the pharynx (see Chapter 14). It's joined to the tongue and the pharynx by the *palatoglossal* and *palatopharyngeal arches.* Clumps of lymphoid tissue called the *palatine tonsils* are located between these arches.

The soft palate works with the tongue (see the next section) to produce movements that help you swallow and force food into the esophagus. It also rises during swallowing to close off the opening between the oropharynx and the nasopharynx to prevent food and liquid from entering your nose. These five muscles also help with swallowing:

- ✔ *Tensor veli palatini:* This muscle originates on the sphenoid bone and the cartilage of the pharyngotympanic tube (see the later section "Moving into the middle ear") and inserts onto the palatine aponeurosis. It's innervated by the *nerve to the medial pterygoid* (CN V_3) and tenses the soft palate and opens the pharyngotympanic tube when yawning or swallowing.

- ✔ *Levator veli palatini:* Originating on the pharyngotympanic tube and part of the temporal bone, this muscle inserts onto the palatine aponeurosis. It's innervated by the *pharyngeal branch of the vagus nerve* (CN X). It elevates the soft palate during yawning or swallowing.

- **Palatoglossus:** This muscle originates on the palatine aponeurosis and inserts on the side of the tongue. It's innervated by the pharyngeal branch of the vagus nerve and elevates the posterior part of the tongue while drawing the soft palate to the tongue.

- **Palatopharyngeus:** Originating on the hard palate and palatine aponeurosis, this muscle inserts into the thyroid cartilage and the lateral wall of the pharynx. It's innervated by the pharyngeal branch of the vagus nerve and tenses the soft palate and pulls the pharynx toward the oral cavity during swallowing.

- **Musculus uvulae:** This muscle originates on the posterior nasal spine of the palatine bone and palatine aponeurosis and inserts into the mucosa of the uvula. It's innervated by the pharyngeal branch of the vagus nerve, and it pulls the uvula upward.

Sticking out your tongue

The *tongue* (refer to Figure 13-3) is a muscular organ that is quite mobile. It helps you speak, taste food and move it around in your mouth, and yes, even show your obnoxious side (when you stick out your tongue at someone). We note the areas and muscles of the tongue in the following sections.

The areas of the tongue

When the mouth is closed, the relaxed tongue takes up most of the space inside the oral cavity. The tongue is basically muscles surrounded by a mucous membrane. It has several parts:

- **Root:** This posterior one-third of the tongue is attached to the floor of the oral cavity. It has a bumpy appearance due to lymphoid nodules.

- **Body:** The mobile anterior two-thirds of the tongue is the body.

- **Apex:** The apex is the tip of the tongue.

- **Dorsum:** This part is the surface of the tongue. The *terminal sulcus* and the *foramen cecum* mark the area where the root and the body meet. It also has a *midline groove* that divides the tongue into left and right halves.

- **Inferior surface of the tongue:** This part has a thin transparent membrane. A large fold of mucosa, called the frenulum, can be seen running down the midline. The ducts of the submandibular salivary glands (see the next section) are found at the base of the frenulum.

The anterior part of the tongue contains a large number of *lingual papillae:*

- ✔ *Vallate papillae:* These papillae (small, rounded protuberances) lie just anterior to the terminal sulcus and contain *taste buds* and *lingual glands* that secrete serous fluids.

- ✔ *Foliate papillae:* These small folds along the sides of the tongue contain taste buds.

- ✔ *Filiform papillae:* These papillae cover a large portion of the dorsum. They're thread-like and sensitive to touch but do not contain taste buds.

- ✔ *Fungiform papillae:* These mushroom-shaped papillae appear as red spots. They're most concentrated on the apex and sides of the tongue. They also contain taste buds.

The tongue can sense five types of sensations with its papillae: sweet, salty, sour, bitter, and umami, which is a savory meaty flavor.

The muscles of the tongue

The tongue has a lot of movement due to eight pairs of muscles. They're divided by the *lingual septum.* Four pairs are intrinsic (only in the tongue and not attached to bone), and four pairs are extrinsic (they originate from outside the tongue). All the muscles of the tongue, except for the palatoglossus, are innervated by the hypoglossal nerve (CN XII). The palatoglossus is innervated by the pharyngeal plexus (CN X).

Following are the intrinsic muscles:

- ✔ *Superior longitudinal muscle:* This muscle originates on the submucosal fibrous layer and the septum and inserts into the margins of the tongue and mucous membrane. It curls the tongue upward and also shortens it.

- ✔ *Inferior longitudinal muscle:* Originating in the root of the tongue and on the hyoid bone (see Chapter 14), this muscle inserts into the apex. It curls the tongue downward and shortens it.

- ✔ *Transverse muscle:* This muscle originates on the septum and inserts on the lateral margins of the tongue. It narrows and protrudes the tongue.

- ✔ *Vertical muscle:* This muscle originates on the submucosal fibrous layer of the dorsum and inserts on the inferior surfaces of the borders of the tongue. It flattens and broadens the tongue.

Here are the extrinsic muscles:

- ✔ *Genioglossus:* This fan-shaped muscle originates on the mandible and inserts onto the entire dorsum of the tongue and the hyoid bone. It protrudes the tongue and assists with other movements.

- ✔ *Hyoglossus:* This thin muscle originates on the hyoid bone and inserts onto the inferior and lateral parts of the tongue. It depresses and shortens the tongue.

- ✔ *Styloglossus:* This small, triangular muscle originates on the styloid process of the temporal bone and inserts onto the posterior parts of the tongue. It retrudes (pulls back) the tongue and curls its sides.

- ✔ *Palatoglossus:* This crescent-shaped muscle originates on the palatine aponeurosis and inserts onto the posterolateral part of the tongue. It elevates the posterior part of the tongue and depresses the soft palate.

Making spit in the salivary glands

Salivary glands produce *saliva,* a clear fluid that keeps mucous membranes moist, lubricates foods while you chew, starts the digestion of starches, and helps prevent tooth decay. The mouth has the following salivary glands:

- ✔ *Parotid glands:* These salivary glands are the largest. They're located between the rami of the mandible and the mastoid processes of the temporal bone (described in Chapter 12). They empty saliva into the vestibule via the *parotid ducts.*

- ✔ *Sublingual glands:* These glands lie in the floor of the oral cavity between the mandible and genioglossus muscle. Their *sublingual ducts* open into the floor of the oral cavity near the *plica fimbriatae,* which are lingual folds found on either side of the frenulum.

- ✔ *Submandibular glands:* These glands are located along the body of the mandible. The *submandibular duct* is found between the mylohyoid and the hyoglossus muscles of the tongue and empties through small papilla on either side of the frenulum.

Tapping into the temporomandibular joint

The *temporomandibular joint* is a modified-hinge type of synovial joint (see Chapter 3 for more about joints) made up of the condylar process of the mandible (jawbone) and the mandibular fossa of the temporal bone, which are described in Chapter 12. The surfaces of the joint are lined with fibro-cartilage, which is unusual for a synovial joint — most are lined with hya-line cartilage. The joint has an *articular disc* in the middle of the joint cavity. The temporomandibular joint allows you to open and close your mouth and allows for elevation, depression, protrusion, retrusion (moving backward), and lateral movements of the jaw.

The muscles that move the temporomandibular joint are called the muscles of mastication (chewing). They include the following:

✔ **Temporalis:** This muscle originates on the temporal fossa of the temporal bone (see Chapter 12) and inserts on the coronoid process and anterior part of the ramus of the mandible (also discussed in Chapter 12). It's innervated by the mandibular nerve (CN V_3), and it elevates and retracts the mandible.

✔ **Masseter:** This muscle originates on the inferior and medial part of the maxillary process of the zygomatic bone and the zygomatic arch (these bones are discussed in Chapter 12). It inserts onto the angle of the jaw and the lateral part of the ramus of the mandible. It's innervated by the mandibular nerve and elevates the mandible.

✔ **Lateral pterygoid:** This muscle has two heads that originate in two places: The superior head originates on the greater wing of the sphe-noid, and the inferior head originates on the lateral pterygoid plate of the sphenoid bone (you'll find these bones in Chapter 12). The superior head inserts on the joint capsule and the articular disc. The inferior head inserts on the condyloid process of the mandible. The lateral pterygoid muscles protract (move forward) the mandible when both the left and right contract together. When one lateral pterygoid contracts, it swings the jaw to the contralateral (opposite) side. It is innervated by the mandibular nerve.

✔ **Medial pterygoid:** This muscle also has two heads. One head originates on the lateral pterygoid plate and the pyramidal process of the palatine bone, and the other head originates on the tuberosity of the maxilla. Both heads insert onto the medial part of the ramus of the mandible. It's innervated by the mandibular nerve, and it works with the masseter to elevate the mandible.

The fibrous layer of the joint capsule (the connective tissue surrounding the joint) has a thickened portion, called the *lateral ligament,* that strengthens the joint laterally. The *stylomandibular ligament* runs from the styloid process of the temporal bone to the angle of the mandible. The *sphenomandibular ligament* runs from the sphenoid bone to the lingula of the mandible.

Noting nerves

The oral cavity and everything in it get both sensory and motor nerves from branches of several cranial nerves (see Chapter 12 for details about cranial nerves):

- *Greater and lesser palatine nerves* and *nasopalatine nerves* (**CN V$_2$**): Supply the roof and palate

- *Lingual nerve* (**CN V$_3$**): Serves the floor of the mouth and senses touch and temperature for the anterior two-thirds of the tongue

- *Chorda tympani nerve* (**CN VII**): Part of the facial nerve; contains taste fibers from the anterior two-thirds of the tongue

- *Buccal nerve* (**CN V$_3$**): Provides sensory innervation to the skin and mucosa of the cheek

- *Dental plexuses:* Formed by branches of the *superior* (CN V$_2$) and *inferior alveolar nerves* (CN V$_3$); supply the teeth

- *Lingual, palatine, nasopalatine,* and *superior alveolar nerves:* Supply the gingivae

- *Hypoglossal nerve* (**CN XII**): Innervates the muscles of the tongue (except for the palatoglossus)

- *Glossopharyngeal nerve* (**CN IX**): Supplies general sensory and taste for the posterior one-third of the tongue

- *Internal laryngeal nerve* (**CN X**): Branches supply general sensation to a small part of the posterior part of the tongue

- *Postsynaptic parasympathetic secretomotor fibers:* Run to the serous glands from the *submandibular ganglion* that hangs from the lingual nerve

- *Great auricular nerve:* Innervates the parotid gland; comes from the cervical plexus

- *Auriculotemporal nerve* (**CN V$_3$**): Provides sensory innervation to the parotid gland

- *Glossopharyngeal nerve* (**CN IX**): Provides presynaptic parasympathetic fibers to the otic ganglion; postsynaptic parasympathetic fibers from the otic ganglion are secretomotor (stimulate the gland to secrete saliva) to the parotid gland

- *Presynaptic secretomotor fibers:* Fibers from the chorda tympani synapse with postsynaptic fibers of the submandibular ganglion that innervate submandibular and sublingual salivary glands

Viewing blood vessels

The organs and structures of the oral cavity and its structures require a fair amount of blood flow, coming from the following branches of the external carotid artery (see Chapter 14):

- **Superior labial branches of the facial arteries** and **infraorbital arteries:** Supply blood to the upper lip

- **Inferior branches of the facial arteries** and **mental arteries:** Supply the lower lip

- **Superior alveolar arteries (from the maxillary artery):** Supply blood to the upper teeth

- **Inferior alveolar arteries (from the maxillary artery):** Supply the lower teeth

- **Greater** and **lesser palatine arteries:** Supply the palate

- **Branches of the lingual artery:** Supply blood to the tongue

    - *Dorsal lingual arteries:* Supply the posterior part of the tongue

    - *Deep lingual artery:* Supplies the anterior part of the tongue and communicates with the dorsal arteries at the apex

    - *Sublingual artery:* Supplies the sublingual gland and the floor of the oral cavity

- **Branches of the external carotid** and **superficial temporal arteries:** Supply the parotid salivary glands

- **Submental arteries:** Supply the submandibular glands and sublingual glands

Veins of the oral cavity generally follow the arteries and have the same names. The veins of the palate drain into the *pterygoid venous plexus.* The lingual veins of the tongue drain into the internal jugular vein.

Sorting through lymphatics

Lymph from the upper lip, teeth, lateral parts of the anterior part of the tongue, and gingivae drains into the submandibular lymph nodes. Lymph from the lower lip and apex of the tongue drains into the submental lymph nodes. (You can read about these lymph nodes in Chapter 12.)

Lymph from the medial anterior portion of the tongue drains into the inferior deep cervical lymph nodes, and the posterior portion of the tongue drains into the superior deep cervical lymph nodes. (Chapter 14 discusses these lymph nodes.)

The parotid glands drain their lymph into the superficial and deep cervical lymph nodes. The submandibular glands drain lymph into the deep cervical lymph nodes.

Entering the Ear

The two ears allow you to hear sounds and wear really cool earrings. Actually, there's more to an ear than the external part you see on the sides of your head; most of the structures lie inside the middle ear and the inner ear. Some of those structures allow you to hear, and others keep you steady on your feet. Discover the ear and its makeup in the following sections.

Examining the external ear

The *external ear* includes the auricle as well as the external acoustic meatus, also known as the ear canal, which ends at the tympanic membrane separating the external ear from the middle ear.

The *auricle* (or *pinna*) is the part of the ear that you see — it helps transfer sound waves to the external acoustic meatus — and it's also visible in Figure 13-4. It's covered with skin and it has the following landmarks:

- ✔ *Concha:* The deepest depression, just posterior to the opening of the meatus
- ✔ *Helix:* The elevated cartilaginous margin around the posterior and superior part of the auricle
- ✔ *Lobule:* The ear lobe, containing fibrous tissue, fat, and blood vessels
- ✔ *Tragus:* The small projection that lies anterior to the meatus

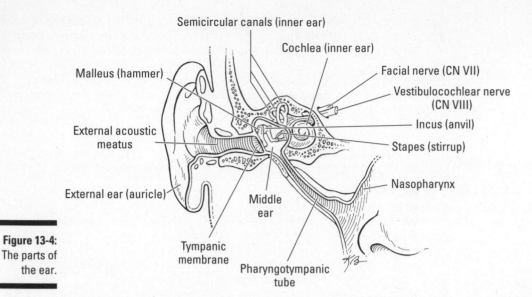

Semicircular canals (inner ear)

Cochlea (inner ear)

Malleus (hammer)

Facial nerve (CN VII)

Vestibulocochlear nerve
(CN VIII)

External acoustic
meatus

Incus (anvil)

Stapes (stirrup)

Nasopharynx

External ear (auricle)

Middle
ear

Figure 13-4:
The parts of
the ear.

Tympanic
membrane

Pharyngotympanic
tube

Sound waves enter the ear through the *external acoustic meatus.* The opening is visible in Figure 13-4. A normal meatus is about 2 or 3 centimeters long, and it meets the tympanic membrane. The lateral part of the meatus is cartilaginous, and the deeper parts are bony. It's lined with skin that contains *ceruminous* and *sebaceous glands,* which produce *cerumen,* or earwax.

The *tympanic membrane* (or eardrum) is a thin oval membrane about 1 centimeter in diameter. The external side is covered with thin skin, and the internal side is covered with mucous membrane.

If you look at the tympanic membrane with an otoscope in a normal, healthy ear, you see a cone of light on the membrane going anteriorly and inferiorly. Superior to the cone of light, you see the *flaccid part* that has fewer fibers than the rest of the membrane, which is called the *tense part.*

Moving into the middle ear

The *middle ear* takes up the space behind the tympanic membrane, inside the temporal bone (refer to Figure 13-4). The space is called the *tympanic cavity,* and it has two parts: the *tympanic cavity proper* directly behind the membrane and the *epitympanic recess,* which is located just above the membrane.

The tympanic cavity is connected to the nasopharynx anteriorly and medially by the *pharyngotympanic tube* (also called the Eustachian tube) and posteriorly and superiorly by the *mastoid antrum,* a cavity in the mastoid process of the temporal bone, by the aditus to the mastoid antrum. The tympanic cavity is lined with mucous membrane and has the following six walls:

- ✔ *Tegmental wall:* This roof is formed by the *tegmen tympani,* which is part of the temporal bone (see Chapter 12).

- ✔ *Jugular wall:* This floor is formed by a bone that separates the middle ear from the internal jugular vein (see Chapter 14).

- ✔ *Membranous wall:* This lateral wall is formed mostly by the tympanic membrane and the bony wall of the epitympanic recess.

- ✔ *Labyrinthine wall:* This medial wall separates the middle ear from the inner ear. It includes the *promontory of the labrynthine wall* and the *oval* and *round windows.*

- ✔ *Carotid wall:* This anterior wall separates the tympanic cavity from the carotid canal and artery. It has the opening for the pharyngotympanic tube and the canal for the tensor tympani muscle.

- ✔ *Mastoid wall:* This posterior wall has an opening called the *aditus to the mastoid antrum* that connects the tympanic cavity (epitympanic recess) to the mastoid air cells (sinus).

The tympanic cavity is home to the auditory ossicles and muscles as well as the chorda tympani and the tympanic plexus of nerves (both of which we cover later in this chapter). The *auditory ossicles* are a chain of mobile bones that cross the tympanic cavity from the tympanic membrane to the oval window on the labrynthine wall. Their function is to transmit sound from the air of the external acoustic meatus (see the preceding section) to the fluid in the labyrinth. The ossicles are small bones covered with mucus membrane, but unlike other bones, they have no periosteum (refer to Figure 13-4):

- ✔ *Malleus:* Also known as the *hammer,* this bone is attached to the tympanic membrane. It has a rounded *head* superiorly, a *neck* that lies against the flaccid part of the tympanic membrane, and a *handle* that's embedded in the membrane. The head articulates (forms a joint) with the incus.

- ✔ *Incus:* This bone is also known as the *anvil.* It articulates with both the malleus and the stapes. Its body lies in the epitympanic recess (along with the head of the malleus), and a *long limb* lies parallel to the handle of the malleus. A *short limb* is connected to the posterior wall of the tympanic cavity. The *lenticular process* of the long limb articulates with the stapes.

- ✔ *Stapes:* The base of the this bone (also known as the *stirrup*) is attached to the oval window.

The main muscles of the tympanic cavity include the following:

✔ **Tensor tympani:** This muscle originates superior to the pharyngotympanic tube, the sphenoid, and the temporal bone and inserts into the handle of the malleus. It tenses the tympanic membrane and dampens the movements of the ossicles to prevent ear damage from loud sounds. It is innervated by the trigeminal nerve (CN V_3).

✔ **Stapedius:** This muscle is found in the *pyramidal eminence* on the posterior wall of the tympanic cavity. Its tendon inserts onto the neck of the stapes. Like the tensor tympani, it helps to dampen loud sounds. It is innervated by the facial nerve (CN VII).

The *pharyngotympanic tube* (refer to Figure 13-4) has both a bony and cartilaginous section and is lined with mucous membrane. The function of the tube is to equalize pressure between the middle ear and the air pressure outside the body. Its diameter is controlled by the *levator veli palatini* that pushes on one wall when it contracts and the *tensor veli palatini* muscles that pull on the other wall.

Diving deeper into the inner ear

The *inner ear* houses the *vestibulocochlear organ* that maintains balance and receives sound from the middle ear. It has two parts: the bony labyrinth and the membranous labyrinth.

The bony labyrinth

The *bony labyrinth* contains the *otic capsule,* which is denser than the surrounding temporal bone. It contains fluid called perilymph and three cavities, called the cochlea, vestibule, and semicircular canals:

✔ **Cochlea:** Pictured in Figure 13-4, the *cochlea* is a shell-shaped opening with a *cochlear duct,* which is important for hearing. It has a *spiral canal* that begins at the vestibule and turns around a bony core called the *modiolus,* which has canals for blood vessels and branches of the cochlear nerve. It opens into the subarachnoid space (see Chapter 12) via the *cochlear aqueduct.* It has a *round window* and a *secondary tympanic membrane.*

✔ **Vestibule:** This small, oval chamber contains the *utricle* and the *saccule* along with parts of the vestibular labyrinth. An oval window is on its lateral wall. The *vestibular aqueduct* runs to the posterior surface of the temporal bone.

✔ **Semicircular canals:** These three canals open up into the vestibule. Each is semicircular in shape and has a swelling called the *bony ampulla.* You can find the semicircular canals in Figure 13-4.

The membranous labyrinth

The *membranous labyrinth* is within the bony labyrinth. It contains fluid called *endolymph* and is surrounded by the perilymph that fills the bony labyrinth. The membranous labyrinth includes the *vestibular labyrinth,* which contains is the *utricle* and the *saccule* (two vestibular sacs), three semicircular ducts in the semicircular canals, and the *cochlear labyrinth* (duct of the cochlea). These structures and fluids are involved in both balance and hearing.

The *internal acoustic meatus* is a canal that runs laterally within the temporal bone. It houses the *vestibulocochlear nerve* (CN VIII; refer to Figure 13-4), which divides into its vestibular and cochlear divisions.

Keeping an ear out for nerves and vessels

The nerves that supply the ear include the following:

- ✔ *Great auricular nerve* and *auriculotemporal nerve* (CN V$_3$): Discussed in Chapter 12, these nerves supply the skin of the auricle with a little help from the facial nerve. The auriculotemporal nerve also supplies a portion of the external acoustic meatus and the external surface of the tympanic membrane.

- ✔ *Auricular branch:* This branch of the vagus nerve (CN X) innervates part of the external surface of the tympanic membrane.

- ✔ *Glossopharyngeal nerve* (CN IX): This nerve innervates the linings of the middle ear and the pharyngotympanic tube.

The *posterior auricular artery* and the *superficial temporal artery* supply blood to the auricle. The *ascending pharyngeal artery*, the *middle meningeal artery,* and the *artery of the pterygoid canal* provide blood to the pharyngotympanic tube. Blood is drained from the ear by veins that accompany the arteries.

Lymphatic fluid from the auricle is drained into the *superficial parotid lymph nodes* (described in Chapter 12), *mastoid lymph nodes* located near the mastoid process, and deep cervical lymph nodes (see Chapter 14).

The Skin (Cross Section)

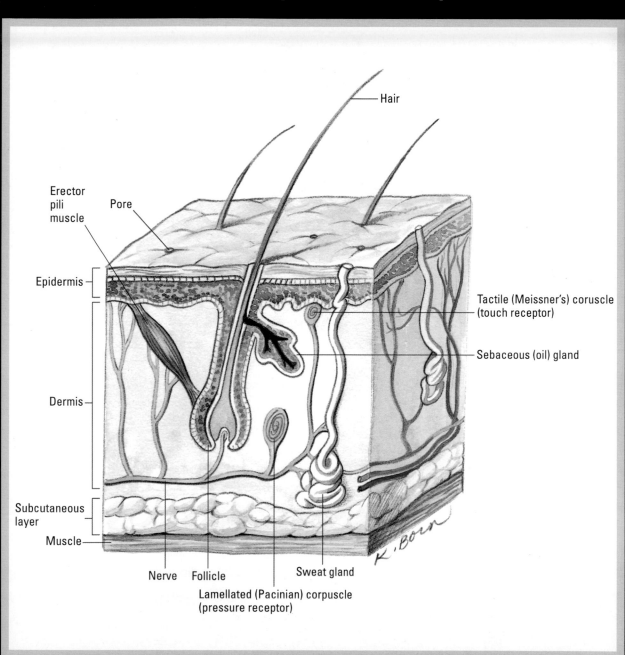

Hair

Erector pili muscle

Pore

Epidermis

Tactile (Meissner's) coruscle (touch receptor)

Sebaceous (oil) gland

Dermis

Subcutaneous layer

Muscle

Nerve

Follicle

Sweat gland

Lamellated (Pacinian) corpuscle (pressure receptor)

K. Born

Your body's largest organ is your skin (known clinically as *integument*). It includes the outer covering that protects your inside parts from the elements and from microorganisms. See Chapter 3 for details.

The Major Bones of the Skeletal System

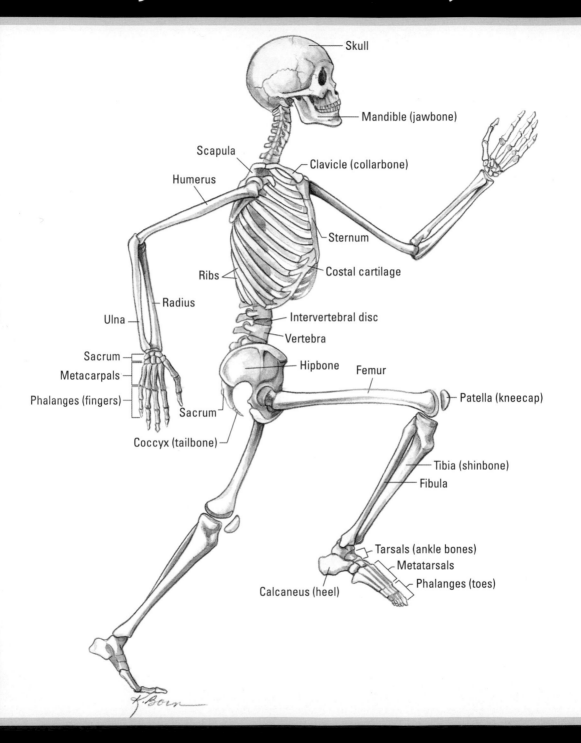

The bones of the skeleton form the body's basic framework. See Chapter 3 for details.

The Muscular System

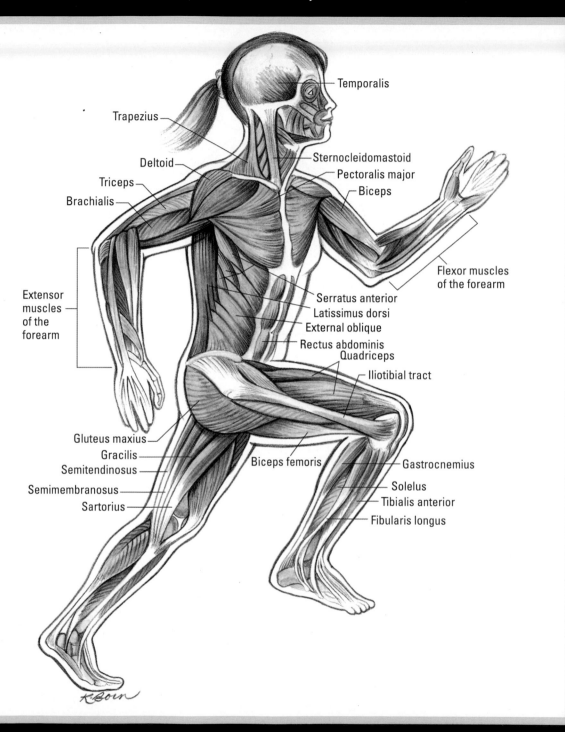

Temporalis

Trapezius

Deltoid

Triceps

Brachialis

Sternocleidomastoid

Pectoralis major

Biceps

Extensor
muscles
of the
forearm

Flexor muscles
of the forearm

Serratus anterior

Latissimus dorsi

External oblique

Rectus abdominis

Quadriceps

Iliotibial tract

Gluteus maxius

Gracilis

Semitendinosus

Semimembranosus

Sartorius

Biceps femoris

Gastrocnemius

Solelus

Tibialis anterior

Fibularis longus

K. Boin

More than 600 muscles provide movement throughout your body. Three different types of muscle exist: skeletal muscle, cardiac muscle, and smooth muscle. See Chapter 3 for details.

The Nervous System

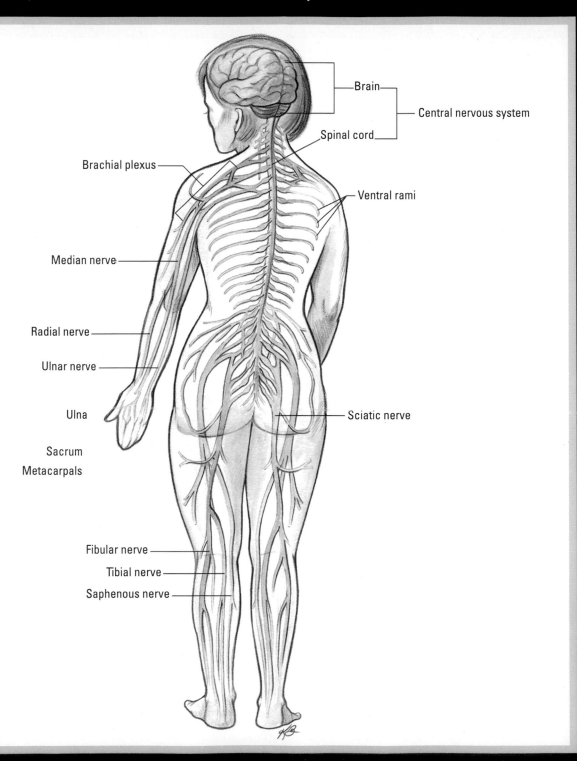

Brain

Central nervous system

Spinal cord

Brachial plexus

Ventral rami

Median nerve

Radial nerve

Ulnar nerve

Ulna

Sciatic nerve

Sacrum

Metacarpals

Fibular nerve

Tibial nerve

Saphenous nerve

The nervous system is your body's control center. The structures of the nervous system include the brain, the spinal cord, and nerves that reach every part of your body. See Chapter 3 for details.

The Sympathetic and Parasympathetic Nervous Systems

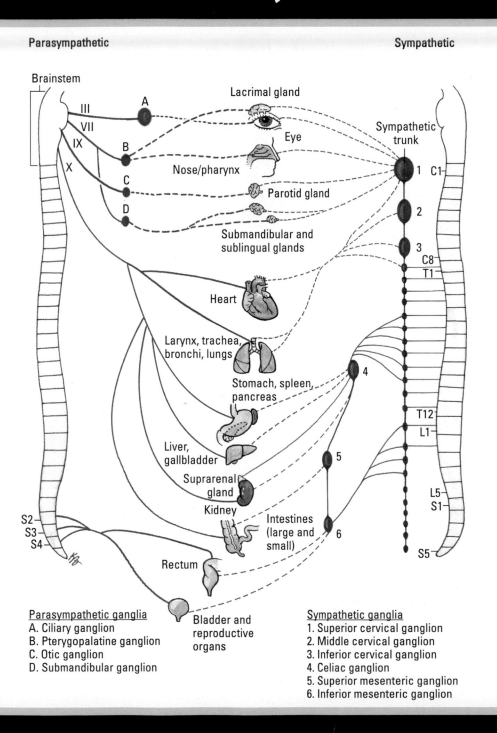

Parasympathetic

Sympathetic

Brainstem

III
VII
IX
X

A

B

C

D

Lacrimal gland

Eye

Nose/pharynx

Parotid gland

Submandibular and
sublingual glands

Heart

Larynx, trachea,
bronchi, lungs

Stomach, spleen,
pancreas

Liver,
gallbladder

Suprarenal
gland

Kidney

Rectum

Intestines
(large and
small)

S2
S3
S4

Bladder and
reproductive
organs

Sympathetic
trunk

C1

1

2

3

4

5

6

C8
T1

T12
L1

L5
S1

S5

Parasympathetic ganglia
A. Ciliary ganglion
B. Pterygopalatine ganglion
C. Otic ganglion
D. Submandibular ganglion

Sympathetic ganglia
1. Superior cervical ganglion
2. Middle cervical ganglion
3. Inferior cervical ganglion
4. Celiac ganglion
5. Superior mesenteric ganglion
6. Inferior mesenteric ganglion

The sympathetic nervous system prepares the body for emergency situations, also known as fight-or-flight reactions. The parasympathetic nervous system helps you rest and digest. See Chapter 3 for details.

The Heart

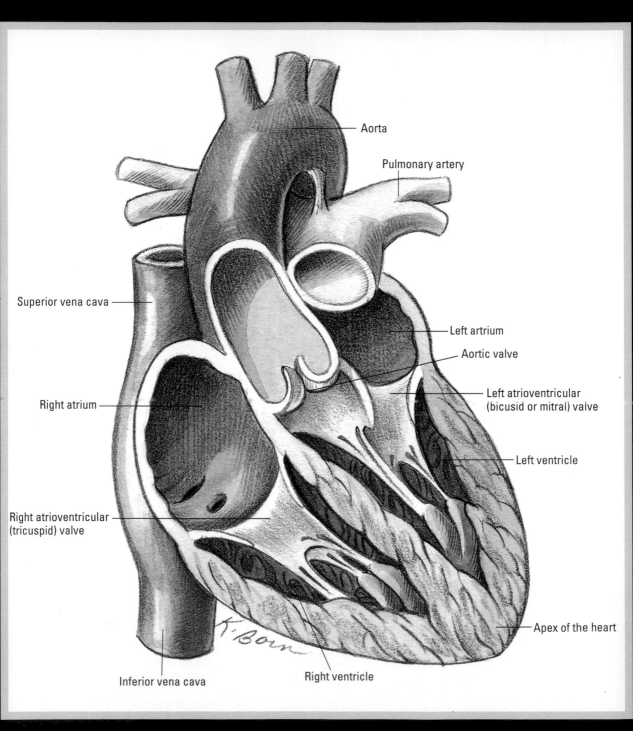

The heart is a muscular four-chambered pump that beats constantly to keep blood flowing to the rest of your body, from your head to your toes. It's part of the cardiovascular system; see Chapters 4 and 8 for details.

The Arteries of the Cardiovascular System

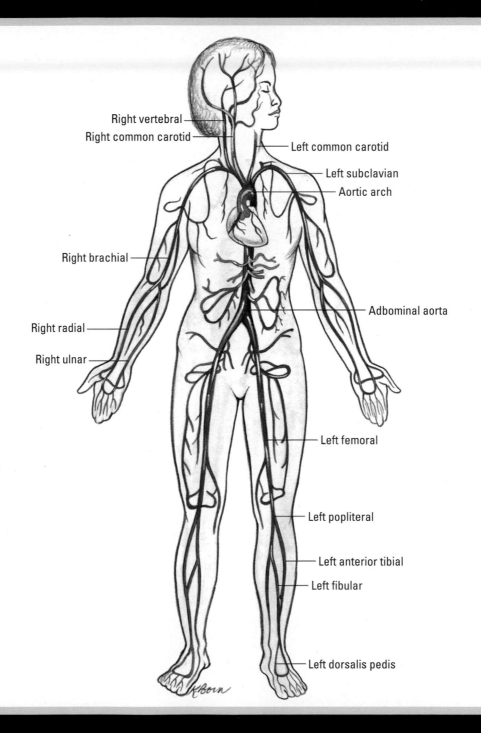

Right vertebral

Right common carotid

Left common carotid

Left subclavian

Aortic arch

Right brachial

Adbominal aorta

Right radial

Right ulnar

Left femoral

Left popliteral

Left anterior tibial

Left fibular

Left dorsalis pedis

K Born

Arteries are the blood vessels that take blood away from the heart; they're part of the cardiovascular system. See Chapter 4 for details.

The Veins of the Cardiovascular System

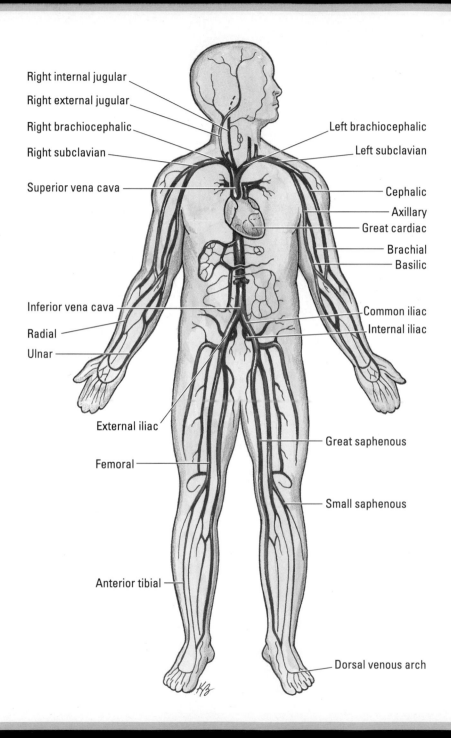

Right internal jugular

Right external jugular

Right brachiocephalic

Right subclavian

Superior vena cava

Inferior vena cava

Radial

Ulnar

External iliac

Femoral

Anterior tibial

Left brachiocephalic

Left subclavian

Cephalic

Axillary

Great cardiac

Brachial

Basilic

Common iliac

Internal iliac

Great saphenous

Small saphenous

Dorsal venous arch

Veins are the blood vessels that return blood to the heart; they're part of the cardiovascular system. See Chapter 4 for details.

The Respiratory System

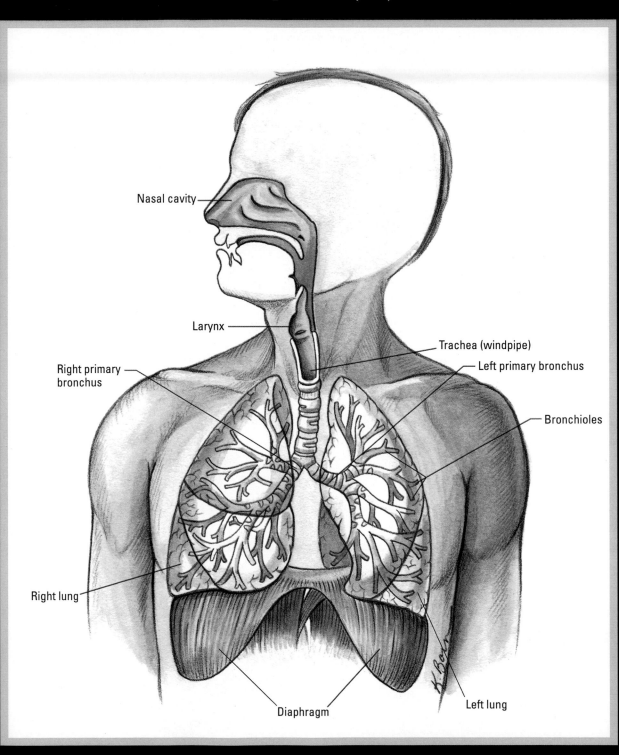

By breathing air in and out via the respiratory system, oxygen gets into the lungs and bloodstream, and carbon dioxide gets out. See Chapter 4 for details.

The Structure of a Respiratory Membrane

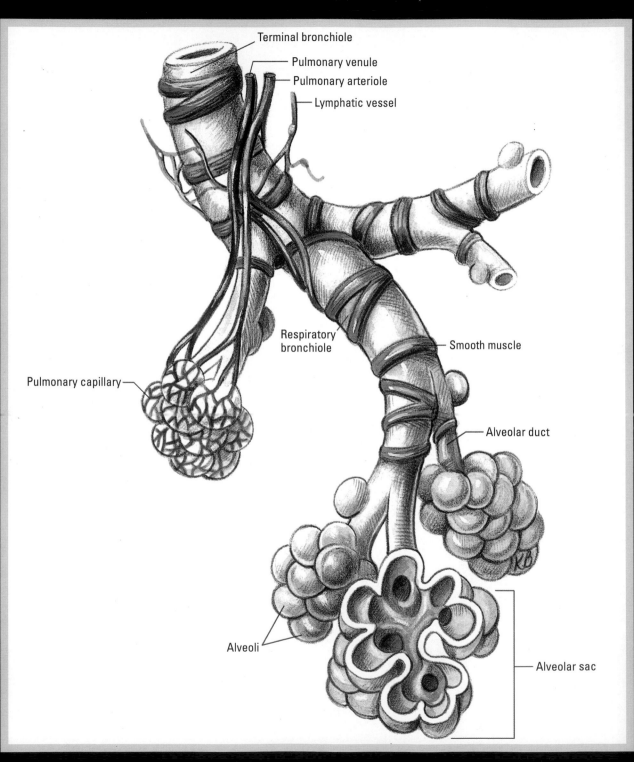

Terminal bronchiole

Pulmonary venule

Pulmonary arteriole

Lymphatic vessel

Respiratory bronchiole

Smooth muscle

Pulmonary capillary

Alveolar duct

Alveoli

Alveolar sac

The bronchi of the respiratory system form branches that eventually end in terminal bronchioles. Each terminal bronchiole divides into many respiratory bronchioles where the exchange of gases takes place in the alveoli. See Chapters 4 and 8 for details.

The Lymphatic System

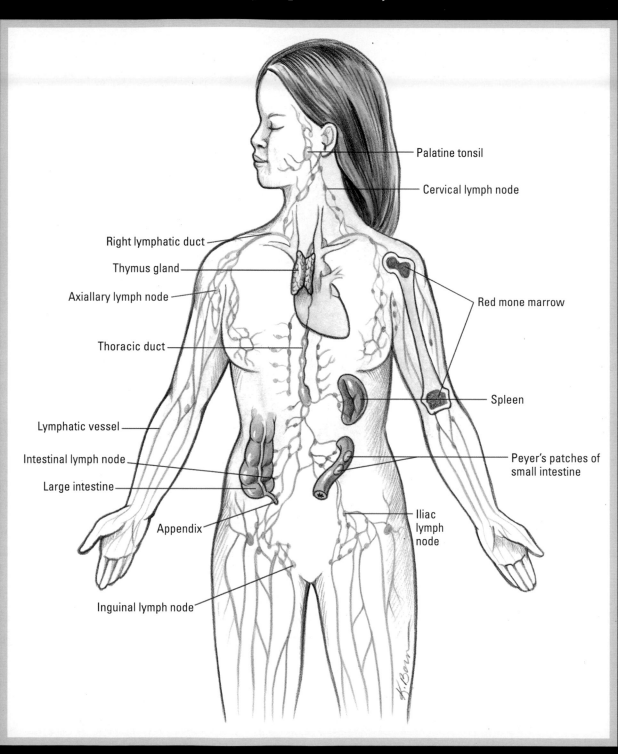

Palatine tonsil

Cervical lymph node

Right lymphatic duct

Thymus gland

Axiallary lymph node

Red mone marrow

Thoracic duct

Spleen

Lymphatic vessel

Intestinal lymph node

Peyer's patches of small intestine

Large intestine

Appendix

Iliac lymph node

Inguinal lymph node

The lymphatic system helps maintain your body's fluid balance and transport some fats. It also works along with the rest of the immune system to fight infections. See Chapter 5 for details.

The Digestive System

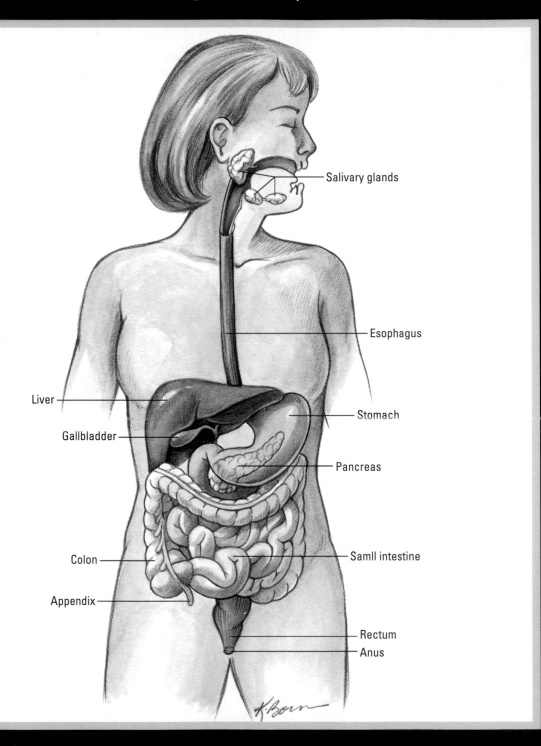

The digestive system takes food into your body, breaks it down into macronutrients and micronutrients, and then absorbs those nutrients so the rest of your body can use them as fuel and raw materials for building tissues and structures. See Chapter 6 for details.

The Urinary System

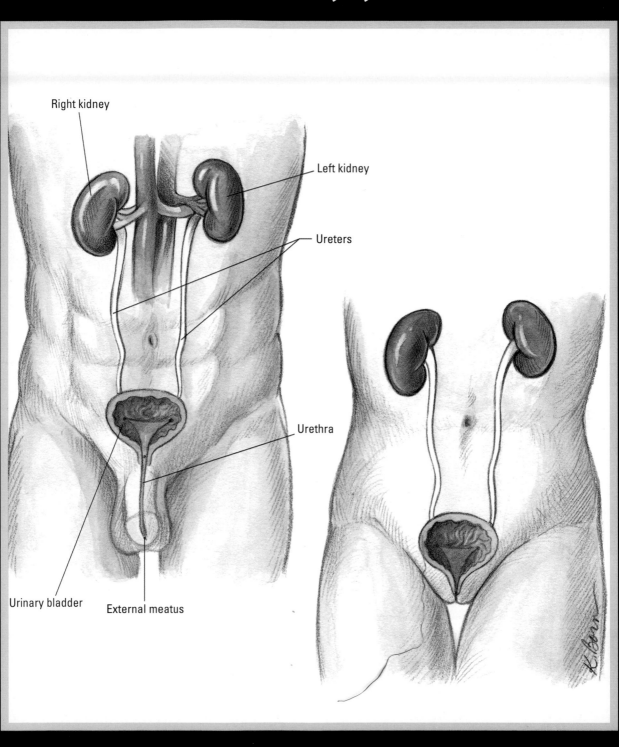

The urinary system filters waste from the blood and produces urine in the kidneys; then it removes the urine from the body. See Chapter 6 for details.

The Kidney

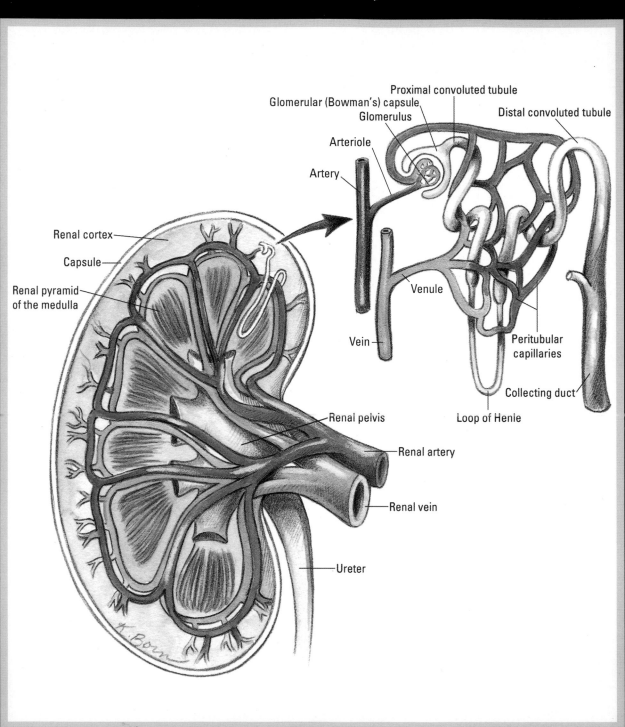

The kidneys filter the blood and form urine, which is transported to the urinary bladder by the ureters; they're part of the urinary system. See Chapters 6 and 10 for details.

The Endocrine System

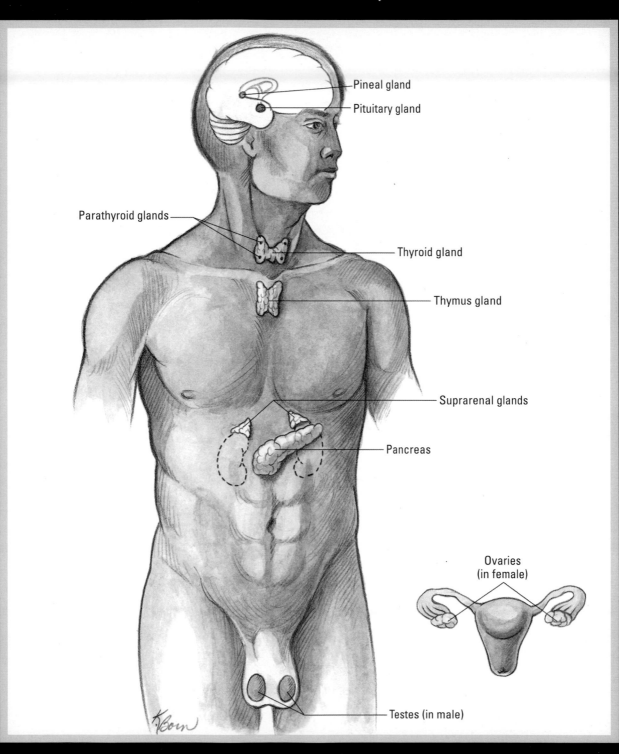

Pineal gland

Pituitary gland

Parathyroid glands

Thyroid gland

Thymus gland

Suprarenal glands

Pancreas

Ovaries
(in female)

Testes (in male)

The endocrine system is made up of glands that produce hormones and release them into the blood. Hormones cause certain reactions to occur in specific tissues. See Chapter 6 for details.

The Reproductive System (Female and Male)

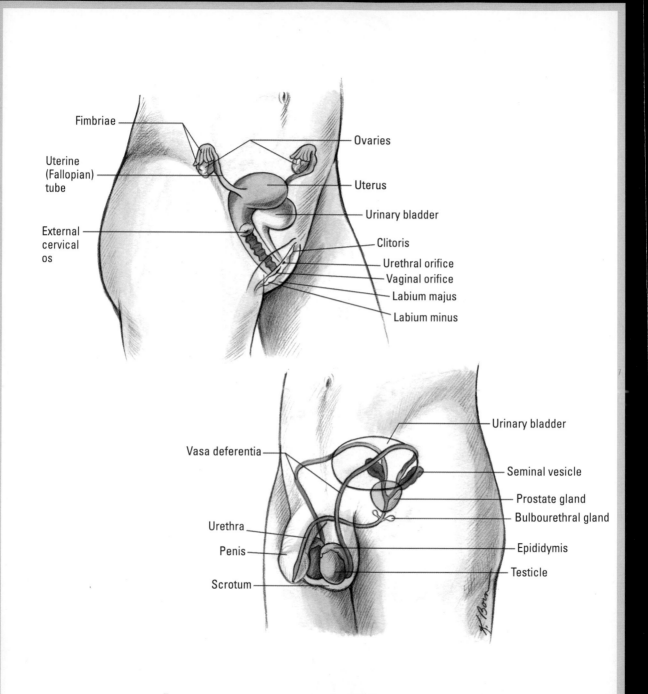

Female reproductive organs include ovaries and the uterine tubes that carry eggs into the uterus; male reproductive organs include the penis and various glands and ducts. See Chapter 11 for details.

Chapter 14

It's Neck and Neck

K nowledge of the neck anatomy is necessary to examine the musculoskeletal, nervous, respiratory, digestive, endocrine, lymphatic, and
cardiovascular systems. After all, the neck is much more than a pedestal
for the head. It has a lot going on inside, so we divide the parts into two
groups, the superficial structures and the deep structures. After we cover the
muscles, nerves, and blood vessels of both structures, we discuss the organs
housed in the neck and the skin and surface anatomy.

Sizing Up the Superficial Structures: Muscles, Nerves, and Blood Vessels

The superficial structures of the neck include mostly muscles, blood vessels,
and nerves that either work in the neck or travel through the neck to get to
the head or the trunk.

The superficial structures are located in two triangles: the anterior triangle
of the neck, and the posterior triangle of the neck. We break these triangles
down for you in the following sections.

Dividing the triangles: The sternocleidomastoid

The *sternocleidomastoid* muscle (SCM) is visible on either side of the neck (see Figure 14-1). It separates the posterior triangle of the neck from the anterior triangle of the neck. It's attached to the sternum and clavicle (breastbone and collarbone) and the mastoid process of the temporal bone of the skull.

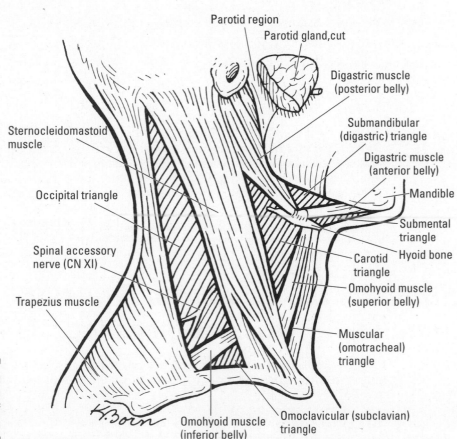

Parotid region

Parotid gland, cut

Digastric muscle (posterior belly)

Submandibular (digastric) triangle

Digastric muscle (anterior belly)

Mandible

Submental triangle

Hyoid bone

Carotid triangle

Omohyoid muscle (superior belly)

Muscular (omotracheal) triangle

Omoclavicular (subclavian) triangle

Omohyoid muscle (inferior belly)

Sternocleidomastoid muscle

Occipital triangle

Spinal accessory nerve (CN XI)

Trapezius muscle

Figure 14-1: The triangles of the neck.

The sternocleidomastoid muscle has two portions (somewhat like two prongs): the sternal head and the clavicular head. The sternal head originates on the manubrium (the upper part of the sternum; see Chapter 7), and the clavicular head originates on the medial part of the clavicle (see Chapter 16). The space between the two heads is called the *lesser supraclavicular fossa.* The two heads join together as they move upward and insert onto the mastoid process of the temporal bone (the easily palpated bony bump located just behind and below the ear; see Chapter 12).

Contracting one sternocleidomastoid muscle tilts your head to that side and can rotate the head in the opposite direction. Contracting both at the same time flexes the neck and extends the head. The spinal accessory nerve (CN XI) provides the efferent (motor) innervation, and the afferent (sensory) innervation comes from the C3 and C4 spinal nerves.

Going back to the posterior triangle of the neck

The borders of the posterior triangle of the neck are formed by the trapezius muscle posteriorly, the sternocleidomastoid muscle anteriorly, and the omohyoid muscle inferiorly. The roof is formed by fascia, and the floor is formed by the splenius capitus, levator scapulae, and scalene muscles. In the following sections, you explore the muscles, nerves, and blood vessels of the posterior triangle.

Muscles of the posterior triangle of the neck

This triangle is home to parts of several muscles:

- ✔ *Splenius capitis* (discussed in Chapter 15 with the other intrinsic back muscles)
- ✔ *Levator scapula* (covered with the shoulder girdle in Chapter 16)
- ✔ *Anterior, middle,* **and** *posterior scalenes* (discussed later in this chapter)

Nerves in the posterior triangle of the neck

You find several nerves in the posterior triangle of the neck, too. You can locate some of these nerves in Figure 14-2:

- ✔ *Spinal accessory nerve (cranial nerve XI)*
- ✔ *Roots of the brachial plexus*
- ✔ *Suprascapular nerve*
- ✔ *Cutaneous branches of the cervical plexus:*
    - • *Lesser occipital nerve*
    - • *Great auricular nerve*
    - • *Transverse cervical nerve*
    - • *Supraclavicular nerve*
- ✔ *Phrenic nerve*

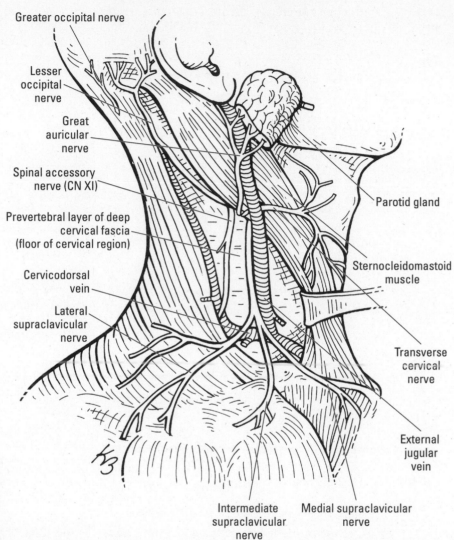

Greater occipital nerve

Lesser occipital nerve

Great auricular nerve

Spinal accessory nerve (CN XI)

Prevertebral layer of deep cervical fascia (floor of cervical region)

Cervicodorsal vein

Lateral supraclavicular nerve

Parotid gland

Sternocleidomastoid muscle

Transverse cervical nerve

External jugular vein

Intermediate supraclavicular nerve

Medial supraclavicular nerve

Figure 14-2: Posterior triangle of the neck.

Blood vessels of the posterior triangle of the neck

The posterior triangle of the neck has several veins and arteries (you can see some of them in Figure 14-2):

- *External jugular vein*
- *Subclavian vein*
- *Brachiocephalic vein*

✔ *Cervicodorsal vein*

✔ *Suprascapular artery*

✔ *Occipital artery*

✔ Part of the *subclavian artery*

Understanding the anterior triangle of the neck

The anterior triangle of the neck, or the front of the neck, is bordered by the sternocleidomastoid muscle, the midline of the neck from the chin to the manubrium, and the bottom of the mandible (jawbone). You can see the anterior cervical triangle in Figure 14-1.

Muscles of the anterior triangle of the neck

Many muscles are located in the anterior triangle of the neck, and they're classified according to their relationship to the hyoid bone. The hyoid bone is a horseshoe-shaped bone located in the anterior part of the neck below the chin. It serves as an anchor for muscles that help you swallow and move your tongue.

✔ *Hyoid muscles:* Located above (suprahyoid) and below (infrahyoid) the hyoid bone, these muscles move the hyoid bone and larynx (more about the larynx later in this chapter).

✔ *Suprahyoid muscles:* These muscles connect the hyoid bone to the cranium (see Chapter 12). They form the floor of the mouth and assist the larynx during speaking. Following are the four suprahyoid muscles:

• The *mylohyoid* originates on the mylohyoid line of the mandible and inserts onto the body of the hyoid. It elevates the hyoid, the floor of the mouth, and the tongue.

• The *geniohyoid* originates on the inferior mental spine of the mandible and inserts onto the body of the hyoid. It pulls the hyoid anteriorly and superiorly and shortens the floor of the mouth.

• The *stylohyoid* originates on the styloid process of the temporal bone and inserts onto the body of the hyoid. It elevates and retracts the hyoid to elongate the floor of the mouth.

• The *digastric* has two portions. The anterior belly originates on the mandible, and the posterior belly originates on the temporal bone of the skull. The digastric inserts onto the body and the greater horn of the hyoid. It works with the infrahyoid muscles to depress the mandible against resistance and elevates the hyoid.

✔ *Infrahyoid muscles:* These muscles are below the hyoid bone. They provide a base for the tongue and help stabilize the hyoid during swallowing and speaking.

- The *omohyoid* originates on the superior border of the scapula (shoulder blade) and inserts onto the inferior border of the hyoid. It depresses and retracts the hyoid.

- The *sternohyoid* originates on the manubrium and medial end of the clavicle and inserts onto the body of the hyoid. It depresses the hyoid after elevation during swallowing.

- The *sternothyroid* originates on the posterior surface of the manubrium (superior part of the sternum) and inserts onto the thyroid cartilage. It depresses the hyoid and larynx.

- The *thyrohyoid* originates on the thyroid cartilage and inserts onto the inferior border of the body and greater horn of the hyoid. It depreses the hyoid and elevates the larynx.

Nerves

Two cranial nerves, the vagus and glossopharyngeal, have branches in the anterior cervical triangle (you can read about the cranial nerves in Chapter 13). Two more nerves are located here:

✔ The *transverse cervical nerve* innervates the skin over the anterior triangle of the neck.

✔ The *hypoglossal nerve* travels to the tongue.

Blood vessels of the anterior triangle of the neck

The anterior triangle of the neck is also home to a couple of well-known blood vessels, plus a few more. *Carotid arteries* include the *common carotid artery* and the *internal* and *external carotid arteries.* The common carotid artery travels upward within the *carotid sheath* and then forks into the internal and external carotid arteries.

Several arteries branch off the external carotid artery (you can see some of them in Figure 14-3):

✔ *Superior thyroid artery:* Provides blood flow to the thyroid gland and the larynx

✔ *Ascending pharyngeal artery:* Supplies blood to the pharyngeal wall (we discuss the pharynx later in "Speaking of the pharynx, larynx, and trachea")

✔ *Lingual artery:* Takes blood to the tongue (see Chapter 12)

✔ *Facial artery:* Supplies blood to parts of the face

✔ *Occipital artery:* Takes blood to the back of the scalp (see Chapter 12)

✔ *Posterior auricular artery:* Supplies the scalp and the auricle (the external ear; see Chapter 12)

✔ *Superficial temporal artery:* Also sends blood to the scalp

✔ *Maxillary artery:* Goes up to the skull and supplies blood to the middle areas of the face

The *internal jugular vein* is formed as the dural venous sinuses leave the skull through the internal jugular foramen. It continues inferiorly until it joins the subclavian vein to form the brachiocephalic vein.

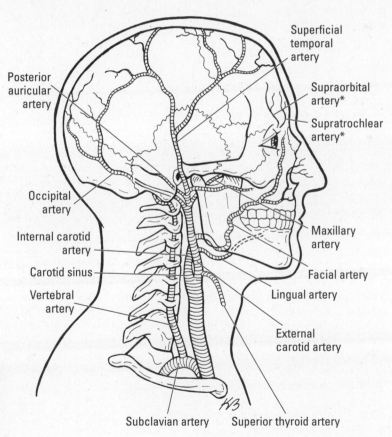

Figure 14-3:
Some arteries of the neck.

*Branches of the internal carotid artery

The carotid body

The anterior triangle of the neck has an interesting bit of tissue called the *carotid body*. You can find it near the bifurcation of the common carotid artery (the place where it splits into the internal and external carotid arteries). Near the bifurcation of the common carotid artery is also a small dilation (widened area) of the internal carotid artery, called the *carotid sinus* (which you can see in Figure 14-3). The carotid sinus has baroreceptors that detect changes in blood pressure. When they're stimulated, they cause a slowing of heart rate and a decrease in blood pressure. The carotid sinus is innervated by cranial nerves IX and X.

The carotid body is a *chemoreceptor,* which is a sensory receptor that monitors chemical changes in the blood. The carotid body monitors the amounts of oxygen and carbon dioxide in the blood, and when the amount of oxygen starts to get too low, it triggers a response that changes your heart rate and breathing rate. It's innervated by cranial nerves IX and X.

Neck Deep: Diving into the Deep Structures

Underneath the superficial triangles lurk the deep structures of the neck. More muscles are located in the deep structures, which makes sense if you think about all the different directions you can move your neck. You also find more blood vessels and nerves. We cover all the bits and pieces of the deep structures in this section.

Flexing the neck: The prevertebral muscles

The seven *cervical vertebrae* form the bony framework of the neck (we cover their anatomy along with the rest of the spine in Chapter 15). The cervical vertebrae have a lot of joints that allow for movement in several directions, so lots of corresponding muscles help move the neck. The muscles that flex the neck are located anterior and lateral to the cervical vertebrae. The muscles that extend and rotate the neck are located posterior to the vertebrae and work like the intrinsic muscles of the back, so they're covered in Chapter 15.

Prevertebral muscles run in front of the cervical vertebrae, and they contract generally to flex the neck and bow the head. You can see them in Figure 14-4:

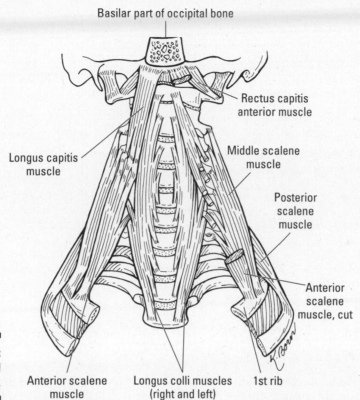

Basilar part of occipital bone

Rectus capitis anterior muscle

Longus capitis muscle

Middle scalene muscle

Posterior scalene muscle

Anterior scalene muscle, cut

Figure 14-4:
Prevertebral muscles.

Anterior scalene muscle

Longus colli muscles (right and left)

1st rib

✔ *Longus capitis:* This muscle originates on the occipital bone at the base of the skull and inserts onto the transverse processes (slender lateral projections) of the 3rd, 4th, 5th, and 6th cervical vertebrae.

✔ *Longus colli:* This muscle originates on the anterior bodies of the top three cervical vertebrae and the transverse processes of the 3rd, 4th, 5th, and 6th cervical vertebrae. It inserts onto the bodies of the 5th, 6th, and 7th cervical vertebrae and the 1st, 2nd, and 3rd thoracic vertebrae and the transverse processes of the 3rd, 4th, and 5th cervical vertebrae.

✔ *Rectus capitis anterior:* This muscle originates on the base of the cranium and inserts onto the anterior surface of the 1st cervical vertebra.

✔ *Anterior scalene:* This muscle originates on the transverse processes of the 3rd, 4th, 5th, and 6th cervical vertebrae and inserts onto the 1st rib.

The *lateral prevertebral muscles* run more along the sides of the neck. They generally work to laterally flex the neck (tilt your head to one side). You can see some of them in Figure 14-4, too:

- ✓ *Splenius capitis:* This muscle originates on the spinous processes (bumps you can feel on the midline of the back) of the 1st, 2nd, 3rd, 4th, 5th, and 6th thoracic vertebrae and on the nuchal ligament (see Chapter 15). It inserts onto the mastoid process of the temporal bone.

- ✓ *Rectus capitis lateralis:* Originating on the occipital bone, this muscle inserts onto the transverse processes of the 1st cervical vertebra.

- ✓ *Middle scalene:* This muscle originates on the transverse processes of the 4th, 5th, 6th, and 7th cervical vertebrae and inserts onto the 1st rib.

- ✓ *Posterior scalene:* This muscle originates on the transverse processes of the 4th, 5th, and 6th cervical vertebrae and inserts onto the 2nd rib.

Rooting around the root of the neck

The *root* of the neck is the area where the neck attaches to the thorax (the part of the trunk between the neck and the abdomen, including the chest). It's home to several important nerves and blood vessels that pass between the head, neck, thorax, and upper extremities.

Nerves

Quite a few nerves reside in the root of the neck:

- ✓ *Vagus nerves:* These cranial nerves (see Chapter 12) travel in the carotid sheath with the internal jugular vein and common carotid arteries before moving into the thorax.

- ✓ *Phrenic nerves:* These nerves arise from the 3rd, 4th, and 5th cervical nerves and descend into the thorax to innervate the diaphragm (see Chapter 7).

- ✓ *Cervical portion of the sympathetic trunks:* These trunks are located to the front and sides of the cervical vertebrae. They contain the *superior, middle,* and *inferior cervical sympathetic ganglia* (nerve clusters; see Chapter 3 for more info on ganglia).

  - The *superior cervical ganglion* is at the level of the 1st or 2nd cervical vertebrae. It contributes fibers to the *internal carotid plexus.* Some fibers form the *superior cervical cardiac nerve* that runs to the heart.

  - The *middle cervical ganglion* is located near the thyroid artery at the level of the 6th cervical vertebra. It has fibers that serve the heart through the *middle cervical cardiac nerve* and *periarterial plexuses* that serve the thyroid.

  - The *stellate ganglion* (or *cervicothoracic ganglion*) is formed from the inferior cervical ganglion fusing with the 1st thoracic ganglion. It's located near the 7th cervical vertebra. Some of the nerve fibers of the stellate ganglion form the *inferior cervical cardiac nerve,* which services the heart.

Blood vessels

Here are the main arteries in the root of the neck:

✔ *Brachiocephalic trunk:* This artery branches off the arch of the aorta (see Chapter 8) just behind the manubrium. It moves to the right and divides into the right common carotid and right subclavian arteries.

✔ *Right* and *left subclavian arteries:* The right subclavian branches off the brachiocephalic trunk, and the left subclavian starts from the arch of the aorta. Both arteries have several branches:

   • The *vertebral artery* runs through the *foramina* (openings) of the transverse processes of the first six cervical vertebrae. (See Chapter 15 for details on the vertebrae.)

   • The *internal thoracic artery* runs into the thorax.

   • The *thyrocervical trunk* has several branches: the *suprascapular artery,* which supplies blood to the muscles on the back of the scapula (see Chapter 16), and the *cervicodorsal trunk,* which branches off into the *dorsal scapular* and *superficial cervical arteries* (sometimes the dorsal scapular artery branches off the subclavian artery). The *dorsal scapular artery* supplies the levator scapulae and rhomboid muscles of the upper back. The *inferior thyroid artery* also stems from the thyrocervical trunk. It supplies blood to the thyroid and parathyroid glands and the larynx, plus it sends blood to muscles of the neck.

   • The *costocervical trunk* gives rise to *superior intercostal* and *deep cervical arteries.*

Veins accompany the arteries in the root of the neck. They return blood to the heart from the head (you can see some of these veins in Figure 14-5):

✔ *External jugular vein:* This vein drains blood from the scalp and face and empties into the subclavian vein lateral to the internal jugular vein.

✔ *Anterior jugular vein:* This vein drains blood from superficial submandibular veins and drains to the external jugular vein or the subclavian vein.

✔ *Left* and *right anterior jugular veins:* These two veins join to form the *jugular venous arch.*

✔ *Subclavian vein:* This vein begins near the 1st rib and joins the internal jugular vein in the anterior cervical triangle where it forms the *brachiocephalic vein.* This area is called the *venous angle.*

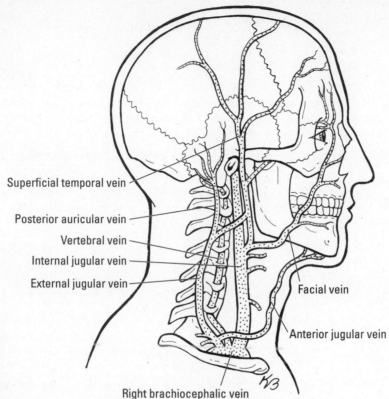

Superficial temporal vein

Posterior auricular vein

Vertebral vein

Internal jugular vein

External jugular vein

Facial vein

Anterior jugular vein

Right brachiocephalic vein

Figure 14-5:
Some veins
of the neck.

Homing In on the Neck Organs

Several organs are found in the neck. We start in this section by discussing the thyroid and parathyroid glands, and then we move on to the organs that help you breathe and talk.

Front and center: Thyroid and parathyroid glands

The thyroid gland is located in the anterior portion of the neck, in front of the trachea's 2nd, 3rd, and 4th C-shaped cartilaginous pieces and below the larynx (more about them in the next section). It's made up of two *lobes,* left and right, that are connected by an *isthmus* and covered by a fibrous capsule and then by a fascial capsule.

The thyroid gland helps regulate metabolism (the chemical reactions that convert food into energy) by producing two hormones called *thyroxine* and *triiodothyronine*. It also produces thyrocalcitonin, which helps regulate the levels of calcium in your blood.

The thyroid gets its blood supply from the superior and inferior thyroid arteries. Its nerve supply comes from the superior, middle, and inferior cervical sympathetic ganglia. Lymphatic fluid from the thyroid drains into the deep cervical lymph nodes (discussed in the upcoming section "Locating lymphatic vessels and nodes").

Four *parathyroid glands* are nestled behind the thyroid gland (two on each side) and are covered with the same fascial capsule as the thyroid. The top two *superior parathyroid glands* are located at the level of the bottom of the cricoid cartilage. The *inferior parathyroid glands* are near the bottom of each thyroid lobe.

Parathyroid anatomy is unpredictable. Although having four parathyroid glands is common, the number can vary from two to six or even more. Even the location of the glands is variable. Although they're usually located behind the thyroid, they can be in the lower regions of the neck and even the thorax.

Parathyroid glands produce *parathyroid hormone* that stimulates the breaking down of bone to increase calcium levels in the blood. It also helps you absorb more calcium from the foods you eat.

The parathyroid arteries typically branch from the inferior thyroid artery. However, the superior parathyroid glands may also be supplied by branches of the superior thyroid artery. The parathyroid veins drain into the thyroid veins. Lymph flows to the deep cervical and paratracheal nodes.

Speaking of the pharynx, larynx, and trachea

The pharynx, larynx, and trachea all help you breathe and speak. We cover these structures in the following sections. The esophagus travels through the neck (from the oropharynx) on its way to the thorax and into your abdomen. We include it in our discussion of the abdominal organs in Chapter 10.

The pharynx

The pharynx is the region posterior to the nasal cavity, oral cavity, and larynx that extends from the base of the skull inferiorly until it becomes continuous with the esophagus.

The pharyngeal muscles include an external layer: the *superior, middle,* and *inferior constrictor muscles.* They constrict the pharynx to force food toward the esophagus when swallowing. Under this layer lies another layer of muscles: the *palatopharyngeus, stylopharyngeus,* and *salpingopharyngeus.* They elevate the larynx and shorten the pharynx when you speak and when you swallow.

The pharynx is divided into three regions: the nasopharynx (behind the nasal cavity), the oropharynx (behind the mouth), and the laryngopharynx, which leads to the trachea (see Figure 14-6 for some parts of the pharynx):

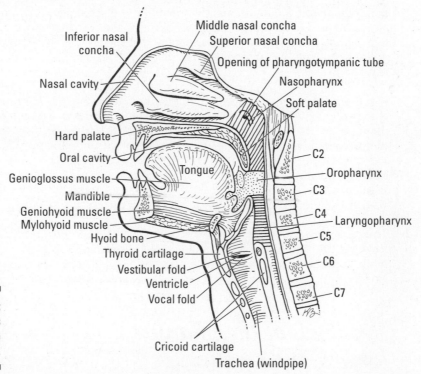

Figure 14-6:
Some parts
of the
pharynx.

✔ **Nasopharynx:** The nose opens into the *nasopharynx* via openings called *choanae.* It contains *pharyngeal tonsils,* which are collections of lymphoid tissue. The auditory tube, or *pharyngotympanic tube* (see Chapter 13), opens into the nasopharynx. It's accompanied by the *salpingopharyngeal fold,* which is a fold of mucous membrane.

✔ **Oropharynx:** The *oropharynx* begins where the oral cavity ends. The base of the tongue forms the floor, and the *palatoglossal* and *palatopharyngeal arches* form the lateral walls. The palatoglossal arch is a fold of mucosa that runs from the soft palate to the tongue. The palatopharyngeal arch is a fold of mucosa posterior to the palatoglossal arch that attaches from the soft palate to the pharyngeal wall. *Palatine tonsils* are found in the *tonsilar sinuses* between the arches. The soft palate (see Chapter 12) forms the roof.

✔ **Laryngopharynx:** The *laryngopharynx* lies behind the larynx (coming up next in this chapter). Its walls are formed by the thyroid cartilage and the middle and inferior pharyngeal constrictor muscles. The *piriform fossa* is a depression in the mucous membrane on each side of the inlet.

Blood flow to the pharynx is supplied by the tonsillar artery and branches of the maxillary and lingual arteries (see Chapter 12). The maxillary nerve, glossopharyngeal nerve, and vagus nerve (again, see Chapter 12) provide nerve supply. Lympthatic fluids drain into the deep cervical nodes (which we cover later in "Locating lymphatic vessels and nodes").

The larynx (voice box)

The larynx, commonly called the voice box, is the organ that contains the vocal folds (vocal cords) that allow your voice to be heard. It lies at the levels of the 4th, 5th, and 6th cervical vertebrae. In the following sections, we discuss ligaments and membranes, the vocal folds, and the muscles, blood vessels, and nerves of the larynx.

Ligaments and membranes

The framework of the larynx is made up of cartilage held together by membranes and ligaments. You can see these structures in Figure 14-7:

✔ **Thyroid cartilage:** The *thyroid cartilage* is the largest structure in the larynx. It is made up of two pieces of hyaline cartilage (see Chapter 3) that meet in the front and middle to form the *laryngeal prominence,* or Adam's apple. The posterior portion of the cartilage forms two horns, the *superior horn* and the *inferior horn.*

✔ **Cricoid cartilage:** The *cricoid cartilage* is ring shaped and is the only complete ring in the entire airway. The posterior portion is taller than the anterior part of the ring. It sits below the thyroid cartilage.

✔ **Arytenoid cartilages:** Two *arytenoid cartilages* are small, pyramid-shaped cartilages that sit atop the cricoid cartilage at the back of the larynx. Each has the following parts:

   • An *apex* that articulates with (joins with) the corniculate cartilage

   • A *base* that articulates with the cricoid cartilage

   • A *vocal process* attached to the vocal ligament

   • A *muscular process* that attaches to the *posterior* and *lateral cricoarytenoid muscles*

A. Lateral view

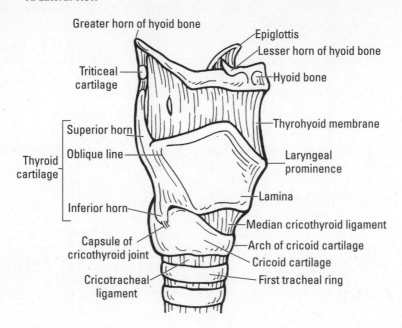

Greater horn of hyoid bone

Epiglottis

Lesser horn of hyoid bone

Triticeal cartilage

Hyoid bone

Thyrohyoid membrane

Superior horn

Oblique line

Laryngeal prominence

Thyroid cartilage

Inferior horn

Lamina

Median cricothyroid ligament

Capsule of cricothyroid joint

Arch of cricoid cartilage

Cricoid cartilage

Cricotracheal ligament

First tracheal ring

B. Posterior view

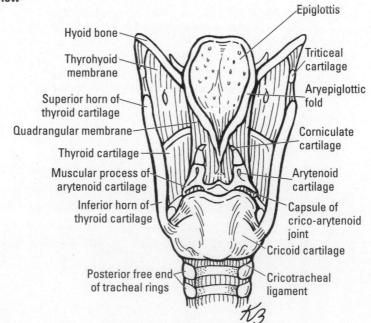

Epiglottis

Hyoid bone

Thyrohyoid membrane

Triticeal cartilage

Superior horn of thyroid cartilage

Aryepiglottic fold

Quadrangular membrane

Corniculate cartilage

Thyroid cartilage

Muscular process of arytenoid cartilage

Arytenoid cartilage

Inferior horn of thyroid cartilage

Capsule of crico-arytenoid joint

Cricoid cartilage

Posterior free end of tracheal rings

Cricotracheal ligament

Figure 14-7: The larynx and associated ligaments and membranes.

- **Corniculate cartilages:** Two small *corniculate cartilages* articulate with the arytenoid cartilage, and two small *cuneiform cartilages* are found in the *aryepiglottic folds.*

- **Epiglottis:** The *epiglottis* is a piece of elastic cartilage (see Chapter 3) covered with a mucous membrane. It's found behind the tongue, and it attaches to the back of the thyroid cartilage.

- **Thyrohyoid membrane:** The *thyrohyoid membrane* connects the thyroid cartilage to the hyoid bone. Part of it thickens to form the *thyrohyoid ligament.*

- **Cricotracheal ligament:** The *cricotracheal ligament* runs between the cricoid cartilage and the first ring of the trachea (see the later section "The trachea").

- **Quadrangular membrane:** The *quadrangular membrane* runs between the epiglottis and the arytenoid cartilages. Part of the inferior free edge forms the *vestibular ligament,* which is part of the *vestibular folds.*

- **Median cricothyroid ligament:** The *median cricothyroid ligament* attach the cricoid cartilage to the thyroid cartilage.

An emergency airway puncture involves placing a hollow needle into the throat of a person who is choking and for whom other methods to assist with breathing have failed. It's technical name is *cricothyrotomy,* and it's performed on the median cricothyroid ligament.

The cavity of the larynx includes the *vestibule* between the inlet and the vestibular folds, the *middle region* between the vestibular folds and vocal folds, and the *lower region* between the vocal folds and the cricoid cartilage.

Vocal folds (vocal cords)

The vocal folds (or vocal cords) produce the sounds you make when talking, singing, or shouting. Each fold is made up of a *vocal ligament* and *vocalis muscles.*

Vocal folds produce the tones that come from the larynx. The gap between them is called the *rima glottidis.*

The shape of the rima glottidis changes depending on what the vocal folds are doing. The rima is narrow during normal breathing, but it's much wider during forced respiration. When you speak, the folds are close together and form a slit.

Men tend to have deeper voices due to longer vocal folds.

Muscles, blood vessels, and nerves of the larynx

In the larynx, the *oblique arytenoid muscles* narrow the laryngeal inlet, and *thyroepiglottic muscles* widen it. They both also move the vocal folds, along with the *cricothyroid muscles, thyroarytenoid, lateral cricothyroid, posterior cricothyroid,* and *transverse arytenoid muscles.*

All of the intrinsic muscles of the larynx except the cricothyroid are innervated by the recurrent laryngeal nerve (via the inferior laryngeal nerve). The cricothyroid muscle is innervated by the external laryngeal nerve, a branch of the superior laryngeal branch of the vagus nerve. The internal laryngeal nerve, a branch of the superior laryngeal branch of the vagus nerve, provides sensory innervation to the larynx above the vocal cords. Sensory innervation inferior to the vocal cord comes from the inferior laryngeal nerve.

Blood supply to the larynx is from the superior thyroid artery and the inferior thyroid artery.

The trachea

The *trachea,* a fibrocartilaginous tube, runs from the larynx into the thorax, where it splits into the right and left main bronchi. (The bronchi are discussed in Chapter 8, and you can turn to Chapter 3 to find out about fibrocartilage.) The trachea tube is made up of *tracheal rings,* but the rings aren't complete; they're C-shaped with the open edges up against the esophagus. That gap is covered by the *trachealis muscle.*

Locating lymphatic vessels and nodes

Most of the superficial parts of the neck drain lymphatic fluid into the *superficial cervical lymph nodes* that run alongside the external jugular vein. From there, the lymph moves into the *inferior cervical lymph nodes. Deep cervical lymph nodes, jugulo-omohyoid nodes,* and *jugulodigastric nodes* run with the internal jugular vein. The *infrahyoid node* is located near the hyoid bone. Lymphatic vessels from the deep cervical nodes come together to form the *jugular lymphatic trunks* that drain into the thoracic duct and the right lymphatic duct (see Chapter 8).

Surrounding the Neck: Skin and Surface Anatomy

The neck is covered by the *subcutaneous tissue of the neck,* or superficial fascia, just under the skin. It has nerves, blood vessels, lymphatic vessels, lymph nodes, and fat. A large, thin muscle called the *platysma* covers the front of the neck just underneath this fascia.

The deep cervical fascia includes three layers, which allow the organs, muscles, and deep lymph nodes to move and slide against each other when you breathe or swallow:

- ✔ *Investing layer:* This most superficial layer of cervical fascia surrounds the entire neck. It also covers the trapezius and sternocleidomastoid muscles.

- ✔ *Pretracheal layer:* This thin layer is attached to the upper part of the neck and to the laryngeal cartilage. It covers the thyroid and parathyroid glands and infrahyoid muscles.

- ✔ *Prevertebral layer:* Another thick layer of fascia, this layer passes behind the pharynx and esophagus but in front of the vertebral column and prevertebral muscles.

You can see the trachea, hyoid bone, and thyroid gland located beneath the skin. The Adam's apple (thyroid cartilage) may be visible, especially in males, and is easy to palpate (examine by touch).

You can locate the thyroid cartilage with your fingertips fairly easily. If you then move your fingers downward, you can locate the thyroid gland and the tracheal rings below that. Asking the patient to swallow as you palpate may make locating the thyroid gland a little bit easier because it moves upward when swallowing.

If you move your fingers laterally from the thyroid out toward the sternocleidomastoid muscle, you can feel the pulsations of the carotid artery.

Chapter 15

Back to Back

*B*ack pain (especially lower-back pain) is a common reason for people to seek medical care. Back pain can be caused by too much leaf raking or snow shoveling or by traumatic injuries, but sometimes back pain is a symptom of a serious disorder. Several sources of pain are possible, including muscle strains, ligament sprains, nerve-root impingement (pressure on the nerve root), joint arthritis, and other disorders of the bones and meninges (coverings of the spinal cord).

In this chapter, we examine the anatomy of the back, including the typical and not-so-typical vertebrae, the muscles that move and support (and occasionally ache), the spinal cord and its nerve roots, and the tissues that provide blood flow and lymphatic drainage. The vertebrae of all sections of the spine are commonly described together, so we include the spinal portion of the neck in this chapter as well, and we show you how to assess the surface anatomy of the back.

Stacking Up the Vertebral Column

The spine is made up of bones called *vertebrae,* so the spine is more properly referred to as the *vertebral column.* The vertebral column keeps your body upright but also offers the flexibility to move around. In addition, your vertebral column houses and protects the spinal cord, but it has openings to allow spinal nerve roots through.

As you find out in the following sections, some general characteristics are shared by all vertebrae, but we also have a few atypical vertebrae to explore. You also get the scoop on the joints along the vertebral column.

Analyzing a typical vertebra

Most vertebrae are more or less the same, although they have a few differences of sizes and shapes. (The cervical region has two atypical vertebrae that defy the norm, and we discuss them in the later section "Cervical, thoracic, and lumbar vertebrae.")

A typical vertebra is made up of an anterior vertebral body and a posterior vertebral arch.

- ✔ **Vertebral body:** The vertebral body is fairly large, especially in a *lumbar* vertebra (in other words, a vertebra found in the lower back; see "Putting the vertebrae into groups" for more about this area of the vertebral column). The vertebral bodies support the weight of your body.

- ✔ **Vertebral arch:** The vertebral arch is made up of two *pedicles* (one on each side of the vertebra) that project posteriorly from the vertebral body. Posteriorly, each pedicle is attached to a *lamina,* and the two laminae merge together in the midline forming the arch. The vertebral arch and body form the vertebral foramen.

In the following sections, we discuss the bony projections of the vertebral arch and the various openings that allow nerves and blood vessels through.

Bony processes

A typical vertebral arch has seven bony *processes* (projections of bone that stick out from the arch): one *spinous process,* two *transverse processes,* and four *articular processes.*

- ✔ **Spinous** and **transverse processes:** These processes work as levers and serve as attachment sites for back muscles (we talk about these muscles later in this chapter).

  - Each spinous process projects posteriorly from the point where the laminae merge on the vertebral arch.

  - The transverse processes project laterally from the pedicle/lamina junctions.

The spinous processes are easy to find — right down the center of the back. You can usually see them, or at least you can *palpate* (medically examine by touch) them because very little fat accumulates over the vertebral column.

- ✔ **Articular processes:** These processes form joints between successive vertebrae. The superior and inferior articular processes arise from the same junctions as the transverse processes (one superior and one inferior process on each side), and each process has an articular surface called a *facet.* The inferior processes of each typical vertebra form synovial joints (see Chapter 4) called *zygapophysial joints,* with the superior processes of the vertebra below.

Whew! Who knew that one bone could have so many parts?

Openings for nerves and blood vessels

The opening formed between the vertebral body and the vertebral arch is called the *vertebral foramen,* which forms the *vertebral canal* when all the vertebrae are stacked on top of each other. This canal is home to the spinal cord, which we discuss later in "Spying on the spinal cord and nerves."

The pedicles of a vertebral arch have notches on their superior and inferior surfaces. These notches combine with the notches of the pedicles on adjacent vertebrae to form the *intervertebral foramina,* the openings between the vertebrae where the blood vessels and spinal nerves pass to and from the spinal cord and the vertebral column. (We talk about the blood vessels and spinal nerves in more detail later in this chapter.)

Spina bifida is a congenital birth defect in which the vertebral arch doesn't develop properly, leaving an opening posterior to the spinal cord. A mild form, called *spina bifida occulta,* is hidden under the skin (but may present with a small tuft of hair over the surface) and usually has no symptoms. *Spina bifida cystica* is more severe, causing a visible herniation of the meninges protruding from the infant's back. Getting an adequate intake of folate (a B vitamin) or folic acid supplements before and during pregnancy can reduce the risk of the disorder.

Putting the vertebrae into groups

The vertebral column consists of 33 vertebrae located in five regions: 7 cervical, 12 thoracic, 5 lumbar, 5 sacral, and 4 coccygeal. Each region has unique characteristics.

Fractures of the vertebrae are often due to forceful compression and/or flexion as a result of a traumatic accident such as a bad car accident. Diving into a shallow pool or lake can result in a compression fracture when the diver hits his or her head on the pool floor or lake bottom.

Cervical, thoracic, and lumbar vertebrae

The first three regions of the vertebral column are shown in Figure 15-1. The seven *cervical vertebrae* (C1–C7) are found in the posterior region of the neck and include two atypical and five typical vertebra. Twelve *thoracic vertebrae* (T1–T12) form the most posterior part of the thoracic cage, and five *lumbar vertebrae* (L1–L5) form the lower back:

  ✔ **Atypical cervical vertebrae (C1–C2):** These vertebrae are also called the *atlas* (C1) and the *axis* (C2).

- The atlas doesn't have a vertebral body or a spinous process; it has two *lateral masses* connected by a *posterior arch* and an *anterior arch.* The superior portion of each lateral mass has an articular surface that *articulates* (forms a joint) with the skull and a similar surface inferiorly that articulates with the axis.

- The axis has a superiorly pointing projection called *the odontoid process* (or sometimes called the *dens*). The atlas pivots around the odontoid process.

✔ **Typical cervical vertebrae (C3–C7):** These vertebrae have bodies that are smaller than the other types, and the vertebral foramina are large and triangular in shape. The spinous processes are shorter and *bifid* (split into two projections) on the 3rd, 4th, and 5th vertebrae. The superior facets face upward and backward, and the inferior facets face downward and forward. Each transverse process includes a *foramen transversarium,* which allows passage of the vertebral artery and vein.

✔ **Thoracic vertebrae (T1–T12):** These 12 vertebrae have medium-sized bodies that are heart shaped with small vertebral foramina (see Figure 15-2). The spinous processes are quite long; in fact, some slope inferiorly to the level of the vertebra below. Most thoracic vertebrae have *costal facets* on the transverse processes that articulate with the ribs (see Chapter 7), with the exception of T11 and T12, which don't have those facets. The superior facets face backward but more laterally than the cervical vertebrae. The inferior facets face forward and medially.

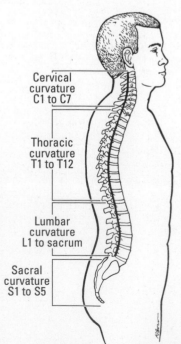

Figure 15-1:
Most vertebrae are grouped into three regions: cervical, thoracic, and lumbar.

Cervical curvature C1 to C7

Thoracic curvature T1 to T12

Lumbar curvature L1 to sacrum

Sacral curvature S1 to S5

A. Superior view

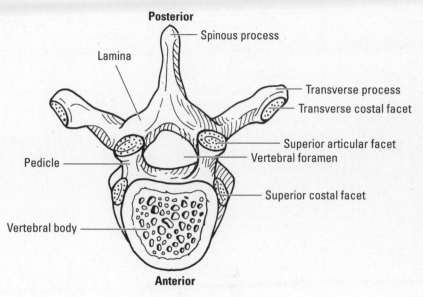

Posterior

Spinous process

Lamina

Transverse process

Transverse costal facet

Superior articular facet

Vertebral foramen

Pedicle

Superior costal facet

Vertebral body

Anterior

B. Lateral view

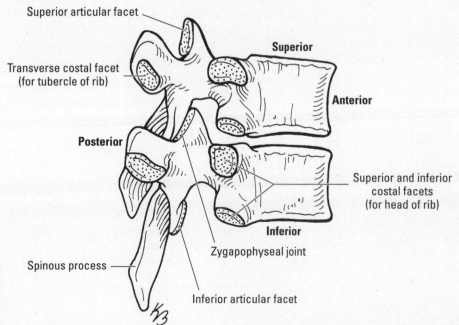

Superior articular facet

Superior

Anterior

Transverse costal facet
(for tubercle of rib)

Superior and inferior
costal facets
(for head of rib)

Posterior

Inferior

Spinous process

Zygapophyseal joint

Inferior articular facet

Figure 15-2:
The thoracic
vertebrae.

✔ **Lumbar vertebrae (L1–L5):** These vertebrae are large and have kidney-shaped bodies with short, rectangular spinous processes. The transverse processes are long and slender. The superior facets face medially, and the inferior facets face laterally.

The sacrum and the coccyx

Five partial vertebrae (S1–S5) in the sacral region fuse to form the wedge-shaped *sacrum* (refer to Figure 15-1). The broad superior surface serves as a base of the vertebral column. The narrow inferior surface of the sacrum forms a joint with the coccyx. What's that, you ask? The *coccyx,* or tailbone, hangs inferiorly from the sacrum. It's formed from the fusion (or partial fusion) of three to five small vertebrae.

The *median sacral crest* is formed by the fused spinous processes and is palpable under the skin. The *sacral canal* is formed from the vertebral foramina of the sacral segments and contains the sacral and coccygeal spinal roots.

Connecting with the vertebral joints

The joints of the vertebral column include the joints between the bodies of adjacent vertebrae and joints between the adjacent vertebral arches. Two types of joints in the neck are given special attention because they're different from other joints: the *atlanto-occipital joints* and the *atlanto-axial joints* in the upper cervical region. These joints between the first two cervical vertebrae and the cranium permit a greater degree of movement than the rest of the vertebral column. The vertebrae also articulate (form a joint) with the ribs (in Chapter 7) and the hip bones (in Chapter 19).

Getting old isn't easy, and your bones may not help. Aging or injuries may result in the growth of *osteophytes* (also called bone spurs), which are bony projections that occur in the joint spaces. These growths result in osteoarthritis, a disease that can cause pain and loss of mobility of the vertebral joints.

Atlanto-occipital joints: Joining the head and the atlas

Atlanto-occipital joints are synovial joints (moveable joints surrounded by a joint capsule; flip to Chapter 3) located between the occipital condyles (see Chapter 12) and the superior articular surfaces of the lateral masses of the atlas (which we describe in the earlier section "Cervical, thoracic, and lumbar vertebrae"). You have two atlanto-occipital joints, which allow you to nod your head. They're held in place by the *anterior and posterior atlanto-occipital membranes,* which help prevent excessive movement of the joints.

Atlanto-axial joints: Joining the atlas and axis

The three atlanto-axial joints are also synovial joints. One is found between the dens (odontoid process) of the axis (2nd cervical vertebra) and the anterior arch of the atlas (1st cervical vertebra), and two are located between the lateral masses of the 1st cervical vertebra and the superior articular facets of the 2nd cervical vertebra.

The following four ligaments stabilize these joints:

- *Apical ligament:* Connects the dens (odontoid process) to the foramen magnum of the occipital bone (see Chapter 12 for information on the skull)

- *Alar ligaments:* Connect the dens (odontoid process) to the lateral margins of the foramen magnum

- *Cruciate ligament:* Attaches the dens (odontoid process) to the anterior arch of the atlas and the body of the axis to the foramen magnum of the occipital bone

- *Tectorial membrane:* Starts at the skull and becomes the posterior longitudinal ligament (you find out more about the posterior longitudinal ligament in the next section)

Intervertebral joints: Joining other vertebrae to each other

Intervertebral joints, which connect adjacent vertebrae, include both synovial and cartilaginous joints.

- *Intervertebral synovial joints:* These joints are found between the superior and inferior facets of adjoining vertebral arches. They are supported by the following ligaments:

  - The *interspinous ligament* runs between the spinous processes.

  - The *supraspinous ligament* connects the tips of the spinous processes and forms the strong *nuchal ligament* that runs posterior to the cervical spine.

  - *Intertransverse ligaments* connect the adjacent transverse processes, and the *ligamentum flavum* connects the laminae of adjoining vertebrae.

- *Intervertebral cartilaginous joints:* A fibrocartilaginous joint is formed between the adjacent vertebral bodies with *fibrocartilaginous intervertebral discs* located between the bodies. Each disc is made up of a gelatinous mass, the *nucleus pulposus,* which is surrounded by the *annulus fibrosus* (which is made up of tough fibrous layers).

  - *Anterior* and *posterior longitudinal ligaments* run in bands down the anterior and posterior surfaces of the vertebral bodies from the skull to the sacrum. They help to stabilize the vertebral column.

Disc herniations, or slipped discs, occur when the nucleus pulposus penetrates into or through the annulus fibrosus. The herniations cause back and limb pain because the bulging disc puts pressure on the nerve roots.

Cervical sprains and strains, also called *whiplash injuries,* may damage the ligaments and intervertebral discs along with the muscles of the neck and upper back.

Sacral joints

The sacrum articulates with the hip bones (see Chapter 19) to form the *sacroiliac joints.* The superior surface of the sacrum has two superior facets that articulate with the inferior articular processes of the 5th lumbar vertebra.

The sacrococcygeal joint is formed between the coccyx and the sacrum. It has an intervertebral disc and is stabilized by *sacrococcygeal ligaments.*

Studying the Spinal Cord and Meninges

The spinal cord serves as an information pathway between your brain and the peripheral nerves that serve the rest of your body. It's quite delicate and requires a lot of protection. Your spinal cord has three coverings and is sheltered in the vertebral column.

Spying on the spinal cord and nerves

The vertebral canal (see the earlier section "Analyzing a typical vertebra") is home to the spinal cord, which extends from the brainstem down into the lumbar portion of the vertebral column. It begins as an extension of the medulla oblongata (see Chapter 12) and runs inferiorly to around the 1st or 2nd lumbar vertebra, where it terminates as the *conus medullaris.*

The spinal cord has two enlarged areas, the cervical enlargement and the lumbosacral enlargement:

- The *cervical enlargement* gives rise to the spinal nerves that exit this portion of the cord and form the *brachial plexus,* which innervates the upper extremities (see Chapters 16, 17, and 18).

- The *lumbosacral enlargement* includes spinal nerves that form the *lumbar and sacral plexuses,* which innervate the lower extremities (see Chapters 19, 20, and 21).

Speaking of spinal nerves: You have 31 pairs of spinal nerves that leave the spinal cord to innervate various structures throughout the body. They're categorized by regions: 8 cervical, 12 thoracic, 5 lumbar, 5 sacral, and 1 coccygeal. (We discuss these regions of the vertebral column in the earlier section "Putting the vertebrae into groups.")

Each spinal nerve is formed from the convergence of _posterior_ and _anterior nerve roots._ The cell bodies of the anterior nerve roots are located in the _anterior horns of gray matter_ in the spinal cord, and the cell bodies of posterior nerve roots are located as a mass of cell bodies called the _spinal ganglia_ (posterior root ganglia) outside of the cord. The anterior nerve roots contain motor fibers, and the posterior nerve roots contain sensory fibers (see Chapter 4 for more about the nervous system). The spinal nerve roots merge to form spinal nerves (spinal nerves contain both sensory and motor fibers) where they leave the vertebral canal.

Just past the point where the nerve roots merge, each spinal nerve divides into a _posterior ramus_ and an _anterior ramus._ The posterior ramus innervates the skin and deep back muscles, and the anterior ramus innervates the rest of the trunk and the extremities. The rami (like the spinal nerves) are mixed (contains both sensory and motor fibers). The _recurrent meningeal branch of the spinal nerves_ innervates most of the vertebral column; however, the zyg-apophysial joints are innervated by _the medial branches of the posterior rami._

The spinal cord tapers into a conical-shaped _conus medullaris_ and actually ends around the level of the 2nd lumbar vertebra, so the nerve roots that emerge past that point become quite long because they have to extend down to exit the intervertebral foramens in the remaining lumbar and sacral levels. The collection of those spinal roots resembles a horse's tail, so it's referred to as the _cauda equina._

The spinal nerve roots may be impinged by arthritic osteophytes or by disc herniations. Pressure on the posterior nerve roots causes pain in the back and in any extremity served by the nerve roots being affected. Pressure on anterior nerve roots results in motor weakness. A patient with nerve-root impingement of one of the lumbar spinal nerve roots due to a herniated disc may feel pain and tingling in the buttock, hip, and leg. Nerve-root impingement in the neck can cause pain and weakness in the arm and forearm.

Coverings and cushions: Understanding the meninges and cerebrospinal fluid

The spinal cord is surrounded by three _meninges_ (membranes) and cerebrospinal fluid. The meninges also cover the brain (see Chapter 12). Together the meninges and cerebrospinal fluid help to protect the spinal cord and the spinal nerve roots (see Figure 15-3). Here are the three meninges:

✔ *Dura mater:* This fibrous, outermost layer of the meninges forms a tough *dural sac* that's separated from the vertebrae by an *extradural space.* The dural sac ends at the 2nd sacral vertebra. In fact spinal blocks (type of anesthetic) are given between the 2nd lumbar and the 2nd sacral vertebrae because only the cauda equina is located there, not the spinal cord. Dura mater also covers the nerve roots with *dural root sheaths.*

✔ *Arachnoid mater:* This more-delicate meninx forms the middle layer. It's separated from the dura mater by a thin layer of cells called the *dura-arachnoid interface.*

✔ *Pia mater:* The pia mater is a vascular membrane that covers the spinal cord and is separated from the arachnoid mater by the *subarachnoid space,* which is filled with cerebrospinal fluid. It also covers the nerve roots and spinal blood vessels.

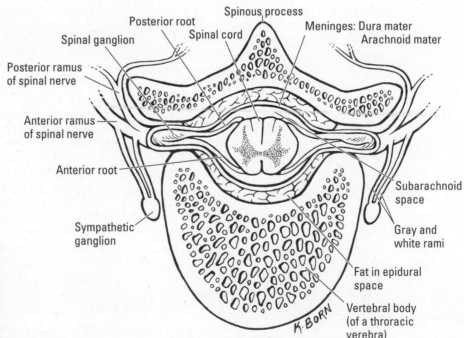

Figure 15-3: The meninges and spinal cord.

The spinal cord is held in place by the *filum terminale,* a slender extension of dural linings that run from the conus medullaris (end of the spinal cord) to the coccyx (tailbone). In addition, 21 pairs of *denticulate* ligaments attach the spinal cord to the arachnoid mater and dura mater. These ligaments are formed from pia mater.

Cerebrospinal fluid is formed mainly by the *choroid plexuses* of the brain (see Chapter 12). It circulates over the brain and down around the spinal cord, where it cushions the spinal cord and removes waste products before it passes into the blood stream.

Flexing Your Back Muscles

Your back requires strong muscles to keep you upright and move those vertebrae (and the rest of you) around. Back muscles are divided into two specific groups, as you find out in the following sections: the extrinsic muscles that are associated with upper extremity and shoulder movement, and the intrinsic muscles that deal with movements of the vertebral column. Several small muscles in the cervical (neck) area of the vertebral column are also important.

Shouldering the load: The extrinsic muscles

Superficial extrinsic muscles connect your upper extremities to the trunk, and they form the V-shaped musculature associated with the middle and upper back. They include the *trapezius, latissimus dorsi, levator scapulae,* and the *rhomboids.* Because their job is to move the upper extremities, we cover them in detail in Chapter 16.

Intermediate extrinsic muscles include the *serratus posterior superior* and *inferior.* Most of their function is involved with respiration (see Chapter 3), and we cover them with the thoracic cage in Chapter 7.

Twisting and turning: The intrinsic muscles

Intrinsic muscles, which stretch all the way from the pelvis to the cranium, help to maintain your posture and move the vertebral column. They're divided into three groups: the superficial layer, the intermediate layer, and the deep layer. The muscles in all of the layers are innervated by the posterior rami of spinal nerves. We discuss all three layers in the following sections.

Injuries of the intrinsic back muscles often occur while using improper lifting technique. You can protect the back muscles by bending from the hip and knee when you lift objects from the ground.

The superficial layer

Thick *splenius* muscles form the superficial layer of muscles and are located on the lateral and posterior portions of the neck. They laterally flex, rotate, and extend your head and neck. Bodies have two kinds of splenius muscles:

- ✔ *Splenius capitis muscles:* These muscles originate from the nuchal ligament and spinous processes of the 7th cervical vertebra and the upper thoracic vertebrae. They run superiorly to the mastoid processes of the temporal bone (see Chapter 12).

- ✔ *Splenius cervicis muscles:* These muscles originate with the splenius capitis but insert onto the transverse processes of the upper cervical vertebrae.

The intermediate layer

The *erector spinae* muscles (also called the *sacrospinalis* muscles) lay on either side of the vertebral column, running from the lumbosacral area superiorly to various places along the ribs and up to the base of the skull (see Figure 15-4). Their job is to extend the vertebral column and maintain the normal curvature (posture) of the vertebral column. The erector spinae muscles, detailed in the following list, all originate from the posterior sacrum, sacroiliac ligaments, sacral and lumbar spinous processes, and iliac crest (see Chapter 19):

- ✔ *Iliocostalis muscles:* These muscles run superiorly where they insert onto the angles of the ribs and the transverse processes of the lower cervical vertebrae.

- ✔ *Longissimus muscles:* These muscles travel superiorly to their insertions on the ribs, the transverse processes of the thoracic and cervical vertebrae, and the mastoid process of the temporal bone.

- ✔ *Spinalis muscles:* These muscles run superiorly to insert on the spinous processes of the upper thoracic vertebrae and to the cranium.

The deep layer

Underneath the intermediate intrinsic back muscles is another layer of muscles that help to support posture and assist the intermediate muscles in moving the spine. The *deep intrinsic muscles* are smaller than the erector spinae muscles, and none of them traverse more than six vertebral segments (refer to Figure 15-4).

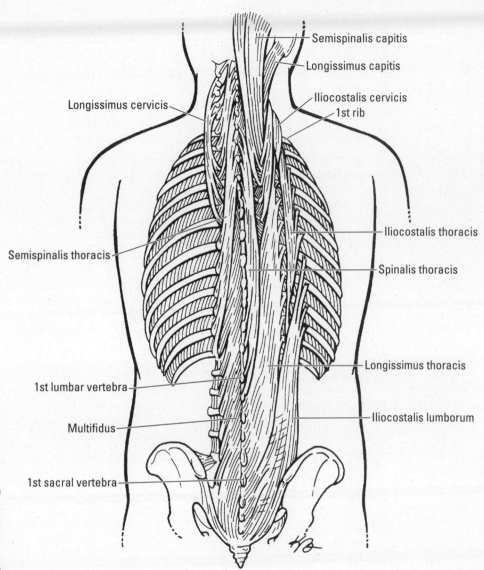

Semispinalis capitis

Longissimus capitis

Iliocostalis cervicis
1st rib

Longissimus cervicis

Iliocostalis thoracis

Semispinalis thoracis

Spinalis thoracis

Longissimus thoracis

1st lumbar vertebra

Iliocostalis lumborum

Multifidus

1st sacral vertebra

Figure 15-4:
Selected
intrinsic
muscles.

✔ *Semispinalis muscles:* This group is the most superficial of the deep intrinsic muscles. These muscles run from the midthoracic spine superiorly through the cervical spine. They have three divisions *(thoracis, cervicis,* and *capitis)* that originate from the transverse processes of the 4th cervical vertebra through the 10th, 11th, or 12th thoracic vertebra. The fibers travel superiorly for about four to six segments each and attach on spinous processes and the occipital bone.

✔ *Multifidus muscles:* These short, triangular muscles originate in various places but always travel superiorly and medially for two to four segments and attach on the spinous processes.

✔ *Rotatores muscles:* The rotatores lie underneath the multifidus muscles. They originate from the transverse processes of a single vertebra and travel superiorly to insert into the spinous process of the vertebra one or two segments superior to it. The rotatores help with rotation and *proprioception* (knowing how your body is positioned).

Even smaller minor deep intrinsic muscles, the *interspinales, intertransversarii,* and the *levatores costarum,* assist in proprioception and movement along the vertebral column.

Nodding your head: The suboccipital muscles

The suboccipital region includes the posterior part of the 2nd cervical vertebra (the axis, in the neck) to the area inferior to the occipital region of the head (see Chapter 12). Four small muscles located on each side of the suboccipital region help with posture and assist with extension and rotation of the head (see Figure 15-5):

✔ *Rectus capitis posterior muscles:* These two muscles insert onto the occipital bone; the *rectus capitis posterior major* originates at the spinous process of the 2nd cervical vertebra (the axis) and the *rectus capitis posterior minor* originates from the posterior arch of the 1st cervical vertebra (the atlas).

✔ *Obliquus muscles:* These two muscles complete the suboccipital quartet. The *obliquus capitis inferior* travels from the spinous process of the 2nd cervical vertebra to the transverse process of the 1st cervical vertebra, and the *obliquus capitis superior* has its origin at the transverse process of the 1st cervical vertebra and inserts onto the occipital bone.

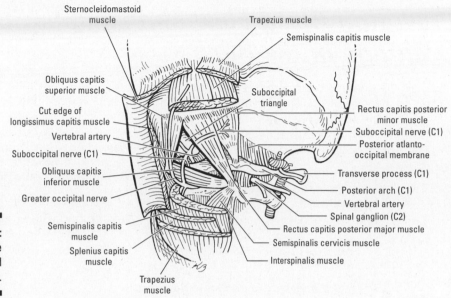

Sternocleidomastoid muscle

Trapezius muscle

Semispinalis capitis muscle

Obliquus capitis superior muscle

Suboccipital triangle

Cut edge of longissimus capitis muscle

Vertebral artery

Suboccipital nerve (C1)

Obliquus capitis inferior muscle

Greater occipital nerve

Rectus capitis posterior minor muscle

Suboccipital nerve (C1)

Posterior atlanto-occipital membrane

Transverse process (C1)

Posterior arch (C1)

Vertebral artery

Spinal ganglion (C2)

Rectus capitis posterior major muscle

Semispinalis cervicis muscle

Interspinalis muscle

Semispinalis capitis muscle

Splenius capitis muscle

Trapezius muscle

Figure 15-5: The suboccipital muscles.

When back pain doesn't come from the back

When you see a patient with back pain, it's probably due to irritation or injury of the soft tissues we cover in this chapter. But sometimes the problem isn't in the back; it's in another area. This phenomenon is called *referred pain,* and it can make the diagnosis a bit confusing. The most common example of referred pain is the ache that is often felt in the left shoulder and arm in a person who is suffering from a heart attack.

The back has its share of referred pain areas. A patient with gallstones may feel the pain just below his or her right scapula (shoulder blade), or someone suffering with a kidney stone may feel pain on either flank. And although men suffering from myocardial infarctions feel pain in the left shoulder, women in the midst of a heart attack may feel only some pain between the scapulae.

When a patient comes in with back pain, no history of injury or overuse, and no indication of arthritic changes, referred pain is a possibility.

Providing Blood Flow and Lymphatic Drainage in the Back

The spinal cord, vertebral column, back muscles, and supporting tissues need to be maintained via blood vessels. Lymphatic vessels serve the area as well.

The spinal cord needs blood to function properly. The arterial supply comes from *anterior* and *posterior spinal arteries* that stem from the vertebral arteries. The veins serving the spinal cord drain into the vertebral venous plexuses that form inside the vertebral canal.

Blood flow to the vertebral column is provided by the following arteries:

✔ Branches of the *vertebral arteries* and *ascending cervical arteries* in the neck

✔ *Posterior intercostal arteries* in the thorax

✔ *Subcostal* and *lumbar arteries* in the abdomen

✔ *Iliolumbar* and the *lateral* and *medial sacral arteries* in the pelvis

Blood is transported away from the vertebral column by the *spinal veins,* which form venous plexuses inside and outside of the vertebral canal. The *intervertebral veins* collect blood from the venous plexuses and empty into the *vertebral veins of the neck* and *segmental veins in the trunk.* The veins of the vertebral plexuses don't have valves, so they can allow the spread of neoplastic (cancerous) cells.

Deep lymphatic vessels follow the spinal veins and drain into the *deep cervical, posterior mediastinal, lateral aortic,* and *sacral nodes* (see Chapters 8, 10, and 14). The superficial lymphatic vessels in the neck drain into the *cervical nodes* (see Chapter 14), lymph in the trunk above the level of the iliac crests drains into the *axillary nodes* (see Chapter 16), and lymph from below the iliac crests drains into *superficial inguinal nodes* (see Chapter 11).

Assessing the Surface Anatomy of the Vertebrae and Back Muscles

Examining the surface anatomy of the back includes inspecting the skin (see Chapter 5), noting the symmetry (or asymmetry) of the back and its muscles, and assessing the curvatures of the spine. Knowing what landmarks to look for can help you locate potential problem areas for patients with back pain.

Looking for curves in the spine

When you examine a patient from behind, the spine should be in a straight vertical line. *Scoliosis* is an abnormal lateral curvature and rotation of the spine. It can be mild and not cause any symptoms at all, or it can be quite severe and painful.

When you look at a standing person from the side, you should see four curves:

✔ The neck (cervical region) and low back (lumbar region) should have curves that are concave posteriorly; in other words, they curve in toward the front of your body.

✔ The mid back (thoracic region) and sacral portion of the spine should have curves that are convex posteriorly; in other words, they curve outward, away from the front of your body.

These curves help to provide flexibility and strength to the spine.

You may see a couple of conditions related to excessive curvature:

✔ *Scoliosis* is an abnormal lateral curvature and rotation of the spine.

✔ *Kyphosis* (dowager's hump, or hunchback) is due to an excessively curved thoracic region of the vertebral column. Osteoporosis (loss of bone density), especially in elderly women, can result in kyphosis.

✔ *Lordosis* is an excessive curve in the lumbar region. It may be caused by disease of the vertebral column or by an increase in weight in the abdominal region. It is common during the later stages of pregnancy.

Scoliosis is usually diagnosed in the tween or early teen years and is more common in girls than in boys. Treatment for scoliosis starts with observation as long as the curve remains below 25–30 degrees. If the curve gets worse, a brace may be used, depending on the age of the person. Severe scoliosis, with a 45 degree curve or higher, may require surgery.

Seeing bones on the back's surface

A bony bump called the *occipital protuberance* is at the midline of the base of the skull, just above the neck. Running directly below the occipital protuberance and down the middle of the neck is the *nuchal groove* that you can feel with your fingers. The *nuchal ligament* covers the palpable spinous processes of the cervical vertebrae in the neck.

The most prominent bump in the midline of the back, near the base of the neck, is usually the spinous process of the 7th cervical vertebra, although for some people it may be the 1st thoracic vertebra. Some, and possibly all, of the spinous processes of the thoracic and lumbar vertebrae are visible when a patient bends forward. The transverse processes aren't visible, but they can be palpated on either side of the spinous processes.

The *iliac crests* of the hip bones (see Chapter 19) should be level while the patient is standing and can be used as landmarks to draw an imaginary horizontal line to locate the level of the 4th lumbar vertebra. Inferior to that line, you may also see two dimples on either side of the sacrum, just over the sacroiliac joints (between the sacrum and the hip bones — find out more in Chapter 19).

The median sacral crest is a vertical bony ridge in the midline of the sacrum. You can palpate the *sacral* hiatus and the tip of the coccyx at the superior part of the *intergluteal cleft* (see Chapter 19).

Viewing the back muscles

In the midline of the back you can see the *posterior median furrow,* which lies over the spinous processes of the vertebral column. The erector spinae muscles run on either side of the furrow. You may be able to see (or at least palpate) them as two bulges on either side of the furrow.

Some of the extrinsic back muscles are visible in the lateral thoracic portions of the back, including the trapezius, rhomboid, and latissimus dorsi muscles that help to attach the upper extremities to the axial skeleton. The trapezius muscles form a diamond-like shape over the upper back, and the latissimus dorsi give the back its V-shape. The positions of the *scapulae* are also visible (see Chapter 16).

Part IV
Moving to the Upper and Lower Extremities

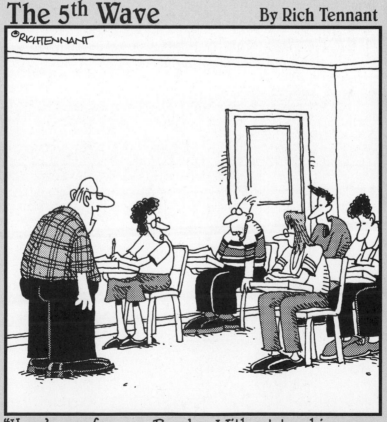

The 5th Wave — By Rich Tennant

"Here's one for you, Bender. Without touching your head, how many bones are there in a numbskull?"

In this part . . .

Your extremities give you movement and the ability to move from place to place. They allow you to walk your dog, drive a car, play a video game, hug your kids, and lift a box. Part IV is all about the upper and lower limbs. We explain the anatomy of the shoulders, arms, and hands and then move on to the hips and thighs, the rest of the leg, and the feet.

Chapter 16

Shouldering the Load: The Pectoral Girdle and the Arm

In This Chapter

▶ Identifying the bones and joints that make up the shoulder

▶ Reviewing the muscles and tissues

▶ Looking for landmarks and locating the structures under the skin

The most proximal part of the upper extremity is the shoulder, or pectoral girdle (remember that a *girdle* is a structure that surrounds something; *pectoral* refers to the chest). Its joints allow for a great amount of movement for the arm that's attached to it. You'll want to know the anatomy of the pectoral girdle in case a patient has sustained a shoulder injury or suffers from a medical disorder like arthritis (a degenerative disease of the joints).

This chapter reviews the anatomy of the pectoral girdle and arm, including the bones and joints, muscles, nerves, and blood vessels.

Boning Up on the Shoulder and the Arm

The bony structures of the shoulder include the pectoral girdle and one arm bone (see Figure 16-1). These bones have some interesting landmarks, including various bumps and projections. The shoulder and arm bones can be broken or dislocated by traumatic injuries, so in the following sections we get you up to speed on their anatomy.

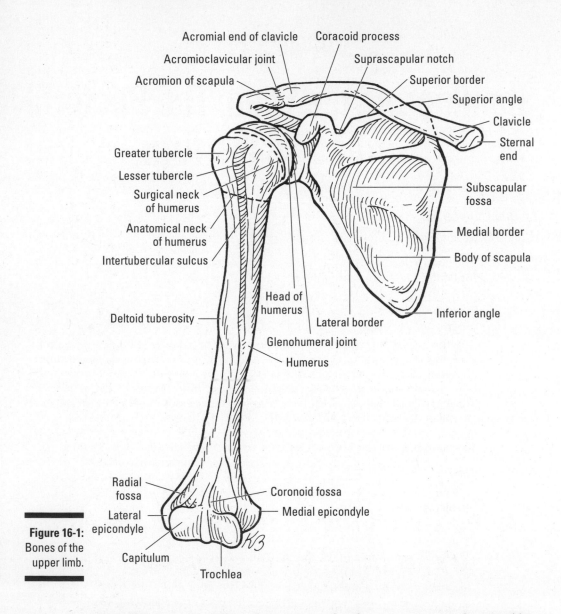

Acromial end of clavicle

Coracoid process

Acromioclavicular joint

Suprascapular notch

Acromion of scapula

Superior border

Superior angle

Clavicle

Sternal end

Greater tubercle

Lesser tubercle

Surgical neck of humerus

Anatomical neck of humerus

Intertubercular sulcus

Subscapular fossa

Medial border

Body of scapula

Head of humerus

Deltoid tuberosity

Lateral border

Inferior angle

Glenohumeral joint

Humerus

Radial fossa

Coronoid fossa

Lateral epicondyle

Medial epicondyle

Figure 16-1: Bones of the upper limb.

Capitulum

Trochlea

Looking at the bones of the pectoral girdle

The two bones of the shoulder, the clavicle and the scapula, comprise the pectoral girdle.

Clavicle: The collarbone

The *clavicle,* or collarbone, lies horizontally at the root of the neck. It's a long, thin bone that curves outward at the middle of your body and curves inward on the end where it goes to the shoulder. It's easy to see and *palpate* (medically examine by touch) in most people (refer to Figure 16-1).

The clavicle articulates (forms a joint) with the manubrium (see Chapter 7) and with the scapula, so it's described as having two ends: the *sternal end,* which attaches to the manubrium, and the *acromial end,* which joins the scapula. You can see these ends in Figure 16-1. The *conoid tubercle* is found on the bottom of the acromial end of the clavicle.

The clavicle is a common site for fractures (in fact, it's the most commonly fractured bone in the body), which usually happens when a person stretches out her hand to prevent a fall. When the hand contacts a hard surface, the force goes through the arm and up into the shoulder to the clavicle. Falling directly on the shoulder may result in a fracture, too.

Scapula: The shoulder blade

The *scapula* is easy to locate on the upper back; it's the large bone that runs on the surface of the 2nd and 7th ribs. It has a flat, triangle-shaped *body.* The anterior surface of the body faces the ribs and has a large subscapular fossa (indentation).

The posterior surface has a horizontal projection near the top called the *spine of the scapula* that ends at the top of the shoulder at the *acromion* (refer to Figure 16-1). The spine divides the posterior surface of the scapula into a *supraspinous fossa* and an *infraspinous fossa.*

The pear-shaped *glenoid cavity* is located at the upper and outer part of the scapula. The *coracoid process* is located just above the glenoid cavity, and it projects forward and upward. You can see the coracoid process in Figure 16-1.

It's not funny, but it's humerus

The arm contains one sturdy bone, the *humerus.* In this chapter, we take a look at the end that attaches to the shoulder. The anatomy of the distal portion (or the part farthest away from its attachment to the body) is presented in Chapter 17, where we discuss the forearm.

The spherical-shaped *head* is at the proximal end of the humerus, which joins the shoulder girdle. Just below the head you find the *anatomic neck,* which is a slightly narrower portion of the bone. *Greater* and *lesser tubercles* are right below the anatomical neck and are separated by the *intertubercular sulcus* (*bicipital groove*). The *shaft,* or the longer middle portion of the humerus, joins the proximal part at the *surgical neck.* The shaft has two important landmarks, the *deltoid tuberosity* and the *spiral groove.*

Joining the Parts

The shoulder and arm bone are joined together by ligaments (see Chapter 3). The joints allow the shoulder to move your arm up and down, in circles, in front, and toward the back. In the following sections, we describe the joints of the pectoral girdle.

Collaring the sternoclavicular joint

The *sternoclavicular joint* is formed by the articulation (joining of two bones) of the sternal end of the clavicle with the manubrium of the sternum (see Chapter 7). It's a strong joint, but it also allows mobility of the pectoral girdle.

The sternoclavicular joint is a synovial joint that has an articular disc (see Chapter 3 for more on the anatomy of joints) and is surrounded by the *joint capsule.* The sternoclavicular joint is held together by a few ligaments:

- ✔ **Anterior** and **posterior sternoclavicular ligaments:** These ligaments reinforce the joint in the front and back.

- ✔ **Interclavicular ligament:** This ligament runs between the sternal ends of the two clavicles across the tops of the joints.

- ✔ **Costoclavicular ligament:** This ligament attaches the bottom of the sternal end of the clavicle to the 1st rib.

Reviewing the acromioclavicular joint

The *acromioclavicular joint* is a synovial joint formed by the articulation of the acromial end of the clavicle with the acromion of the scapula. The acromioclavicular joint allows the scapula to rotate on the clavicle.

The acromioclavicular joint includes a wedge-shaped articular disc and is surrounded by a fibrous joint capsule. It's stabilized by the *coracoclavicular ligament,* which is composed of the *conoid ligament* and the *trapezoid ligament* and extends from the coracoid process of the scapula to the acromial end of the clavicle. The conoid ligament runs from the coracoid process to the conoid tubercle on the clavicle, and the trapezoid ligament runs from the coracoid process to the inferior part of the clavicle.

Hanging on to the humerus

The *glenohumeral joint* joins the head of the humerus to the glenoid cavity. It's a ball-and-socket joint (see Chapter 3) that allows for a wide range of movement for the arm.

Because the glenohumeral joint is a ball-and-socket joint, you can adduct (move your arm toward the midline of your body), abduct (move your arm away from the midline), extend your arm backward, or flex your arm forward. You can also rotate your arm medially (internally) or laterally (externally) and circumduct the arm (make a circle-like movement).

Imagine your arm hanging down by your side with your elbow bent (so your forearm is parallel to the floor). If you move your forearm and hand toward the midline of your body, you're medially rotating your arm in the glenohumeral joint. If you move your forearm and hand out away from your body in the opposite direction, then you're laterally rotating the arm at the glenohumeral joint.

The glenoid cavity is lined with a ring-shaped piece of cartilage called the *labrum,* which forms a lip that helps the head of the humerus fit into the cavity a little more securely. Three ligaments help stabilize the joint:

- *Coracohumeral ligament:* This ligament connects the base of the coracoid process to the front of the greater tubercle of the humerus.

- *Transverse humeral ligament:* This ligament runs between the greater and lesser tubercles and forms a canal with the intertubercular sulcus (bicipital groove). The bicipital tendon runs through this canal. (We look at the bicipital tendon and the biceps brachii that it belongs to in the next chapter.)

- *Coracoacromial ligament:* This ligament runs between the acromion and the coracoid process. This structure is also called the *coracoacromial arch.*

These ligaments can't stabilize the glenohumeral joint alone. Additional support is provided by the muscles of the rotator cuff (which we discuss later in this chapter).

The following two bursae (see Chapter 3) form cushions between the tendons and bones of the glenohumeral joint:

- ✔ *Subacromial bursa:* Also called the *subdeltoid bursa,* this bursa is found between the acromion, the coracoacromial ligament, and the deltoid muscle and the supraspinatus muscle (discussions of those muscles are coming up in this chapter).

- ✔ *Subscapular bursa:* This bursa is between the scapula and the tendon of the subscapularis muscle (also coming up in this chapter).

Sniffing around the Axilla (Armpit)

The axilla, or underarm (or, less delicately put, the armpit) is that indentation formed under the area where your arm attaches to your shoulder. Blood, lymph vessels, and nerves going to and from the arm pass through the axilla. The structure of the axilla and its blood vessels are the subject of the following sections.

Forming the apex, the base, and the walls

The size and shape of the axilla is defined by six features:

- ✔ *Apex:* Formed by the *cervicoaxillary canal;* bounded by the clavicle, the 1st rib, and the top of the scapula

- ✔ *Base:* Formed by the skin that stretches from the arm to the thoracic cage; forms the indentation known as the *axillary fossa*

- ✔ *Anterior wall:* Made up of the pectoralis major and minor (more on those muscles later in this chapter), forming the *anterior axillary fold*

- ✔ *Posterior wall:* Made up of the subscapularis, latissimus dorsi, and teres major muscles (all coming up later this chapter), forming the *posterior axillary fold*

- ✔ *Medial wall:* Formed by the thoracic cage and the serratus anterior (see Chapter 7)

- ✔ *Lateral wall:* Made by the intertubercular sulcus (bicipital groove) of the humerus

Tracking the axillary artery and vein

The *axillary artery* branches from the subclavian artery (see Chapter 14) as it passes over the 1st rib. It ends near the bottom of the scapula. The axillary artery is divided into three parts: first, second, and third:

- ✔ *First part of the axillary artery:* Goes from the lateral border of the 1st rib to the medial border of the pectoralis minor; has one branch, the *superior thoracic artery*

- ✔ *Second part of the axillary artery:* Runs behind the pectoralis minor; has two branches: the *thoracoacromial artery* and the *lateral thoracic artery*

- ✔ *Third part of the axillary artery:* Extends from the lateral border of the pectoralis minor to the lower border of the teres major; has three branches: the *subscapular artery* and the *anterior* and *posterior circumflex humeral arteries*

The *axillary vein* is formed by the union of the *accompanying brachial veins* and the *basilic vein.* It runs up alongside the axillary artery and becomes the subclavian vein (see Chapter 14) around the level of the 1st rib. Check out Figure 16-4 later in this chapter to see some arteries of this region.

Moving the Shoulder and the Arm

The shoulder is an amazing thing. Its bones and joints allow you to move your arm in many different directions so that you can lift things up, push things away, or execute the many motions the shoulder makes when you throw a ball overhand.

The muscles that provide the movement for the shoulder and upper arm include the anterior muscles in the front, the posterior muscles in the back, and the shoulder muscles that are sort of in between. Keep reading for more on these muscle groups.

Taking a look at the anterior muscles

Four *anterior pectoral muscles* move the pectoral girdle and arm from the front (see Figure 16-2):

✔ ***Pectoralis major:*** This muscle has two *heads,* or sections of muscle tissue, and covers much of the front of the thoracic cage. The *clavicular head* attaches to the medial portion of the clavicle. The *sternocostal head* attaches to the sternum and first six costal cartilages (see Chapter 7). It inserts into the lateral lip of the intertubercular groove of the humerus. The pectoralis major flexes, adducts, and medially rotates the humerus.

✔ ***Pectoralis minor:*** This muscle is found in the anterior wall of the axilla, underneath the pectoralis major. It attaches to the 3rd through 5th ribs and the coracoid process of the scapula. It helps to stabilize the scapula.

✔ ***Subclavius:*** This small, round muscle is located just below the clavicle. It anchors and holds the clavicle down during movement.

✔ ***Serratus anterior:*** This muscle is attached to the lateral (toward the side of the body, away from the midline) portions of the first eight ribs and the medial border of the scapula. It helps hold the scapula against the back.

An injury to the long thoracic nerve (coming up in this chapter) causes the serratus anterior to lose strength. The result is a winged scapula, so named because the scapula is not held tight against the back and resembles a wing.

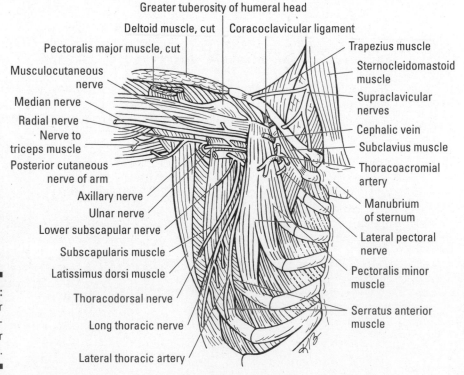

Figure 16-2: Anterior axioap- pendicular muscles.

Greater tuberosity of humeral head

Deltoid muscle, cut   Coracoclavicular ligament

Pectoralis major muscle, cut

Trapezius muscle

Musculocutaneous nerve

Sternocleidomastoid muscle

Median nerve

Supraclavicular nerves

Radial nerve

Cephalic vein

Nerve to triceps muscle

Subclavius muscle

Posterior cutaneous nerve of arm

Thoracoacromial artery

Axillary nerve

Ulnar nerve

Manubrium of sternum

Lower subscapular nerve

Subscapularis muscle

Lateral pectoral nerve

Latissimus dorsi muscle

Pectoralis minor muscle

Thoracodorsal nerve

Long thoracic nerve

Serratus anterior muscle

Lateral thoracic artery

Moving to the posterior muscles

The *posterior axioappendicular muscles* (or extrinsic back muscles) attach the pectoral girdle to the thoracic wall and posterior thoracic cage (see Chapters 7 and 15).

- ✔ **Trapezius:** This triangular muscle covers the back of the neck and the upper half of the posterior thoracic cage. It attaches to the base of the skull, the nuchal ligament, and spinous processes of the 7th cervical vertebra and all 12 thoracic vertebrae (see Chapter 15), and runs to the clavicle, the acromion, and the spine of the scapula. The trapezius has three portions: the *superior part* elevates the scapula, the *middle part* retracts the scapula, and the *inferior part* depresses the scapula while lowering the shoulder.

- ✔ **Latissimus dorsi:** This V-shaped muscle covers much of the thoracic wall below the trapezius. It attaches to the spinous processes of the bottom six thoracic vertebrae, the iliac crest (see Chapter 15), the thoracolumbar fascia, and the bottom four ribs (see Chapter 7). It also attaches to the humerus. The latissimus dorsi extends, adducts, and medially rotates the humerus.

- ✔ **Levator scapulae:** This muscle runs deep to the sternocleidomastoid and trapezius muscles (see Chapter 14). It attaches to the transverse processes of the first four cervical vertebrae and the medial side of the scapula. It raises the scapula upward and rotates the glenoid cavity downward.

- ✔ **Major** and **minor rhomboids:** These muscles run underneath the trapezius, from the spinous processes of the 7th cervical vertebra through the 5th thoracic vertebra to the scapula. They pull the scapula toward the vertebral column.

Shaping up the shoulder muscles

Six *scapulohumeral muscles* attach to the scapula and the humerus, all working to move the glenohumeral joint:

- ✔ **Deltoid:** This muscle gives the shoulder its rounded shape. It originates at the outer third of the clavicle and the acromion and spine of the scapula and inserts into the deltoid tuberosity on the humerus. It has three sections. The *anterior part* flexes and medially rotates the humerus. The *middle part* abducts the humerus. And the *posterior part* extends and laterally rotates the humerus.

What causes shoulder pain?

Patients who complain of shoulder pain commonly have problems that fall into one of four categories: inflammation of soft tissues, instability, osteoarthritis, or fractures.

- Inflammation often affects the rotator cuff. Such conditions include *bursitis,* which is inflammation and swelling of the bursa, and *tendinitis,* which is the inflammation of the tendons that attach muscles to the bones. Tendons can also tear either partially or completely away from the bone. Shoulder impingement can occur when the acromion presses on the rotator-cuff tendons and the subacromial bursa as the arm is lifted.

- Instability includes partial or complete shoulder dislocations that happen when the head of the humerus is forced out of the glenoid cavity. This dislocation is usually due to traumatic injury, but it can also happen from overuse. Dislocations can reoccur if the ligaments, tendons, and muscles are sufficiently damaged.

- Osteoarthritis happens when the cartilage of a joint wears down. It causes pain, swelling, and stiffness and usually worsens over time.

- Fractures usually involve the clavicle, but the humerus is also subject to several types of fractures that can occur at the head, tuberosities, surgical neck, or shaft. The fractures are usually due to traumatic injury.

Shoulder pain can also be due to serious health conditions such as tumors, infection, and problems with the nervous system or referred pain during a heart attack.

- *Teres major:* This muscle originates at the bottom part of the scapula and inserts into the intertubercular groove of the humerus. It adducts and medially rotates the humerus.

- *Supraspinatus:* This muscle originates at the supraspinous fossa of the scapula and inserts into the greater tubercle of the humerus. It helps the deltoid abduct the humerus.

- *Infraspinatus:* Originating at the infraspinous fossa of the scapula, this muscle inserts into the greater tubercle on the humerus. It laterally rotates the humerus.

- *Teres minor:* This muscle originates at the lateral part of the scapula and inserts into the greater tubercle of the humerus. It adducts and laterally rotates the humerus.

- *Subscapularis:* Originating at the subscapular fossa, this muscle inserts at the lesser tubercle of the humerus. It adducts and medially rotates the humerus.

The last four muscles on that list (supraspinatus, infraspinatus, teres minor, and subscapularis) are often referred to collectively as the *rotator-cuff muscles* because their tendons form a cuff around the glenohumeral joint and help to protect and stabilize it.

Maintaining the Tissues

The tissues of the pectoral girdle need oxygen and energy along with nervous supply and lymph drainage. Here's a look at the blood vessels, nerves, and lymphatics that keep your shoulder running.

Acknowledging the nerves and blood supply

The *roots* of the brachial plexus are formed by the ventral rami of the 5th cervical through the 1st thoracic spinal nerves. The roots combine to form three *trunks* (*superior, middle,* and *inferior*). Each trunk splits to form an anterior and a posterior *division*. The divisions combine to form *lateral, posterior,* and *medial cords,* which in turn become nerves that innervate (supply nerve impulses) the structures of the upper extremity. You can find all these nerves in Figure 16-3:

- ✔ *Dorsal scapular* (C5): This nerve originates from the brachial plexus at the 5th cervical root, goes through the middle scalene muscle, and runs to the levator scapulae and rhomboids. It innervates the rhomboids.

- ✔ *Long thoracic* (C5–C7): Formed by branches of the 5th, 6th, and 7th cervical roots, this nerve runs through the middle scalene muscle into the axillary canal and goes to the superficial part of the serratus anterior muscle, which is the muscle it innervates.

- ✔ *Suprascapular* (C5–C6): This nerve arises from the superior trunk of the brachial plexus and runs laterally through the scapular notch to innervate the supraspinatus and infraspinatus muscles and the glenohumeral joint.

- ✔ *Nerve to the subclavius* (C5): This nerve arises from the superior trunk and runs down past the clavicle to innervate the subclavius muscle and the sternoclavicular joint.

- ✔ *Lateral pectoral* (C5–C7): Branching off the lateral cord, this nerve runs to the pectoral muscles. It innervates the pectoralis major, but some fibers form a communicating branch to the medial pectoral nerve that innervates the pectoralis minor.

- ✔ *Medial pectoral* (C8–T1): This nerve arises from the medial cord and descends lateral to the lateral pectoral nerve. It innervates the pectoralis minor and the sternocostal part of the pectoralis major.

- ✔ *Upper subscapular* (C5–C6): This nerve arises from the posterior cord and enters the subscapularis muscle. It innervates the superior portion of the subscapularis.

✔ *Lower subscapular* **(C5–C6):** This nerve branches from the posterior cord and passes inferiorly to innervate the inferior portion of the subscapularis and teres major muscles.

✔ *Thoracodorsal* **(C7–C8):** Arising from the posterior cord, this nerve runs downward and laterally along the posterior axillary wall to the top of the latissimus dorsi muscle, which it innervates.

✔ *Axillary* **(C5–C6):** This nerve arises from the posterior cord and runs through the axillary fossa. It innervates the glenohumeral joint, teres minor, and deltoid muscles.

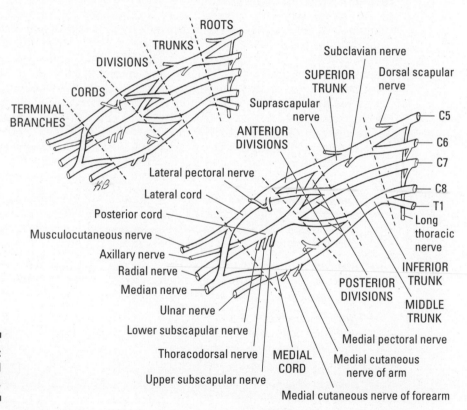

Figure 16-3:
The brachial
plexus.

These branches of the brachial plexus innervate the skin and muscles of the arm and forearm (we describe them in more detail in Chapters 17 and 18):

✔ *Medial cutaneous nerve of the arm* **(C8, T1):** This nerve branches from the medial cord and innervates the skin of the medial arm.

✔ *Medial cutaneous nerve of the forearm* **(C8, T1):** This nerve branches from the medial cord and innervates the skin of the medial forearm.

✔ *Musculocutaneous nerve* (C5–C7): This nerve is a terminal branch of the lateral cord that innervates muscles of the anterior arm and the skin of the lateral forearm.

✔ *Median nerve* (C5–T1): Forming from branches of the lateral and medial cords, this nerve supplies muscles in the anterior forearm, muscles in the hand, and the skin of the lateral palm.

✔ *Ulnar nerve* (C8–T1): This nerve is a terminal branch of the medial cord that innervates muscles in the anterior forearm, muscles in the hand, and the skin of the medial hand.

✔ *Radial nerve* (C5–T1): This nerve is a terminal branch of the posterior cord that innervates the muscle of the posterior arm and posterior forearm, the skin in those regions, and the dorsum of the hand.

Arterial blood flow is provided by branches of the subclavian artery (see Chapter 14) and the axillary artery that runs from the axilla and continues down into the arm as the brachial artery. You can see these arteries in Figure 16-4.

✔ *Internal thoracic:* This artery starts on the first part of the subclavian artery and descends anteriorly and medially. It runs posterior to the clavicle and 1st costal cartilage and forms branches in the thoracic cage (see Chapter 7 for more info).

✔ *Suprascapular:* This artery stems from the thyrocervical trunk (a branch of the subclavian artery) and runs inferiorly and laterally across the anterior scalene muscle, phrenic nerve, subclavian artery, and brachial plexus. Next, it runs posterior and parallel to the clavicle and then laterally to the infraspinous fossa of the scapula.

✔ *Superior thoracic:* This artery starts on the first part of the axillary artery and runs anteriorly and medially along the superior edge of the pectoralis minor and then to the thoracic wall.

✔ *Thoracoacromial:* This artery starts on the second part of the axillary artery and curls around the superomedial edge of the pectoralis minor before dividing into four branches: the *pectoral, deltoid, acromial,* and *clavicular* branches.

✔ *Lateral thoracic:* This artery also starts on the second part of the axillary artery and descends onto the thoracic wall.

✔ *Circumflex humeral:* This artery has two parts (anterior and posterior) that branch off the third part of the axillary artery and anastomose (join together) to encircle the surgical neck of the humerus.

✔ *Subscapular:* This artery also starts on the third part of the axillary artery and descends along the lateral border of the scapula and divides into the circumflex scapular artery and the thoracodorsal artery:

 • *Circumflex scapular:* This branch curves around the lateral border of the scapula and enters the infraspinous fossa before anastomosing with the suprascapular artery.

- *Thoracodorsal:* This branch descends into the latissimus dorsi muscle.

✔ ***Deep brachial artery of the arm:*** This artery starts on the brachial artery and runs along the radial groove of the humerus to the elbow joint.

✔ ***Superior ulnar collateral:*** This artery also starts on the brachial artery and runs to the posterior part of the elbow.

✔ ***Inferior ulnar collateral:*** This artery starts on the brachial artery and runs to the medial part of the elbow.

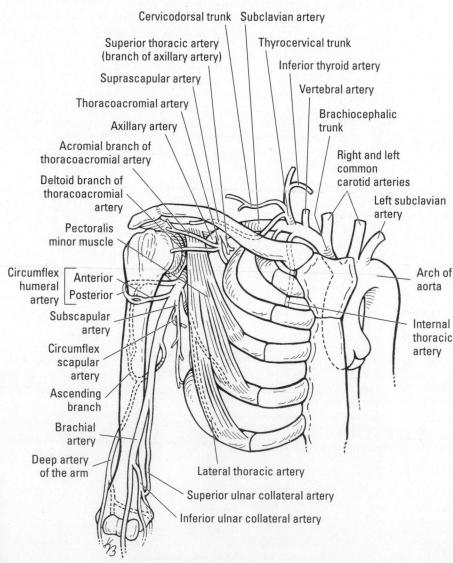

Cervicodorsal trunk Subclavian artery
Superior thoracic artery (branch of axillary artery)
Thyrocervical trunk
Suprascapular artery
Inferior thyroid artery
Thoracoacromial artery
Vertebral artery
Axillary artery
Brachiocephalic trunk
Acromial branch of thoracoacromial artery
Right and left common carotid arteries
Deltoid branch of thoracoacromial artery
Left subclavian artery
Pectoralis minor muscle
Circumflex humeral artery — Anterior / Posterior
Arch of aorta
Subscapular artery
Internal thoracic artery
Circumflex scapular artery
Ascending branch
Brachial artery
Deep artery of the arm
Lateral thoracic artery
Superior ulnar collateral artery
Inferior ulnar collateral artery

Figure 16-4: Arteries of the shoulder.

Venous drainage is provided by deep veins that travel alongside the arteries and by two superficial veins, the *cephalic vein* and the *brachial vein*.

Remembering the lymphatic vessels

The *deltopectoral nodes* are superficial lymph nodes that receive lymph from superficial vessels. The axilla contains five groups of lymph nodes (see Figure 16-5, and see Chapter 5 for more information on the lymphatic system):

- ✔ *Pectoral (anterior) nodes:* This group of nodes is located on the medial wall of the axilla and at the bottom of the pectoralis minor. Lymph from the anterior thoracic wall and breast flows into these nodes.

- ✔ *Subscapular (posterior) nodes:* These nodes lie along the posterior axillary fold. They get lymph from the posterior thoracic wall and scapular area.

- ✔ *Humeral (lateral) nodes:* This group is on the lateral wall of the axilla near the axillary vein. Most of the lymph from the upper extremity flows into these nodes.

- ✔ *Central nodes:* These nodes lie underneath the pectoralis minor. Lymph from the pectoral, subscapular, and humeral nodes flow into the central nodes.

- ✔ *Apical nodes:* These nodes are near the apex of the axilla. They get lymph from the other axillary nodes.

The vessels leaving the apical nodes form the *subclavian lymphatic trunk,* which leads to the right lymphatic duct or the thoracic duct on the left side (see Chapter 8).

Axillary lymph nodes may become enlarged and tender following an infection in the upper extremity.

The axillary nodes are also the most common site for the metastasis, or the spreading, of breast cancer cells. *Sentinel nodes* is the name given to the first lymph nodes into which the tumor drains. With breast cancer, these sentinel nodes are usually the axillary nodes. A biopsy may be performed on these nodes to determine if cancer is spreading. If the biopsy is negative, metastasis is unlikely; if the biopsy is positive, the cancer cells may have spread into more lymph nodes beyond the sentinel nodes.

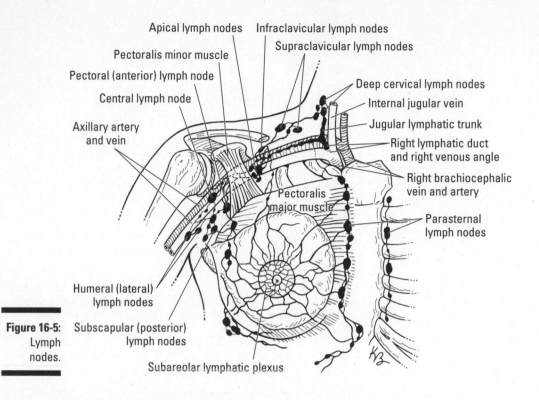

Apical lymph nodes

Infraclavicular lymph nodes

Supraclavicular lymph nodes

Pectoralis minor muscle

Pectoral (anterior) lymph node

Central lymph node

Deep cervical lymph nodes

Internal jugular vein

Jugular lymphatic trunk

Right lymphatic duct and right venous angle

Axillary artery and vein

Pectoralis major muscle

Right brachiocephalic vein and artery

Parasternal lymph nodes

Humeral (lateral) lymph nodes

Figure 16-5: Lymph nodes.

Subscapular (posterior) lymph nodes

Subareolar lymphatic plexus

Covering Your Shoulders and Arms: The Surface Anatomy

Superficial fascia lies just under the skin of the shoulder region, with deep fascia covering muscle tissues. See Chapter 3 for more about fascia.

- ✔ *Pectoral fascia:* Covers the pectoralis major and joins the fascia of the abdominal wall

- ✔ *Clavipectoral fascia:* Runs from the clavicle to cover the *subclavius muscle* and *pectoralis minor*

- ✔ *Suspensory ligament of the axilla:* Comes from part of the clavipectoral fascia and supports the *axillary fascia,* which stems from the pectoral fascia

- ✔ *Deltoid fascia:* Covers the deltoid muscle and attaches to the pectoral fascia anteriorly and the *infraspinous fascia* posteriorly

Cutaneous nerves lie in the subcutaneous layer and innervate the skin of the upper extremity. The cutaneous nerves that supply the shoulder and upper arm come from branches of the cervical plexus (see Chapter 14), the brachial plexus, and intercostal nerves (see Chapter 7):

- ✔ ***Supraclavicular nerves:*** Innervate the skin over the clavicle and superiolateral (upper and outer) portion of the pectoralis major

- ✔ ***Superior lateral cutaneous nerve:*** Innervates the skin over the inferior part of the deltoid and the lateral part of the arm (it's a branch of the axillary nerve)

- ✔ ***Intercostobrachial nerve:*** Innervates the skin on the upper medial part of the arm

The following list gives you an idea of where some of the shoulder structures lie under the skin and notes a few surface landmarks to see:

- ✔ The clavicle is visible and easily palpated just below the neck.

- ✔ The *clavipectoral triangle* is a small depression bordered by the clavicle, the clavicular head of the pectoralis major, and the deltoid muscle.

- ✔ The pectoralis major muscle is seen or palpated on the front of the chest wall.

- ✔ The deltoid muscle gives the shoulder its shape.

- ✔ The latissimus dorsi, teres major, and trapezius form the shape of the upper back.

The triangle *of auscultation* is a small area bordered by the latissimus dorsi inferiorly, the scapula laterally, and the trapezius superiorly. It's a good spot for listening to breathing sounds with a stethoscope. You can find it by palpating the medial border of the scapula — the triangle of auscultation is an area where the muscles are thinner, between the latissimus dorsi and trapezius muscles.

Chapter 17

Bending the Elbow and Focusing on the Forearm

*W*here would humans be without the elbow? It bends the forearm so you can move the things your hands pick up, and it's designed so that you can rotate your forearm just a bit. This chapter looks at the structures of the elbow and the forearm from the inside out.

Forming the Elbow and the Forearm: The Bones

The elbow and the forearm are made up of only three bones. Half of the elbow is formed by the humerus, the lone bone of the arm. The forearm contains two bones; the radius is on the lateral side of the forearm and the ulna is on the medial side. (Think of the anatomical position, described in Chapter 2; the palm of the hand faces forward, so the thumb is on the lateral side of the body and the little finger is medial.) In the following sections, we point you toward the important points on the bones that form the elbow and forearm.

Handling the humerus

The head of the humerus forms the glenohumeral joint of the shoulder with the scapula (see Chapter 16 for more about the proximal and middle parts of the humerus).

The distal end of the humerus (at the elbow) has two prominent bumps: the *medial* and *lateral epicondyles. Medial* and *lateral supraepicondylar ridges* follow the shaft of the humerus down to the epicondyles.

The *condyle of the humerus* forms the elbow joint. The condyle (round prominence at the end of a bone) has a *capitulum* that articulates with the head of the radius, and the *trochlea* articulates with the trochlear notch of the ulna. The *coronoid fossa* is an indentation on the anterior part of the condyle, which leaves room for the coronoid process of the ulna when you flex the elbow. The *radial fossa* is a shallow indentation that accommodates the head of the radius. The *olecranon fossa* is a similar indentation located on the posterior part of the condyle, which leaves room for the olecranon of the ulna when the elbow is straightened out.

Regarding the radius

The *head of the radius* has a concave top that articulates with the capitulum of the humerus. It also articulates with the radial notch of the ulna (which we discuss in the next section). The *neck of the radius* is the narrow portion between the head of the radius and the *shaft of the radius.* The shaft widens as it gets closer to the wrist. The *radial tuberosity* (bony protuberance) is distal to the neck of the radius.

The *distal radial styloid process* articulates with the wrist (see Chapter 18 for more about the portion of the radius that articulates with the wrist).

Understanding the ulna

The proximal end of the ulna has two large projections: The *olecranon* is on the posterior surface, and the *coronoid process* is on the anterior surface. The space between the two projections is called the *trochlear notch.* The trochlea of the humerus fits into the trochlear notch.

The *tuberosity of the ulna* is located distal to the coronoid process. The *radial notch* is a shallow depression found on the lateral side of the coronoid process. The *supinator crest* (prominent ridge) and *supinator fossa* (indentation) are located distal to the coronoid process. The shaft of the ulna is thicker near the elbow and gets thinner as it moves toward the wrist.

The distal portion of the ulna is covered in Chapter 18, where we talk about how it forms the wrist and fits together with the hand bones.

Joining the Elbow and the Forearm

The three bones of the elbow and forearm form two joints in the proximal forearm. The elbow is the main joint that most people can easily recognize. It involves all three bones. The lesser known and somewhat hidden second joint is the radioulnar joint, which involves (can you guess?) the radius and ulna.

Bending the elbow

The *elbow joint* is a synovial hinge joint (see Chapter 3 for more about joints) with two articulations. The trochlea of the humerus articulates with the trochlear notch of the ulna, and the capitulum of the humerus articulates with the head of the radius. The elbow joint is lined by a synovial membrane and is surrounded by a fibrous joint capsule. The joint capsule is supported by collateral ligaments:

- ✔ *Radial collateral ligament:* This ligament runs from the lateral epicondyle of the humerus to the anular ligament of the radius.

- ✔ *Ulnar collateral ligament:* This ligament runs from the medial epicondyle of the humerus to the coronoid process and the olecranon of the ulna. It has three parts: the *anterior, posterior,* and *oblique bands*.

The collateral ligaments and the hinge shape of the elbow joint allow you to flex and extend the elbow. The elbow joint is innervated by the musculocutaneous, radial, and ulnar nerves.

If you look at a person who is standing in the anatomical position, you'll notice the upper extremities are not completely straight. The forearms angle away from the body by about 10 to 15 degrees. This is called the *carrying angle*.

Dislocations of the elbow can happen when a person falls onto an outstretched hand. The force goes up the forearm and drives the ulna posteriorly out of joint.

Reviewing the radioulnar joints

Two separate joints exist between the radius and the ulna. The distal radioulnar joint is down by the wrist, so we discuss it in Chapter 18.

The *proximal radioulnar joint* is a synovial pivot joint that allows the head of the radius to move as it articulates in the radial notch of the ulna. It's lined with a synovial membrane and covered with a fibrous joint capsule. The *anular ligament of the radius* surrounds the head of the radius and holds it in the radial notch. It allows for pronation (turning the palm from facing anteriorly to facing posteriorly) and supination (turning the palm from facing posteriorly back to anterior) of the forearm.

Making the Elbow and Forearm Move: The Muscles

The muscles of the arm are responsible for the movement of your elbow and, by extension, your forearm. In the following sections, we first describe the muscles of the arm, and then we move on to the muscles of the forearm. A lot of the muscles found in forearm also flex and extend your wrist, so we describe those actions in Chapter 18.

The muscles of the arm

Five muscles originate on either the humerus or the scapula (for more details on this bone, flip back to Chapter 16) and insert onto the bones of the forearm to flex and extend the elbow. You can see some of these muscles in Figure 17-1:

- ✔ *Biceps brachii:* This muscle has two heads. The *short head* originates on the coracoid process of the scapula, and the *long head* originates on the supraglenoid tubercle of the scapula. Both heads insert onto the tuberosity of the radius. The muscle is innervated by the musculocutaneous nerve and helps to supinate and flex the forearm.

- ✔ *Brachialis:* This muscle originates on the distal part of the humerus and inserts onto the coronoid process and tuberosity of the ulna. It's innervated by the musculocutaneous nerve and flexes the forearm.

- ✔ *Coracobrachialis:* This muscle originates on the coracoid process of the scapula and inserts on the middle of the medial surface of the humerus. It's innervated by the musculocutaneous nerve and flexes and adducts the arm.

- ✔ *Triceps brachii:* This muscle has three heads. The *long head* originates on the infraglenoid tubercle of the scapula, the *lateral head* originates on the posterior surface of the humerus above the radial groove, and the *medial head* originates on the posterior surface of the humerus just below the radial groove. All three heads insert onto the olecranon of the ulna and are innervated by the radial nerve. The triceps brachii extends the forearm.

- ✔ *Anconeus:* This muscle originates on the lateral epicondyle of the humerus and inserts into the olecranon and posterior surface of the ulna. It's innervated by the radial nerve. It helps extend the forearm and stabilizes the elbow joint.

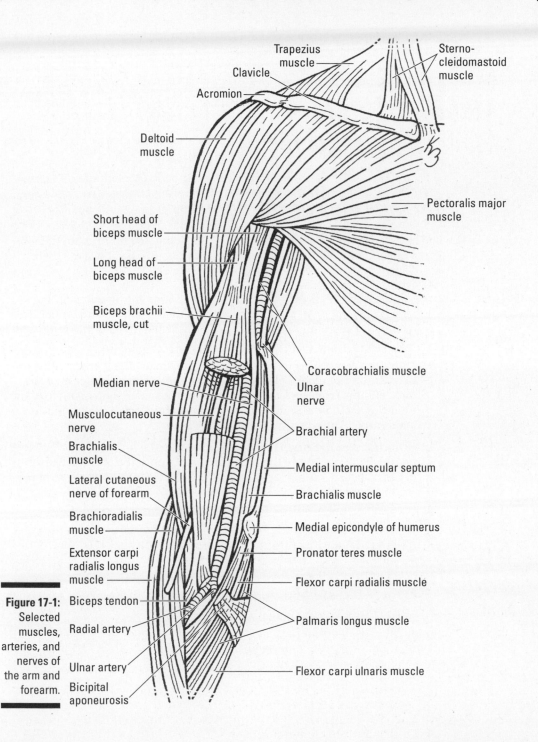

Trapezius muscle

Sterno-cleidomastoid muscle

Clavicle

Acromion

Deltoid muscle

Pectoralis major muscle

Short head of biceps muscle

Long head of biceps muscle

Biceps brachii muscle, cut

Coracobrachialis muscle

Median nerve

Ulnar nerve

Musculocutaneous nerve

Brachial artery

Brachialis muscle

Medial intermuscular septum

Lateral cutaneous nerve of forearm

Brachialis muscle

Brachioradialis muscle

Medial epicondyle of humerus

Extensor carpi radialis longus muscle

Pronator teres muscle

Flexor carpi radialis muscle

Figure 17-1: Selected muscles, arteries, and nerves of the arm and forearm.

Biceps tendon

Radial artery

Palmaris longus muscle

Ulnar artery

Flexor carpi ulnaris muscle

Bicipital aponeurosis

The elbow has three bursae (fluid-filled sacs) tucked in and around the tendons to help them glide over the bones.

- ✔ *Intratendinous olecranon bursa:* Present in the triceps brachii tendon
- ✔ *Subtendinous olecranon bursa:* Located between the olecranon and the triceps tendon
- ✔ *Subcutaneous olecranon bursa:* Located in the connective tissue that lies over the olecranon

The muscles of the forearm

The muscles in the forearm (see Figure 17-2) supinate and pronate the forearm. Remembering which one does which motion is easy, because their actions match their names:

- ✔ *Supinator:* This muscle supinates the forearm. It originates on the lateral epicondyle of the humerus, the radial collateral and anular ligaments, and the ulna. It inserts onto the proximal third of the radius, and it's innervated by the deep branch of the radial nerve.
- ✔ *Pronator teres:* This muscle pronates and flexes the forearm. It has two heads: The *ulnar head* originates on the coronoid process of the ulna, and the *humeral head* originates on the medical epicondyle of the humerus. Both heads insert onto the lateral surface of the radius. It's innervated by the median nerve.
- ✔ *Pronator quadratus:* This muscle pronates the forearm. It originates on the distal portion of the ulna and inserts onto the anterior surface of the radius. It's innervated by the anterior interosseous nerve of the median nerve.

Giving a Nod to the Nerves and Blood Supply

The muscles and joints of the elbow and forearm need nervous supply and blood flow. The major nerves and veins start in your neck and run the length of your arms, often into your hands. You can refer to Figures 17-1 and 17-2 to see some of these nerves and arteries.

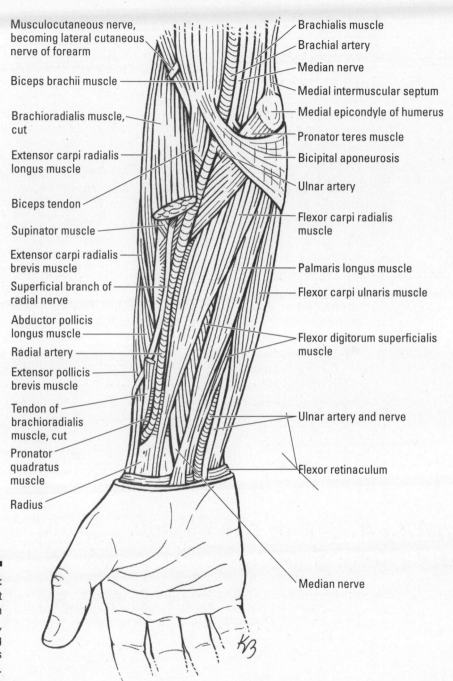

Musculocutaneous nerve, becoming lateral cutaneous nerve of forearm

Biceps brachii muscle

Brachioradialis muscle, cut

Extensor carpi radialis longus muscle

Biceps tendon

Supinator muscle

Extensor carpi radialis brevis muscle

Superficial branch of radial nerve

Abductor pollicis longus muscle

Radial artery

Extensor pollicis brevis muscle

Tendon of brachioradialis muscle, cut

Pronator quadratus muscle

Radius

Brachialis muscle

Brachial artery

Median nerve

Medial intermuscular septum

Medial epicondyle of humerus

Pronator teres muscle

Bicipital aponeurosis

Ulnar artery

Flexor carpi radialis muscle

Palmaris longus muscle

Flexor carpi ulnaris muscle

Flexor digitorum superficialis muscle

Ulnar artery and nerve

Flexor retinaculum

Median nerve

Figure 17-2:
A look at the forearm muscles, including the arteries and nerves.

Nerves

The following nerves branch from the brachial plexus in the neck and travel through the arm to supply the elbow and the forearm. Some of these nerves continue through the forearm to supply the wrist and hand.

- ✔ *Median nerve:* This nerve starts from the brachial plexus and runs from the axilla down alongside the brachial artery (see Chapters 11 and 16). It descends into the cubital fossa (the front of the elbow; read more about the cubital fossa in the "Looking Only Skin Deep: The Surface Anatomy" section at the end of this chapter). It gives off branches that serve the elbow joint and continues down the anterior part of the forearm and into the hand through the carpal tunnel (see Chapter 18).

- ✔ *Ulnar nerve:* This nerve starts from the brachial plexus, passes through the arm medial to the brachial artery, continues posterior to the medial epicondyle of the humerus, and enters the forearm. It travels along the medial part of the forearm until it enters the hand at the wrist (see Chapter 18).

- ✔ *Radial nerve:* This nerve starts from the brachial plexus and runs posterior to the brachial artery and anterior to the long head of the triceps. It curves around the shaft of the humerus and continues toward the cubital fossa. From there it branches into the deep and superficial branches and continues down the lateral part of the forearm to enter the hand (see Chapter 18).

- ✔ *Musculocutaneous nerve:* This nerve runs from the brachial plexus through the anterior part of the arm and becomes the lateral cutaneous nerve of the forearm.

Blood supply

Arteries run from the shoulder down to the wrist with just a few branches given off near the elbow. Superficial and deep veins return blood toward the heart. Following is a brief overview:

- ✔ *Brachial artery:* This artery stems from the axillary artery (see Chapter 16). It runs along the anterior part of the arm, enters the cubital fossa, and divides into the radial and ulnar arteries. It also has the following branches that form arterial anastomoses (joined arteries) that supply the elbow:

  - *Deep artery of the arm (profunda brachii artery)*
  - *Superior ulnar collateral artery*
  - *Inferior ulnar collateral artery*

- ✔ *Ulnar artery:* This artery runs from the cubital fossa down the anterior and medial portion of the forearm until it enters the wrist (see Chapter 18).

- ✔ *Radial artery:* This artery runs from the cubital fossa down the anterior and lateral portion of the forearm until it enters the wrist (see Chapter 18).

- ✔ *Cephalic* and *basilic veins:* These veins provide superficial venous return.

- ✔ *Brachial, radial,* and *ulnar veins:* These veins are deeper. They accompany the arteries of the same names.

Looking Only Skin Deep: The Surface Anatomy

You can easily palpate (medically examine) the olecranon and the epicondyles. The olecranon is the big bony bump that you feel (and probably see) on the back of the elbow. The epicondyles are the prominent bony bumps on either side of the elbow. The biceps and triceps brachii muscles give the fleshy part of the arm its shape.

The *cubital fossa* is a triangular depression on the anterior surface of the elbow. It's bordered by the pronator teres and the brachioradialis muscles. The cubital fossa contains the radial and median nerves, the biceps brachii tendon, and deep veins, and it's the spot where the brachial artery branches into the ulnar and radial artery. You can palpate this area by pressing your fingers into the skin over the anterior section of elbow. It's easiest to do when the arm is relaxed and the elbow slightly bent. The median cubital vein, a common site for venipuncture, runs superficial to the brachial artery and lies just under the skin.

Chapter 18

Shaking Hands and Grabbing the Wrist

....

In This Chapter

▶ Tunneling through the bones and joints of the wrist and hand

▶ Getting to know the muscles, nerves, and blood supply of the wrist and hand

▶ Taking the pulse of the wrist and hand's surface anatomy

....

The wrists and hands are amazing things. Right now you're probably using them to hold this book. You use them to pick up a fork, wave to a friend, or pat your kids on the back (among so many other things!). Understanding the clinical anatomy of the wrists and hands is important because you need them for normal daily activity and hand injuries can be debilitating. In this chapter, we review the wrist and hand, both inside and out. They may be a small part of the body, but you'll find plenty here to look at, with lots of bones, joints, intricate muscles, nerves, and circulatory vessels.

Putting Your Hands (and Wrists) Together

Each hand and wrist has 27 little bones. Think about all the different movements your wrists, hands, and fingers can make, and you can probably understand why they need so many bones: Many bones mean more movement. If they had just a few big bones, your hands wouldn't move well at all and you wouldn't accomplish much in a typical day.

In the following sections, we look at the bones in groups, starting with the wrist bones, and then we move on to the hand bones and the bones that make up your fingers.

When you talk about hands in a clinical setting, your thumb is your first digit, your second digit is your index finger, your middle finger is your third digit, your ring finger is your fourth digit, and your pinkie is your fifth digit.

Starting with the carpal bones

Eight small bones provide strength and a little flexibility to your wrist. They're called *carpal bones,* so sometimes the wrist is referred to as the *carpus.* Most of your wrist movement is between the carpal bones and the radius bone of the forearm (which we discuss in Chapter 17), but some gliding action occurs between carpal bones. (Joints provide this gliding action; we look at these joints later in this chapter.)

The carpals are arranged in two rows of four bones each. Take a look at Figure 18-1 to see how the bones are arranged. Following are the carpal bones in the first row, starting from the lateral side (same side as your thumb, right next to the radius) and working across:

- ✔ *Scaphoid:* Shaped like a little boat; has a *scaphoid tubercle* (bony projection)

- ✔ *Lunate:* Shaped like a crescent moon

- ✔ *Triquetrum:* Shaped like a pyramid

- ✔ *Pisiform:* A small, round bone sitting right on the triquetrum

The next row of carpal bones *articulate* (form joints) with the first row of carpal bones and the metacarpals of the hand. (Don't worry — we talk about the metacarpals next.)

- ✔ *Trapezium:* A four-sided bone

- ✔ *Trapezoid:* A wedge-shaped bone

- ✔ *Capitate:* The largest wrist bone; shaped like a head

- ✔ *Hamate:* Wedge-shaped; similar to the trapezoid but with a bony hook-shaped process (projection of bone) called the *hook of the hamate*

These eight bones can be a little tricky to remember, but we provide a neat little memory device in Chapter 22.

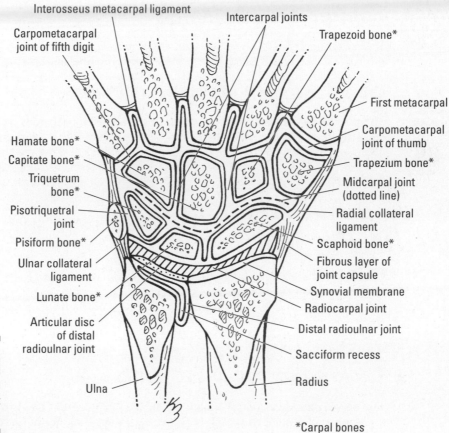

Interosseus metacarpal ligament

Intercarpal joints

Trapezoid bone*

Carpometacarpal joint of fifth digit

First metacarpal

Carpometacarpal joint of thumb

Hamate bone*

Capitate bone*

Trapezium bone*

Triquetrum bone*

Midcarpal joint (dotted line)

Pisotriquetral joint

Radial collateral ligament

Pisiform bone*

Scaphoid bone*

Ulnar collateral ligament

Fibrous layer of joint capsule

Synovial membrane

Lunate bone*

Radiocarpal joint

Articular disc of distal radioulnar joint

Distal radioulnar joint

Sacciform recess

Ulna

Radius

*Carpal bones

Figure 18-1:
Some bones and joints of the wrist and hand.

Moving to the metacarpal bones

Five metacarpal bones make up the structure of the palm of your hand, which is also known as the *metacarpus.* They're easier to remember than the carpals; they're simply named the first through fifth metacarpals. The first metacarpal is on the lateral, or thumb side, of your hand. The fifth metacarpal is on the medial side, just under your pinkie finger.

Each metacarpal has a *base,* which articulates with the carpals, and a *head,* which articulates with the finger bones (clinically known as the *phalanges;* see the next section) to form the knuckles.

Finding the phalanges

The finger and thumb bones are called the *phalanges*. Each thumb has two phalanges: a *proximal phalanx* articulates with the first metacarpal, and a *distal phalanx* forms the tip of the thumb. The rest of the fingers have three phalanges each: proximal, middle, and distal phalanges.

The phalanges are fairly simple bones. Each one has a base on its proximal end (the end closer to the arm), a shaft in the middle, and a head on the distal end (toward the fingertips).

Waving and Wiggling with the Help of Joints

The large number of bones in the hand and wrist makes for a large number of joints, too. In the following sections, we start with a look at the joints that help you move your wrist and wave your hand, and then we move up toward those wiggly fingers.

Looking at the wrist joints

The *distal radioulnar joint* (which you can see in Figure 18-1) allows you to flip-flop each hand at the wrist. It's a synovial joint that allows for a lot of movement (see Chapter 3 for more on synovial and other types of joints); it's formed where the head of the ulna (see Chapter 17) articulates with the ulnar notch of the radius. This joint contains a fibrocartilaginous disc, and it's surrounded by a synovial membrane and fibrous joint capsule. Anterior and posterior ligaments support the joint (in other words, these ligaments are close to the front and to the back of the wrist, respectively). The distal radioulnar joint allows you to *supinate* and *pronate* your hand and wrist (meaning to turn your palm up or down).

The *radiocarpal joint* is a synovial joint that's also found in the wrist (refer to Figure 18-1). The radius articulates with the first row of carpal bones that we describe earlier in this chapter, except for the pisiform. It has a fibrous joint capsule that's attached to that distal end of the radius and the ulna and to the carpal bones. This joint allows you to flex and extend your wrist (bending it forward and backward), circumduct (move in a circle), adduct (move the hand sideways, bringing your little finger closer toward the midline of your body), and abduct (move your hand sideways with your thumb moving away from the midline of the body). Remember that these movements are described for a hand that is in the anatomic position (Chapter 1).

Handing over the hand joints

The *intercarpal joints* are synovial joints formed between the individual bones of the proximal row of the carpal bones, between the individual bones of the distal row of carpal bones, and between the proximal and distal rows (the midcarpal joint). Does that seem confusing? You can see them in Figure 18-1. These joints don't have much movement, just a small amount of gliding between the bones.

The *carpometacarpal joints* are synovial joints between the distal carpal bones and the metacarpals, and the *intermetacarpal joints* are between the metacarpals. The carpometacarpal joint of the thumb (refer to Figure 18-1) is a saddle-shaped joint between the trapezium and the base of the first metacarpal. The joints have a synovial membrane surrounded by fibrous joint capsules. They're supported by anterior, posterior, and *interosseous* (between bone) ligaments. The thumb joint can extend, flex, abduct, adduct, and circumduct. The fifth metacarpal joint is fairly mobile, but the rest don't have much movement.

Pointing to the finger joints

The joints of the fingers include the *metacarpophalangeal joints* and the *interphalangeal joints*. They're all synovial joints with synovial membranes and fibrous joint capsules.

- *Metacarpophalangeal joints:* Connecting the proximal phalanges to the metacarpals are condyloid joints (oval-shaped joint surfaces; see Chapter 3) with strong *palmar* and *collateral ligaments* that allow for movement in different directions (flexion, extension, abduction, adduction, circumduction). You may recognize them as your knuckles.

- *Interphalangeal joints:* These hinge joints (joints that move like the hinge on a door) allow flexion and extension. They join the heads of the phalanges with the bases of the next distal phalanges. Each finger (digits two through five) has one proximal interphalangeal joint and one distal interphalangeal joint. The thumb has only one interphalangeal joint.

Making the Most of Wrist and Hand Muscles

Even with all the bones and joints described in the previous sections, you couldn't do much with your hands and fingers without some muscles. The wrist makes larger movements, and the fingers and thumbs make many fine movements. So you have some longer muscles that run from the forearm (called the *extrinsic muscles*) and lots of little hand and finger muscles (the *intrinsic muscles*). We give you the scoop on all these muscles in the following sections.

Flexing and extending the wrist

In order to use your hands and fingers, you have to be able to bend your wrist. This movement is accomplished by two groups of muscles called the flexors and the extensors.

The flexors

The *flexors* are long muscles that run on the anterior part of the forearm (the anterior compartment) from the elbow down to the hand. The tendons are held in place at the wrist by the *palmar carpal ligament* and the *flexor retinaculum.* The bellies, or "meat," of the muscles are located closer to the elbow, with the tendons running past the wrist. They help give the forearm its shape. Sometimes we just take the easy route and call them the *wrist flexors,* but we list all of them individually for you here. (Some of these muscles flex the fingers and thumbs too, but because they originate on the forearm, we include them here.)

✔ *Flexor carpi radialis:* This wrist muscle originates on the medial epicondyle of the humerus (see Chapter 17) and inserts on the base of the second and third metacarpals. It's innervated by the median nerve and flexes and abducts the hand at the wrist. (We discuss all the nerves that *innervate* — or supply nerve function to — these muscles later in this chapter.)

You can locate the pulse of the radial artery on the lateral side of the anterior wrist by pressing two fingertips just along the flexor carpi radialis.

✔ *Palmaris longus:* This wrist-flexing muscle originates on the medial epicondyle of the humerus and inserts on the distal half of the flexor retinaculum. It's innervated by the median nerve.

✔ *Flexor carpi ulnaris:* This muscle flexes and adducts the hand. It has two heads:

  • The *humeral head* originates at the medial epicondyle of the humerus.

  • The *ulnar head* originates at the olecranon of the humerus.

It inserts on the pisiform, hook of the hamate, and the fifth metacarpal. It's innervated by the ulnar nerve.

✔ *Flexor digitorum superficialis:* This muscle also has two heads:

  • The *humeroulnar head* originates at the medial epicondyle of the humerus and the coronoid process of the ulna.

  • The *radial head* originates at the oblique line of the radius.

The flexor digitorum superficialis inserts on the bodies of the middle phalanges of the fingers, but not the thumb. It's innervated by the median nerve, and it flexes the proximal interphalangeal joints and flexes the proximal phalanges at the metacarpophalangeal joints.

✔ *Flexor digitorum profundus:* This muscle originates at a large part of the proximal and anterior surface of the ulna and the interosseous membrane (see Chapter 17) and inserts at the bases of the distal phalanges of the fingers, but not the thumb. It flexes the distal interphalangeal joints and helps flex the wrist. It's innervated by both the median nerve on the lateral side and the ulnar nerve on the medial side.

✔ *Flexor pollicis longus:* This thumb muscle originates at the anterior surface of the radius and interosseus membrane and attaches to the base of the distal phalanx of the thumb. It's innervated by the anterior interosseus branch of the median nerve and flexes the thumb.

✔ *Pronator quadratus:* This muscle originates on the anterior shaft of the ulna and inserts on the front of the radius. It's innervated by the median nerve, and it pronates the forearm to turn the palm from facing anterior to facing posterior.

You can see some of these muscles in Figure 18-2.

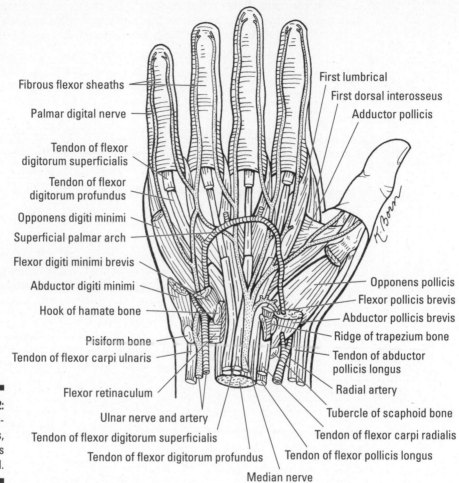

Fibrous flexor sheaths

Palmar digital nerve

Tendon of flexor digitorum superficialis

Tendon of flexor digitorum profundus

Opponens digiti minimi

Superficial palmar arch

Flexor digiti minimi brevis

Abductor digiti minimi

Hook of hamate bone

Pisiform bone

Tendon of flexor carpi ulnaris

Flexor retinaculum

Ulnar nerve and artery

Tendon of flexor digitorum superficialis

Tendon of flexor digitorum profundus

First lumbrical

First dorsal interosseus

Adductor pollicis

Opponens pollicis

Flexor pollicis brevis

Abductor pollicis brevis

Ridge of trapezium bone

Tendon of abductor pollicis longus

Radial artery

Tubercle of scaphoid bone

Tendon of flexor carpi radialis

Tendon of flexor pollicis longus

Median nerve

Figure 18-2:
Some muscles, nerves, and arteries of the hand.

The extensors

The extensors run down the posterior portion of the forearm (the posterior compartment). As with the wrist flexors in the preceding section, the bellies of the muscles are on the forearm and the tendons pass through the wrist and attach to the hand. They're held in place by the *extensor retinaculum*. (Some of these muscles extend fingers or the thumb, but because they originate on the forearm, we include them here.) The extensors are innervated by the radial nerve, which is coming up later in this chapter.

- *Extensor carpi radialis longus:* This muscle originates on the lateral supraepicondylar ridge of the humerus and inserts on the back of the base of the second metacarpal. It extends and abducts the hand at the wrist.

- *Extensor carpi radialis brevis:* Originating on the lateral epicondyle of the humerus, this muscle inserts at the back of the base of the third metacarpal. It extends and abducts the hand at the wrist and supports a clenched fist.

- *Extensor digitorum:* This muscle originates at the lateral epicondyle of the humerus and inserts at the *extensor expansions* of the fingers, but not the thumb. It extends the fingers at the metacarpophalangeal joints.

- *Extensor digiti minimi:* This finger muscle originates at the lateral epicondyle of the humerus and inserts on the extensor expansion of the fifth digit (pinkie finger). It extends the pinkie finger at the metacarpophalangeal joint.

- *Extensor carpi ulnaris:* Originating at the lateral epicondyle of the humerus and the back of the ulna, this muscle inserts on the back of the base of the fifth metacarpal. It extends and adducts the hand at the wrist.

- *Abductor pollicis longus:* Shown in Figure 18-2, this muscle originates at the back of the proximal portions of the ulna, radius, and interosseus membrane. It inserts onto the base of the first metacarpal and abducts and extends the thumb.

- *Extensor pollicis longus:* This thumb muscle originates at the back and middle of the ulna and interosseous membrane. It inserts to the back of the base of the distal phalanx of the thumb and extends that phalanx at the interphalangeal joint. It also extends the metacarpophalangeal and carpometacarpal joints of the thumb.

- *Extensor pollicis brevis:* Another thumb muscle, this one originates at the back of the distal radius and interosseous membrane and inserts onto the back of the base of the proximal phalanx of the thumb. It extends the proximal phalanx of the thumb at the metacarpophalangeal joint and extends the carpometacarpal joint.

- *Extensor indicis:* This muscle originates at the back and distal part of the ulna and interosseus membrane and inserts onto the extensor expansion of the index finger. It extends the index finger and extends the hand at the wrist.

Sticking out your thumb with the thenar muscles

The *thenar muscles* are intrinsic muscles contained within the *thenar compartment,* which is separated from other compartments by fascia (a layer of fibrous connective tissue that covers muscle). These four muscles (which you can see in Figure 18-2) move the thumb.

- *Abductor pollicis brevis:* This muscle originates at the flexor retinaculum and the tubercles on the scaphoid and trapezium bones. It inserts on the lateral side of the base of the proximal phalanx of the thumb. It abducts the thumb and is innervated by the median nerve. (We discuss all the nerves that innervate the thenar muscles later in this chapter.)

- *Flexor pollicis brevis:* This muscle originates and inserts close to the abductor pollicis brevis; however, it flexes the thumb (so it's probably helping you hold this book). It's innervated by the median nerve.

- *Opponens pollicis:* This muscle originates near the two brevis muscles, but it inserts on the lateral side of the first metacarpal. It helps to oppose the thumb (the movement you make when touching the thumb to the pinkie). It's innervated by the median nerve.

- *Adductor pollicis:* This muscle has two heads:

  • The *oblique head* originates at the bases of the second and third metacarpals and associated carpal bones.

  • The *transverse head* originates at the anterior part of the third metacarpal shaft.

  They insert on the medial side of the proximal phalanx of the thumb. The adductor pollicis adducts the thumb (pulls it in next to the fingers) and is innervated by the ulnar nerve.

The thenar muscles form the *thenar eminence,* which is that mound of muscle you can see at the base of the thumb.

Honing in on the hypothenar muscles

The *hypothenar muscles* are intrinsic muscles found in the *hypothenar compartment* and form the *hypothenar eminence* on the medial side of the palm of the hand. They're all innervated by the deep branch of the ulnar nerve (which we discuss later in this chapter), and they move the pinkie finger.

- *Abductor digiti minimi:* This muscle originates at the pisiform and inserts on the medial side of the base of the proximal phalanx of the little finger. It abducts the little finger (that is, pulls it away from the ring finger).

✔ *Flexor digiti minimi:* Originating at the hook of the hamate, this muscle inserts near the abductor digiti minimi. It flexes (curls toward the palm) the proximal phalanx of the little finger.

✔ *Opponens digiti minimi:* This muscle originates at the hook of the hamate and inserts onto the medial border of the fifth metacarpal. It pulls the fifth metacarpal forward and rotates it to oppose the thumb.

Investigating the interosseous muscles and the lumbricals

The third group of intrinsic muscles are the interosseous muscles and the lumbricals; they're found in the hand, and they move the fingers.

✔ *Interosseous muscles:* These seven muscles are innervated by the deep branch of the ulnar nerve (we talk about this nerve and others later in this chapter). They're divided into two groups:

- Four *dorsal interosseous muscles* run between the metacarpals and abduct the fingers (spread them apart). They also flex the metacarpophalangeal joints and extend the interphalangeal joints.

- Three *palmar interosseus muscles* are located on the palmar portion of the second, fourth, and fifth metacarpals. They adduct the fingers (squeeze them together). They also flex the metacarpophalangeal joints and extend the interphalangeal joints.

✔ *Lumbricals:* The lumbricals are located between the metacarpals. The first and second lumbricals are innervated by the median nerve, and the third and fourth lumbricals are innervated by the deep branch of the ulnar nerve. They flex the fingers at the metacarpophalangeal joints and extend the interphalangeal joints.

You can see some interosseus muscles and lumbricals in Figure 18-2.

Knowing the Nerves and Blood Supply of the Wrist and Hand

Busy muscles need plenty of nerve supply and blood flow. As you find out in the following sections, three main nerves (plus all their branches) work the wrist and hand, and many arteries and veins bring blood into and out of the hand.

Getting a handle on carpal tunnel syndrome

Sometimes the median nerve gets squeezed and compressed inside the carpal tunnel area. This pressure causes numbness and tingling in the palm, thumb, and the first two fingers. Eventually the pressure causes sharp shooting pains in your wrist and hand, and it can become more difficult to grab and hold on to things. This pain is known as *carpal tunnel syndrome.* A lot of times it starts at night if your wrist is flexed while you're sleeping. It typically starts in the dominant hand but can occur in both.

Women are more likely to suffer from carpal tunnel syndrome, maybe because the carpal tunnel is smaller in the female wrist. Following are other factors associated with carpal tunnel syndrome:

✔ Having a wrist injury that causes swelling

✔ Hormonal problems with the pituitary gland or thyroid

✔ Fluid retention during pregnancy, PMS, or menopause

✔ Repetitive use of certain types of hand tools

✔ Arthritis in the wrist

Carpal tunnel can be diagnosed by using a couple of orthopedic tests:

✔ The Tinel test is simply tapping your finger on the patient's wrist, right over the median nerve. The test is positive for carpal tunnel syndrome if it causes tingling in the fingers or a shocking sensation, which reproduces the patient's symptoms.

✔ To perform Phalen's test, have the patient force the hands into flexion by holding the arms out in front of the body, bending the wrists, and pressing the backs of the hands together with the fingers pointing downward. The test is positive if symptoms are reproduced within a minute or so.

Diagnosis can be confirmed with nerve conduction tests, which involve placing electrodes on the hand and wrist and measuring the nerve impulses. Carpal tunnel syndrome may be treated by wearing a splint, taking nonsteroidal anti-inflammatory medications for pain relief, and by making changes in the way you work with your wrist. Surgery may be indicated if the other treatments fail.

Getting a feeling for the nerves

REMEMBER

The main nerves you need to know for the wrist and hand come from the *median, ulnar,* and *radial nerves.* These nerves supply the skin, muscles, joints, and other tissues. The nerves allow you to feel what your hands and fingers are touching and help you move those muscles around. You can find these and other nerves in Figure 18-2.

✔ *Median nerve:* The median nerve enters the hand through the *carpal tunnel,* which is a passageway between the tubercles of the scaphoid and trapezium bones laterally and by the pisiform and the hook of the hamate on the medial side. It gives nerve supply to the thenar muscles and the first two lumbricals that we discuss earlier in this chapter, plus it sends sensory fibers to the skin on the lateral part of the palm and to the sides and distal portions of the first three digits.

The *palmar cutaneous branch of the median nerve* branches off before the carpal tunnel. It innervates the middle of the palm.

✓ **Ulnar nerve:** The ulnar nerve comes from under the tendon of the flexor carpi ulnaris and runs through the *ulnar tunnel* (or tunnel of Guyon), which is between the pisiform and the hook of the hamate. The ulnar nerve and its *dorsal cutaneous, palmar cutaneous,* and *superficial branches* innervate the medial portion of the wrist and hand and the medial one and a half digits. The *deep branch of the ulnar nerve* serves the hypothenar muscles that we talk about earlier in this chapter.

✓ **Radial nerve:** The radial nerve has two branches in the forearm: The *deep branch* runs through the posterior part of the forearm, supplying motor innervation to the extensor muscles. The *superficial branch* is a cutaneous nerve that runs under the brachioradialis muscle and passes through the anatomical snuff box, which is a visible depression formed near the base of the thumb by the tendons of the extensor pollicis longus and extensor pollicis brevis muscles. It doesn't innervate any intrinsic hand muscles; instead, it innervates the skin and fascia of the lateral portion of the back of the hand and lateral three and half digits.

Uncovering the arteries and veins

The ulnar and radial arteries carry blood down through the forearm into the wrist, where they *anastomose* (join together) to form arches. These arches, along with several branches, supply blood to the hand and digits.

Here are the arteries that enter the wrist:

✓ **Anterior interosseous artery:** This artery runs from the ulnar artery anterior to the interosseous membrane. It pierces the membrane distally to join the dorsal carpal arch.

✓ **Palmar carpal branch:** This branch runs from the ulnar artery over the anterior part of the wrist under the flexor digitorum profundus tendons.

✓ **Dorsal carpal branch:** This branch runs from the ulnar artery across the back of the wrist under the extensor tendons.

✓ **Palmar carpal branch:** This branch runs from the radial artery across the anterior wrist underneath the flexor tendons.

✓ **Dorsal carpal branch:** This branch runs from the radial artery across the wrist beneath the pollicis and extensor radialis tendons.

These carpal branches of the ulnar arteries join together with the carpal branches of the radial arteries to form two arches in the wrist:

- ✔ *Palmar carpal arch:* The area where the palmar carpal branches of the radial and ulnar arteries meet

- ✔ *Dorsal carpal arch:* Formed by the anastomoses of the dorsal carpal branches of the radial and ulnar arteries

Next up are the arteries and branches that supply blood to the hands and fingers. They also come from the radial and ulnar arteries.

- ✔ *Superficial palmar arch:* This arch is formed by the ulnar artery anastomosing with a superficial branch of the radial artery. It runs in front of the flexor tendons near the middle of the metacarpal bones. (Refer to Figure 18-2 for a picture.)

- ✔ *Deep palmar arch:* This arch is made by the radial artery and a deep branch of the ulnar artery. It runs along the bases of the metacarpals.

- ✔ *Common palmar digitals:* These branches leave the superficial palmar arch to run along the lumbricals to the webbing of the fingers.

- ✔ *Proper palmar digitals:* These branches start from the common palmar digitals and run along the sides of the fingers, but not the thumb.

- ✔ *Princeps pollicis:* This artery starts at the radial artery at the palm and descends to past the first metacarpal to the proximal phalanx of the thumb. There it splits into two branches that run along the sides of the thumb.

- ✔ *Radialis indicis:* This branch arises from the radial artery and runs along the lateral side of the index finger.

The *superficial and deep palmar venous arches* return blood to the heart and are located near the arterial arches. They drain into the deep veins of the forearm (see Chapter 17). *Dorsal digital veins* drain into *dorsal metacarpal veins,* which form the dorsal venous network. This blood drains into the cephalic and basilic veins (see Chapters 16 and 17).

Fitting Like a Glove: The Surface Anatomy of the Wrist and Hand

Earlier in this chapter, we look at the inside of the wrists and hands, so now we check out what's on the outside and just under the surface.

The *fascia of the palm* is thinner over both the thenar and hypothenar eminences. It thickens between the two eminences and forms the *palmar aponeurosis,* a central thickened portion of the deep palmar fascia, and fascial sheaths that surround the fingers. The palmar aponeurosis covers the softer parts of the hand and covers the tendons of those long flexor muscles.

The creases in the skin of the palm are fairly similar in everyone. That's because those are the places where the skin is attached to the deep fascia below.

Here are some landmarks of the wrist and hand surface anatomy:

- ✔ The tendons of the flexor carpi radialis and the palmaris longus are palpable (in other words, you can medically examine them); they're probably visible on the anterior portion of the forearm and wrist. Clenching the fist may make them more prominent.

- ✔ The pisiform bone is palpated just below the hypothenar eminence. It feels like a bony bump on the medial edge of the wrist distal to the moveable part of the wrist.

- ✔ The tendons of extensor digitorum are visible on the back of the hand. They run under the skin from the wrist to the fingers, passing over the knuckles.

- ✔ The head of the ulna may be visible and is palpable on the medial side of the wrist; it's the bony bump on the medial side of the wrist proximal to the moveable part of the wrist.

- ✔ The *anatomical snuff box* is a skin depression bordered by the tendons of the abductor pollicis longus and the extensor pollicis brevis on one side and the extensor pollicis longus on the other side. It's visible and palpable at the base of the thumb. The radial artery and the superficial branch of the radial nerve run through this area.

Chapter 19

Getting Hip to the Hip and the Thigh

*U*nderstanding the anatomy of the pelvic girdle and thighs is important for knowing how people walk and move; you can then diagnose a variety of ailments, especially those related to exercise. This chapter covers the anatomy of the hips and thighs, including the bones, joints, muscles, and neurovascular structures; we also cover a few important surface landmarks for you.

Honing In on Hip and Thigh Bones

The hip bones and the thigh bones (or femurs) are large bones that support your upper body, help you walk around, and support your back when you lift things off the ground. Lucky you — you don't have to memorize too many bones in this region!

The left and right hip (coxal) bones, the sacrum, and the coccyx form the *pelvic girdle,* which is the housing for the pelvic organs. The hip bones also form the socket portion of the hip joint. Each hip bone is made up of three parts — the *ilium,* the *ischium,* and the *pubis.* We cover the hip bones in more detail in Chapter 11.

Breaking down hip fractures

A hip fracture is a break somewhere in the upper part of the femur. It usually occurs from a fall or a direct blow to the hip. People who have osteoporosis, cancer, or certain stress injuries may be at a greater risk for suffering a hip fracture, which may require surgery and a long recovery, especially if the patient is elderly.

Hip fractures are categorized by the location of the fracture (although fractures may occur in more than one area at a time).

✔ **Intracapsular fractures:** Occur at the head and the neck of the femur and usually remain within the joint capsule

✔ **Intertrochanteric fractures:** Occur between the neck and the lesser trochanter and usually cross the area between the two trochanters

✔ **Subtrochanteric fractures:** Occur below the lesser trochanter on the shaft of the femur

The *femur* is the longest and heaviest bone in the human body. It extends from the hip (the proximal end) to the knee (the distal end). Here we talk about the proximal and middle parts, and we cover the distal portion of the femur in Chapter 20, which is all about the knee.

The femur has several important features:

✔ *Head:* A ball-shaped feature at the proximal end of the bone, with a *fovea* (or indentation) for the ligament of the head of the femur

✔ *Neck:* Connects the head to the shaft

✔ *Shaft:* The long part of the bone, with two large projections on the proximal end:

- *Lesser trochanter:* Extends medially from the shaft

- *Greater trochanter:* Extends superiorly and laterally (up and out) from the proximal part of the shaft

✔ *Intertrochanteric line:* A ridge that runs between the trochanters on the anterior (front) side

✔ *Intertrochanteric crest:* Runs between the trochanters on the posterior (back) side of the bone

✔ *Linea aspera:* A long ridge that runs down the back of the shaft

You can see the hip bones and the femur in Figure 19-1.

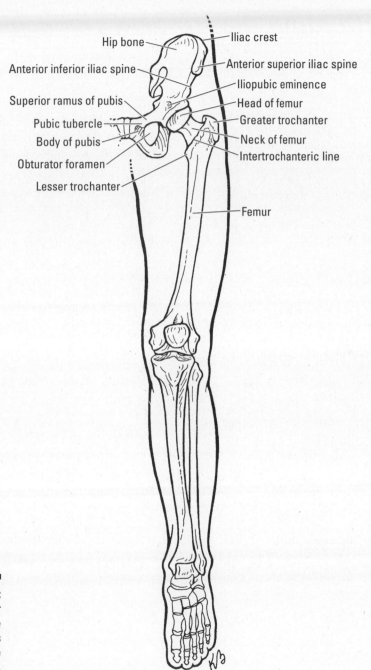

Hip bone

Anterior inferior iliac spine

Superior ramus of pubis

Pubic tubercle

Body of pubis

Obturator foramen

Lesser trochanter

Iliac crest

Anterior superior iliac spine

Iliopubic eminence

Head of femur

Greater trochanter

Neck of femur

Intertrochanteric line

Femur

Figure 19-1:
The anterior view of the hip bones and the femur.

Understanding the Hip and Thigh Joints

Because the hips and thighs don't have many bones, they don't have many joints to look at, either. In the following sections we explore these three joints:

- ✔ *Sacroiliac joint:* Has very little movement; supports the weight of your body

- ✔ *Symphysis pubis:* Also has very little movement; simply joins the hip bones together at the front of your pelvis

- ✔ *Acetabulofemoral joint* **(the hip joint):** Has much more movement and allows you to kick, run, jump, and move your lower extremities in many different directions

Seeking the sacroiliac joint

The *right and left sacroiliac joints* are formed by the sacrum (see Chapter 15) and the iliac bones. They're strong joints that have to bear weight. Each sacroiliac joint is called a *compound joint* because it's made up of two joints: a synovial joint (at the anterior part of the joint), with its joint capsule, and a syndesmosis (at the posterior part of the joint). (See Chapter 3 for more about types of joints.) Unlike most synovial joints, the sacroiliac joint isn't very mobile.

The sacroiliac joints are supported by five ligaments:

- ✔ *Anterior sacroiliac ligaments:* Make up the fibrous joint capsules

- ✔ *Interosseous sacroiliac ligaments:* Transfer the weight of the body through the sacroiliac joints to the femur when you stand or to the ischial tuberosities of the hip bones when you sit

- ✔ *Posterior sacroiliac ligaments:* Extend from the interosseous sacroiliac ligaments

- ✔ *Sacrotuberous* **and** *sacrospinous ligaments:* Support the sacrum and give resiliency to the sacroiliac joints when the vertebral column sustains sudden force

Surveying the symphysis pubis

The *symphysis pubis* is a cartilaginous joint that's formed where the pubic portions of the two hip bones meet anteriorly. This joint has very little movement. It contains a fibrocartilaginous disc called the *interpubic disc,* which is usually larger in women than it is in men.

Two ligaments stabilize the symphysis pubis:

- ✔ The *superior pubic ligament* at the top of the joint
- ✔ The *inferior pubic ligament* along the bottom

Looking at the acetabulofemoral joint

The *acetabulofemoral joint* is the connection of the hip bones with the femur. It's a strong ball-and-socket synovial joint that provides for movement in several different directions. The head of the femur forms the ball, and the cup-shaped *acetabulum* forms the socket. The head of the femur and the *lunate surface of the acetabulum (just inside the rim of the acetabulum)* are covered with cartilage. A fibrocartilagenous rim in the acetabulum forms a lip that increases the depth of the socket. The lip is called the *acetabular labrum.* The joint is lined with a synovial membrane, part of which forms a bursa (a fluid-filled sac) for the obturator externus tendon that we mention in the later section "The medial thigh muscles."

Several ligaments and tissues support this joint:

- ✔ *Transverse acetabular ligament:* This ligament is continuous with the acetabular labrum and helps deepen the socket inferiorly. A fibrous joint capsule attaches to both the hip bone and the transverse acetabular ligament.

- ✔ *Iliofemoral ligament:* This strong Y-shaped ligament is attached to the anterior inferior iliac spine (see Chapter 11) and the acetabular rim and the intertrochanteric line. The iliofemoral ligament prevents hyperextension.

- ✔ *Pubofemoral ligament:* This ligament runs from the obturator crest of the pubic bone (see Chapter 11) to the acetabular joint capsule. It merges with the medial portion of the iliofemoral ligament. It prevents the hip from going too far during abduction (moving the lower extremity away from the midline of the body).

- ✔ *Ischiofemoral ligament:* This ligament runs in a spiral from the acetabular rim to the femur's neck. It supports the joint posteriorly.

- ✔ *Ligament of the head of the femur:* This ligament contains a blood vessel, but it offers little support to the joint.

Swaying Your Hips and Moving Your Thighs with the Help of Muscles

The hips and thighs can move in many different ways due to combinations of lots of muscles. In the following sections, we start with the muscles of the gluteal region. Then we move on to the muscles of the thigh.

Minding the muscles of the buttocks

The gluteal muscles are located on your backside and move your hip. You can see these muscles in Figure 19-2:

- ✔ **Gluteus maximus:** This muscle originates on the posterior gluteal line of the ilium (a curved line that runs from the iliac crest to the greater sciatic notch), the sacrum, the coccyx, and the sacrotuberous ligament (which we mention earlier in this chapter). It inserts onto the *iliotibial tract (band)* of the tensor fasciae latae and the gluteal tuberosity of the femur. It's innervated by the inferior gluteal nerve and extends the thigh (straightens it from a bent or flexed position) and laterally rotates the thigh. (We describe the nerves of the hips and thighs later in this chapter.)

- ✔ **Gluteus medius:** This muscle originates on the ilium between the anterior and posterior gluteal lines and inserts on the lateral portion of the greater trochanter of the femur. It's innervated by the superior gluteal nerve. The gluteus medius abducts and medially rotates the thigh, and it also keeps the pelvis level when the opposite leg is raised.

- ✔ **Gluteus minimus:** This muscle originates between the anterior and posterior gluteal lines of the ilium and inserts onto the anterior surface of the greater trochanter of the femur. It's innervated by the superior gluteal nerve, and it assists the gluteus medius.

- ✔ **Tensor fasciae latae:** This muscle originates on the anterior superior iliac spine and iliac crest (see Chapter 11). It inserts onto the iliotibial tract that inserts into the lateral condyle tibia (see Chapter 20). It's innervated by the superior gluteal nerve and helps to abduct and flex the thigh.

- ✔ **Piriformis:** Originating on the anterior surface of the sacrum, the greater sciatic notch, and the sacrotuberous ligament, this muscle inserts onto the greater trochanter of the femur. It's innervated by the branches of the first two sacral spinal nerves. The piriformis laterally rotates the thigh when the thigh is in extension and abducts the thigh when it's flexed.

- *Obturator internus:* This muscle originates on the ilium and ischium and inserts onto the greater trochanter of the femur. It's innervated by the nerve to the obturator internus and works with the piriformis.

- *Superior* and *inferior gemellus:* The superior gemellus originates on the ischial spine, and the inferior gemellus originates on the ischial tuberosity. They both insert onto the greater trochanter. The superior gemellus is innervated by the nerve to the obturator internus, and the inferior gemellus is innervated by the nerve to quadratus femoris. They work with the piriformis and obturator internus to laterally rotate the thigh in extension and abduct the thigh in flexion.

- *Quadratus femoris:* This muscle originates on the lateral side of the ischial tuberosity and inserts on the intertrochanteric crest of the femur. It's innervated by the nerve to the quadratus femoris, and it laterally rotates the thigh.

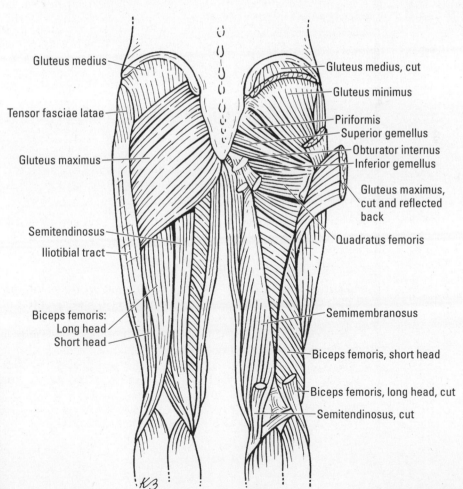

Figure 19-2:
Muscles of the posterior gluteal region and thigh.

Gluteus medius

Tensor fasciae latae

Gluteus maximus

Semitendinosus

Iliotibial tract

Biceps femoris:
Long head
Short head

Gluteus medius, cut

Gluteus minimus

Piriformis

Superior gemellus

Obturator internus

Inferior gemellus

Gluteus maximus, cut and reflected back

Quadratus femoris

Semimembranosus

Biceps femoris, short head

Biceps femoris, long head, cut

Semitendinosus, cut

The muscles that work together to laterally rotate your hip are referred to as the *lateral rotators,* and they include the piriformis, gemellus superior, obterator internus, gemellus inferior, obturator externus, and quadratus femoris. We tell you a mnemonic in Chapter 22 that helps you remember which muscle goes where.

Gluteal bursae contain synovial fluid and help to reduce friction between a muscle and its tendon and bone. The gluteal muscles have three bursa:

- ✔ *Trochanteric bursa:* Lies between the gluteus maximus and the greater trochanter of the femur
- ✔ *Ischial bursa:* Separates the gluteus maximus from the ischial tuberosity
- ✔ *Gluteofemoral bursa:* Lies between the iliotibial band and the origin of the vastus lateralis (see the next section for more about this muscle)

Bursitis is an inflammation of a bursa, and it can result in pain near the joint area. The trochanteric bursa is the mostly commonly affected bursa of the hip joint. *Trochanteric bursitis* can cause pain on the lateral part of the hip, which can radiate down the lateral part of the thigh. The pain is often triggered during activities like running, climbing stairs, or getting up from a seated position.

Turning with the thigh muscles

As you find out in the following sections, the thigh muscles can be divided into three groups:

- ✔ The *anterior thigh muscles,* which extend your leg and flex your thigh
- ✔ The *medial thigh muscles,* which adduct and rotate your thigh
- ✔ The *posterior thigh muscles,* which flex your leg and extend your thigh

The anterior thigh muscles

The muscles of the anterior part of the thigh include the quadriceps group and a few others:

- ✔ *Quadriceps femoris:* This muscle includes four heads that originate in different locations but all share the *quadriceps tendon,* which inserts onto the patella (or kneecap). The continuation of the quadriceps tendon that extends from the patella and inserts onto the tibial tuberosity of the tibia is called the *patellar ligament* (see Chapter 20 for more on the patella and the tibia). All four parts of the muscle are innervated by the femoral nerve (which we describe later in this chapter with other nerves), and they extend the knee. The rectus femoris, however, also flexes the hip.

- *Rectus femoris* forms the middle portion of the quadriceps. It originates at the anterior inferior iliac spine and just above the acetabulum of the hip bone.

- *Vastus lateralis* is the lateral-most head. It originates at the greater trochanter and the linea aspera of the femur.

- *Vastus medialis* is the most medial of the heads. It originates on the intertrochanteric line and linea aspera.

- *Vastus intermedius* lies behind the rectus femoris. It originates on the shaft of the femur.

✔ *Pectineus:* This muscle originates on the superior ramus of the pubis portion of the hip bone (see Chapter 11) and inserts on the pectineal line of the femur. It's innervated by the femoral nerve and adducts and flexes the thigh.

✔ *Sartorius:* Originating on the anterior superior iliac spine, this muscle inserts on the medial surface of the tibia. It's innervated by the femoral nerve, and it flexes, abducts, and laterally rotates the thigh. It also flexes the leg at the knee.

✔ *Iliopsoas:* The iliopsoas is made up of two muscles that flex the thigh. One of those muscles, the psoas major, is also important for posture:

- *Psoas major* originates on the 12th thoracic and the five lumbar vertebrae (see Chapter 15). It inserts onto the lesser trochanter of the femur and is innervated by the first three lumbar spinal nerves.

- *Iliacus* originates on the iliac crest, sacrum, and sacroiliac ligaments. It inserts onto the tendons of the psoas major and the lesser trochanter of the femur. It's innervated by the femoral nerve.

The medial thigh muscles

The muscles of the medial part of the thigh include muscles that bring the thigh toward the midline and rotate it:

✔ *Adductor longus:* This muscle originates on the pubis and inserts onto the middle of the linea aspera of the femur. It's innervated by the obturator nerve and adducts the thigh.

✔ *Adductor brevis:* Originating on the pubis and inserting on the pectineal line and linea aspera of the femur, this muscle is innervated by the obturator nerve. It adducts the thigh.

✔ *Adductor magnus:* This muscle originates on the pubis and the ischial tuberosity. It inserts onto the gluteal tuberosity, linea aspera, and the adductor tubercle of the femur. It's innervated by the obturator nerve and the sciatic nerve. It adducts the thigh and assists in both flexion and extension of the thigh.

✔ *Gracilis:* This muscle originates on the pubis and inserts on the medial tibia. It's innervated by the obturator nerve. It adducts the thigh and flexes the leg at the knee.

✔ *Obturator externus:* Originating at the obturator foramen and membrane of the hip bone, this muscle inserts onto the femur. It's innervated by the obturator nerve and laterally rotates the thigh.

The posterior thigh muscles

The three muscles of the posterior thigh are known as the *hamstring muscles* (visible in Figure 19-2). They extend the thigh from a flexed position and flex the leg.

✔ *Semimembranosus:* The most medial of the three hamstring muscles, this muscle originates on the ischial tuberosity and inserts on the medial condyle of the tibia. It functions with the semitendinosus to extend the thigh and flex and medially rotate the leg. It's innervated by the tibial portion of the sciatic nerve.

✔ *Semitendinosus:* This muscle originates on the ischial tuberosity and inserts onto the superior part of the medial tibia. It's innervated by the tibial portion of the sciatic nerve and extends the thigh and flexes and medially rotates the leg.

✔ *Biceps femoris:* The most lateral of the hamstrings, the biceps femoris has two heads: the long and the short. The long head originates on the ischial tuberosity, and the short head originates on the linea aspera of the femur. They insert onto the lateral side of the fibula. The long head is innervated by the tibial portion of the sciatic nerve, and the short head is innervated by the fibular portion of the sciatic nerve. It extends the thigh and flexes and laterally rotates the leg.

Maintaining the Hip and Thigh Tissues

The joints and muscles of the hips and thighs need nervous input so they can do what your brain wants them to do. The muscles also require a lot of blood flow, which provides oxygen and nourishment, especially when you're physically active. Lymph is also drained away by the lymphatic structures. We delve into the nerves, blood vessels, and lymphatics of the hips and thighs in the following sections.

Knowing the nerves

The following nerves serve the gluteal and thigh regions.

The nerves of the gluteal region and the posterior thigh

You can see some of the following nerves of the gluteal and posterior thigh region in Figure 19-3:

- *Superior clunial nerve* **(L1–L3):** This nerve starts from the 1st through 3rd lumbar spinal nerves (see Chapter 15) and crosses the iliac crest to supply to the skin over the buttocks.

- *Middle clunial nerve* **(S1–S3):** Starting from the 1st through 3rd sacral spinal nerves, this nerve runs to the gluteal region to supply the skin over the buttocks.

- *Inferior clunial nerve:* This nerve branches from the posterior cutaneous nerve of the thigh to the inferior border of the gluteus maximus. It also supplies the skin over the buttocks.

- *Sciatic nerve* **(L4–S3):** This nerve branches from the sacral plexus (see Chapter 15) and passes through the greater sciatic foramen (see Chapter 11) to enter the gluteal region. From there it traverses underneath the biceps femoris and splits into the tibial and common fibular nerves at the knee (see Chapter 20). It innervates the muscles of the posterior thigh.

The sciatic nerve is the longest and widest nerve in the human body and can quite literally cause a pain in the butt when it's compressed by a herniated disc or sometimes by the piriformis muscle. The pain, along with burning, numbness, and tingling sensations, may also be felt in the lower back and down the back of leg on the affected side. This condition is called *sciatica* and can be treated with ice packs, special exercises, and nonsteroidal anti-inflammatory medications. It may also help to avoid sitting positions for long periods of time.

- *Posterior cutaneous nerve of the thigh* **(S1–S3):** Beginning at the sacral plexus, this nerve runs through the greater sciatic foramen and under the gluteus maximus before traveling down the thigh deep to the tensor fasciae latae. It innervates the skin of the buttock, posterior thigh, and calf. It also has a perineal branch that innervates the perineum (see Chapter 11) and upper medial thigh.

- *Superior gluteal nerve* **(L4–S1):** This nerve runs from the sacral plexus through the greater sciatic foramen and between the gluteus medius and minimus. It innervates those two muscles along with the tensor fasciae latae.

✔ *Inferior gluteal nerve* (L5–S2): Running from the sacral plexus though the greater sciatic foramen, this nerve then divides into several branches that innervate the gluteus maximus.

✔ *Nerve to quadratus femoris* (L4–S1): This nerve runs from the sacral plexus through the greater sciatic foramen and innervates the hip joint, inferior gemellus, and quadratus femoris.

✔ *Pudendal nerve* (S2–S4): This nerve runs from the sacral plexus through the greater sciatic foramen and enters the perineum through the lesser sciatic foramen. It innervates the perineum.

✔ *Nerve to obturator internus* (L5–S2): Running from the sacral plexus through the greater sciatic foramen, this nerve enters the lesser sciatic foreman to the obturator internus. It innervates the superior gemellus and obturator internus muscles.

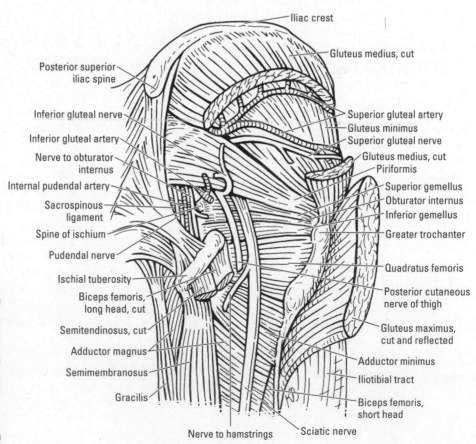

Figure 19-3: The nerves and blood supply of the gluteal region and the posterior thigh.

Iliac crest

Gluteus medius, cut

Posterior superior iliac spine

Inferior gluteal nerve

Inferior gluteal artery

Nerve to obturator internus

Internal pudendal artery

Sacrospinous ligament

Spine of ischium

Pudendal nerve

Ischial tuberosity

Biceps femoris, long head, cut

Semitendinosus, cut

Adductor magnus

Semimembranosus

Gracilis

Superior gluteal artery

Gluteus minimus

Superior gluteal nerve

Gluteus medius, cut

Piriformis

Superior gemellus

Obturator internus

Inferior gemellus

Greater trochanter

Quadratus femoris

Posterior cutaneous nerve of thigh

Gluteus maximus, cut and reflected

Adductor minimus

Iliotibial tract

Biceps femoris, short head

Nerve to hamstrings

Sciatic nerve

The nerves of the anterior and medial thigh

Three nerves run through the region of the anterior and medial thigh:

- *Femoral nerve* (L2–L4): This nerve runs from the lumbar plexus along the psoas major that we describe earlier in this chapter and past the inguinal ligament (see Chapter 9) to enter the femoral triangle. It has branches that innervate the anterior thigh muscles and the hip joint.

- *Obturator nerve* (L2–L4): This nerve runs along the psoas major through the obturator foramen, where it divides into anterior and posterior branches. It innervates the adductor longus, adductor brevis, gracilis, pectineus, obturator externus, and adductor magnus.

- *Saphenous nerve:* This nerve is the terminal cutaneous branch of the femoral nerve. It accompanies the femoral artery and innervates the skin and fascia of the knee, leg, and foot.

Flowing through the arteries and veins

The arteries that provide blood to the hip and the thigh can also be grouped by regions. You can see some of the following arteries of the gluteal and posterior thigh region in Figure 19-3:

- *Superior gluteal artery:* This artery starts from the internal iliac artery (see Chapter 11). It has a superficial branch that enters the gluteal region through the greater sciatic foramen and a deep branch that runs between the gluteus minimus and gluteus medius muscles. The superficial branch supplies blood to the gluteus maximus muscle, and the deep branch supplies blood to the gluteus minimus and medius muscles.

- *Inferior gluteal artery:* Branching off the internal iliac artery, this artery enters the gluteal region through the sciatic foramen to run along the sciatic nerve. It *anastomoses* (a fancy word for *joins*) with the superior gluteal artery and several other arteries. It supplies blood to the gluteus maximus, obturator internus, quadratus femoris, and hamstring muscles.

- *Internal pudendal artery:* This artery branches off the internal iliac artery, enters the gluteal region through the sciatic foramen, and enters the perineum via the lesser sciatic foramen (see Chapter 11). It supplies blood to the external genitalia and parts of the perineum.

- *Perforating arteries:* These arteries branch off the deep femoral artery and provide blood to the hamstring muscles and vastus lateralis.

Following are the arteries of the anterior and medial thigh:

- **Femoral artery:** A continuation of the external iliac artery (see Chapter 11), the femoral artery runs through the femoral triangle and the adductor canal. It then goes on to become the popliteal artery (see Chapter 20). It supplies blood to anterior and medial structures of the thigh.

- **Deep femoral artery (profunda femoris artery):** This artery branches off the femoral artery below the inguinal ligament and runs underneath the adductor longus. It supplies blood to muscles of the thigh.

- **Lateral circumflex femoral artery:** This artery usually starts from the deep femoral artery (but sometimes arises from the femoral artery) and runs deep to the sartorius and rectus femoris muscles. It supplies blood to the anterior part of the gluteal region.

- **Medial circumflex femoral artery:** Typically arising from the deep femoral artery (but sometimes from the femoral artery), this artery runs between the pectineus and iliopsoas muscles to the gluteal region. It supplies blood to the head and neck of the femur.

- **Obturator artery:** This artery branches off the internal iliac artery and runs to the medial part of the thigh. It supplies blood to the obturator externus, pectineus, adductors, and gracilis. It also supplies blood to the muscles near the ischial tuberosities.

Veins return blood from the hip and thigh to the heart. They accompany most of the arteries and have the same names. The most important veins to know are the great saphenous vein and the femoral vein:

- **Great saphenous vein:** This superficial vein travels in the subcutaneous tissue on the anteromedial aspect of the thigh and leg and empties into the femoral vein.

- **Femoral vein:** This vein enters into the pelvic cavity deep to the inguinal ligament, where it becomes the external iliac vein (see Chapter 8).

Looking at the lymphatics

Superficial lymphatic vessels in the thigh follow along with the great saphenous vein and travel up to the *superficial inguinal lymph nodes* located in the inguinal area (see Chapter 11). Lymph drains from these nodes into *external iliac lymph nodes* and the *deep inguinal lymph nodes* of the pelvis.

Lymph from the gluteal region drains into the *gluteal lymph nodes* located next to the gluteal veins (tributaries of the pudendal veins; see Chapter 11) and then into the *iliac lymph nodes* and the *lumbar lymph nodes* of the pelvis.

Summing Up the Surface Landmarks

The hip and thigh are covered with skin and varying amounts of hair. The gluteus maximus gives the buttocks their rounded shape, with the intergluteal cleft separating the two mounds of muscle. Indentations called the *dimples of Venus* may be seen above the buttocks, over the sacroiliac joints.

The quadriceps group of muscles and the hamstring muscles may be visible or palpable under the skin. The hip and thigh area is a common area for adipose tissue (body fat) to accumulate, especially in females.

The femoral artery may be palpated in the *femoral triangle,* which is formed in the anterior and superior part of the thigh. It can be seen as a depression below the inguinal ligament (which runs between the pubic tubercle and the anterior superior iliac spine – see Chapter 11) when the thigh is flexed, abducted, and rotated laterally. It's bounded by the inguinal ligament, the adductor longus muscle, and the sartorius muscle. To find the artery, first palpate the pubis (pubic bone of the pelvis) in the midline of the body. Next, feel for the anterior iliac spine (large bony bump at the anterior of the hip bone; see Chapter 11). The femoral artery is midway between those two structures.

The femoral triangle contains the femoral nerve and the femoral vein. It also is home to deep inguinal lymph nodes.

The *adductor canal* runs from the top of the femoral triangle to the tendon of the adductor magnus. This canal allows nerves and veins to run between the muscles down to the popliteal fossa behind the knee (see Chapter 20).

Chapter 20

Knowing the Knee and the Leg

- -

- -

Without the knee, you'd have a difficult time walking, and you'd have to redesign the recliner in your family room. Knee injuries are the bane of many professional athletes, but knee pain can make life miserable for anybody. The leg is important, too, because it holds on to your foot. In clinical anatomy, the word *leg* refers only to that part between the knee and the ankle. The part above the knee is the *thigh*.

This chapter reviews the bones and joints that make up the knee and leg. Of course, the muscles, nerves, blood vessels, and lymphatics that are part of the knee and leg are important, too. We wrap up with the surface landmarks you need to know.

Logging the Knee and Leg Bones

The bones of the knee and the leg (see Figure 20-1) include the femur, which is the large thigh bone; the tibia and fibula, which are the leg bones between the knee and ankle; and the patella, which is sometimes called the kneecap.

✔ **Femur:** This long bone runs between the hip and the knee. The proximal portion of the femur (which is closer to the trunk) is covered in Chapter 19; here we review the distal portion (which is farther from the trunk). The *medial* and *lateral femoral condyles* protrude from the distal end of the femur (the medial femoral condyle is close to the midline of the body, and the lateral femoral condyle is farther from the midline). Posteriorly, the indented space between the condyles is called the *intercondylar fossa*. Anteriorly, the condyles are joined, forming the smooth patellar surface.

The *linea aspera* is a ridge that runs longitudinally (lengthwise) along the posterior surface of the femur. At its distal end, it diverges into the *medial* and *lateral supracondylar lines* that run toward their respective condyles. These lines serve as attachment points for muscles.

✔ **Tibia:** This long bone is the larger of the two leg bones below the knee. (The distal portion nearest the ankle is covered in Chapter 21.) The proximal end has two projections, called the *medial* and *lateral condyles.* An *intercondylar eminence* with two tubercles (bony prominences) lies between the condyles. The articular surfaces between the condyles and eminence are called the *medial* and *lateral tibial plateaus.* The *tibial tuberosity* (another bony outgrowth) projects anteriorly from the shaft.

Medial tibial stress syndrome (MTSS), better known as "shin splints," is a common condition, especially in people who jog or run frequently. It may be the result of a strained tibialis anterior muscle or feet that pronate too much (in other words, flat feet). Shin splints cause a dull, achy pain in the anterior part of the leg. Treatment for shin splints includes rest, ice on the anterior part of the leg, nonsteroidal anti-inflammatory medications, and arch supports or appropriate shoes.

✔ **Fibula:** This long bone, the thinner of the two leg bones, is located lateral to the tibia. (The distal part of the fibula is covered in Chapter 21.) The proximal part of the fibula has an enlarged head that articulates (forms a joint) with the tibia.

The shafts of the tibia and fibula are connected by an *interosseous membrane.* It's a sheet of connective tissue that fills most of the space between the two bones. The membrane has one opening at the top that allows for passage of blood vessels.

✔ **Patella:** This large sesamoid bone is formed in the tendon of the quadriceps muscle (we tell you more about that muscle later in this chapter; flip to Chapter 3 for details on sesamoid and other types of bones). It's shaped like a triangle, with a thick *base* forming the superior (top) border. The pointed *apex* is at the inferior (bottom) part of the bone. The anterior (front) surface is slightly convex (in other words, the surface curves outward), and the posterior (back) part has *medial* and *lateral articular surfaces* (articular surfaces are joint forming).

Patellofemoral syndrome, or chondromalacia patella, is a painful condition in which the cartilage on the articular surfaces of the patella becomes soft and breaks down. The condition occurs when the patella rubs against the femur due to problems with patellar alignment or excessive physical activity involving the knee. Patellofemoral syndrome is most commonly seen in adolescent and young adult females.

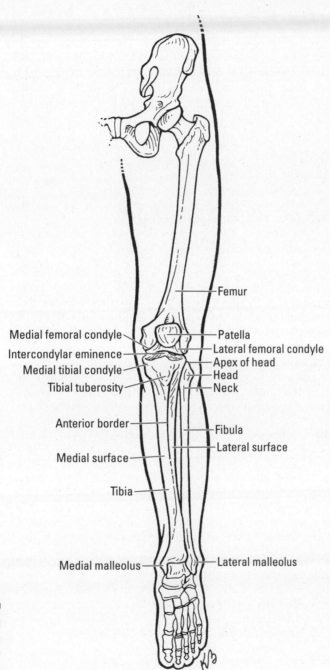

Femur

Medial femoral condyle

Intercondylar eminence

Medial tibial condyle

Tibial tuberosity

Anterior border

Medial surface

Tibia

Medial malleolus

Patella

Lateral femoral condyle

Apex of head

Head

Neck

Fibula

Lateral surface

Lateral malleolus

Figure 20-1:
The bones
of the knee
and leg.

Knocking the Knee Joint

The knee joint is basically a hinge joint that lets you flex and extend the leg, although there is a small amount of gliding movement as well (see Chapter 3 for details on hinge and other types of joints). Although it's a large joint, it isn't as stable as many other joints, so injuring the knee is fairly easy to do (much to the disappointment of many athletes).

In the following sections, we describe the structures in and around the knee joint, including different types of cartilage and ligaments.

Coming up with cartilage and the joint capsule

The knee joint is formed by the articulation of the condyles of the distal femur with the articular surfaces of the proximal tibia (see the previous section for more about these bones). The fibular head also articulates with the lateral part of the tibia. The patella articulates with the patellar surface of the femur, and it rests in the quadriceps tendon and helps protect the knee joint.

The articular surfaces of the main part of the knee joint (technically called the *femorotibial articulations*) are found on the articular surfaces between the condyles of both bones. They're covered with hyaline cartilage. In addition, the knee joint is surrounded by a joint capsule that's made of two layers:

- ✔ An external thin layer of fibrous connective tissue
- ✔ An inner synovial membrane that lines the joint

The *infrapatellar fat pad* lies anterior to the joint capsule but behind the patella. It helps cushion the knee joint.

The infrapatellar fat pad can become pinched between the condyles of the femur and the patella due to direct impact to the knee. The fat pad is quite sensitive, so this pinching can become very painful, especially if the tissue becomes inflamed.

Balancing the menisci

Two crescent-shaped pieces of fibrocartilage called *menisci* are located on the articular surfaces of the tibia (flip to Chapter 3 for the full scoop on fibrocartilage and other types of cartilage). Each meniscus is thinner at the interior part of the knee joint and thicker externally. They work as shock absorbers in the knee and help to balance your weight over the entire joint. You can see the menisci in Figure 20-2.

Assessing arthritis in the knee

The knee is susceptible to a couple types of arthritis:

✔ The knee is commonly affected by *rheumatoid arthritis,* which is an autoimmune disease that damages joint cartilage.

✔ Knees that have been injured are also at a greater risk for developing *osteoarthritis,* which can develop many years after fractures or damage to the ligaments or menisci.

Treatment for arthritis may include medications for pain relief and inflammation, specific exercises, and possibly surgery in severe cases.

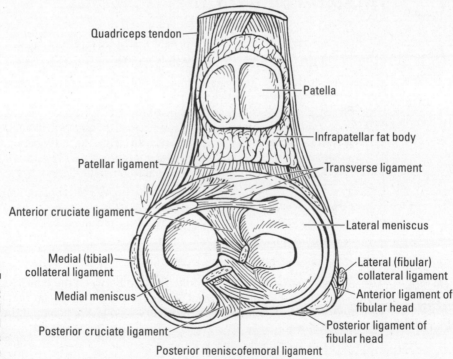

Quadriceps tendon

Patella

Infrapatellar fat body

Patellar ligament

Transverse ligament

Anterior cruciate ligament

Lateral meniscus

Medial (tibial) collateral ligament

Lateral (fibular) collateral ligament

Medial meniscus

Anterior ligament of fibular head

Posterior cruciate ligament

Posterior ligament of fibular head

Posterior meniscofemoral ligament

Figure 20-2: The menisci and ligaments of the knee joint.

Superior view

The *medial meniscus* is shaped like the letter C and is wider at the front than at the back. It's attached to the intercondylar area of the tibia and to the medial (tibial) collateral ligament (see the next section). The *lateral meniscus* is smaller and rounder in shape. It has a little more movement compared to the medial meniscus.

Tearing into menisci

Tearing a meniscus is common and can affect the function of the knee. It's usually caused by a quick twisting or turning movement of the knee while the foot is planted, so it's common in sports. The menisci get thinner with age, so they're also easier for older people to tear.

A minor tear may hurt for two to three weeks and be treated with rest and ice, but a moderate tear can cause pain for years if not treated. Severe tears result in bits of the torn meniscus moving into the joint space, causing the knee to pop, click, catch, or lock into place. A torn meniscus may require surgery to repair the meniscus or trim the edges.

Hanging on with the ligaments

A *ligament* is a type of tissue that stabilizes and strengthens a joint (see Chapter 3 for more about ligaments). The following ligaments help to stabilize the knee joint. (You can see some of them in Figure 20-2.)

- ✔ *Patellar ligament:* This ligament runs from the patellar apex to the tibial tuberosity.

- ✔ *Lateral collateral ligament:* Also known as the *fibular collateral ligament*, this strong, rounded band of ligament runs from the lateral epicondyle of the femur to the lateral part of the head of the fibula. (The *lateral epicondyle* is a bony prominence located proximal to the lateral condyle.)

- ✔ *Medial collateral ligament:* Also called the *tibial collateral ligament*, this strong, flat ligament runs from the medial epicondyle of the femur to the medial surface of the tibia and attaches to the medial meniscus. (The *medial epicondyle* is a bony prominence proximal to the medial condyle.)

- ✔ *Oblique popliteal ligament:* This ligament starts behind the medial condyle of the tibia and runs superiorly and laterally to attach to the posterior part of the joint capsule that we describe earlier in this chapter.

- ✔ *Arcuate popliteal ligament:* This ligament starts from the posterior part of the fibular head and runs superiorly and medially to the posterior part of the knee joint.

- ✔ *Anterior cruciate ligament:* The ACL starts from the anterior part of the intercondylar area of the tibia and runs superiorly, posteriorly, and laterally. It attaches to the posterior, medial side of the lateral condyle of the femur. The ACL prevents the tibia from sliding forward on the femur.

- ✔ *Posterior cruciate ligament:* The PCL starts at the posterior intercondylar area of the tibia and runs superiorly and anteriorly (medial to the ACL) to attach to the anterior part of the lateral side of the medial condyle of the femur. The PCL prevents the tibia from sliding backward on the femur.

- *Coronary ligaments:* These ligaments are part of the joint capsule. They attach the menisci to the tibial condyles.

- *Transverse ligament:* This ligament runs across the anterior intercondylar area and attaches to the menisci anteriorly.

- *Posterior meniscofemoral ligament:* This ligament attaches the lateral meniscus to the posterior cruciate ligament and the medial condyle of the femur.

Bumping up against the bursae

The knee joint contains the following *bursae,* which are fluid-filled sacs that help tendons glide over the bones and other tendons:

- *Suprapatellar bursa:* Between the femur and the quadriceps femoris tendon (we mention this and other muscles later in this chapter)

- *Popliteus bursa:* Between the tendon of the popliteus muscle and the lateral condyle of the tibia

- *Pes anserine bursa:* Between the tendons of the sartorius, gracilis, and semitendinosus muscles (all covered in Chapter 19 on the thigh) and the medial (tibial) collateral ligament (which we discuss later in this chapter)

- *Gastrocnemius bursa:* Between the tendon of the medial head of the gastrocnemius muscle and the joint capsule

- *Semimembranosus bursa:* Between the tendon of the medial head of the gastrocnemius muscle and the tendon of the semimembranosus muscle

- *Subcutaneous prepatellar bursa:* Between the anterior surface of the patella and the skin that covers it

- *Subcutaneous infrapatellar bursa:* Between the tibial tuberosity and the skin

- *Deep infrapatellar bursa:* Between the patellar ligament that we discuss later in this chapter and the anterior part of the tibia

Bursitis of the knee is an inflammation of any of those eight bursae, resulting in pain and tenderness of the knee, swelling, and a warm feeling when you touch the area. The bursae can become irritated by frequent kneeling, direct trauma to the knee, or falling on the knee too often. Bacterial infections and arthritis can also lead to bursitis. Treatment may include medications for pain relief, antibiotics if infection is present, specific exercises, and possibly surgery.

Surveying knee sprains

A *sprain* is an injury to a ligament. Because the knee is fairly vulnerable to injury, knee sprains are fairly common, and most involve the medial or lateral collateral ligaments or the cruciate ligaments (and sometimes a collateral ligament and a cruciate ligament are damaged in the same injury).

Knee sprains are graded on their severity:

✔ A mild sprain is simply a stretched ligament, which usually heals just fine on its own.

✔ A moderate sprain involves some tearing of the ligament. Treatment includes rest, ice, and specific exercises.

✔ A severe sprain may include a complete rupture of a ligament, which usually means surgical repair is necessary.

Kneeling on the patellofemoral joint

The articulation between the femur and the patella (kneecap) is called the *patellofemoral articulation,* and it lies anterior to the joint between the femur and tibia. The *patellar ligament* runs from the apex of the patella to the tibial tuberosity. It's really the distal part of the quadriceps (thigh muscle) tendon, and it helps to guide the movement of the patella during flexion and extension of the knee. Movement of the patella is also stabilized by the *medial* and *lateral patellar retinacula,* which are formed from the patellar tendon and attach to the tibia.

Supervising the superior tibiofibular joint

The *superior tibiofibular joint* isn't technically part of the knee joint, but it's so close to the knee that it's often grouped with it. It's a synovial joint (see Chapter 3 for more about the different types of joints) formed between facets (articular surfaces) on the head of the fibula and the lateral tibial condyle. It's surrounded by a joint capsule and stabilized by the *anterior* and *posterior ligaments of the head of the fibula* (refer to Figure 20-1). The superior tibiofibular joint allows for some gliding movement to occur.

Mastering the Muscles that Affect the Knee and Leg

Most of the muscles that move the knee come from the hip and thigh, whereas most of the muscles of the leg actually move the ankle. We cover the following muscles in more detail in other chapters, but we list them here too, just so you know how they affect the knee and the leg.

Starting with thigh muscles that work with the knee

Some of the muscles that flex and extend the hip also flex and extend the knee. Here's a brief list of the thigh muscles that affect the knee (check out Chapter 19 for more details):

- ✔ *Quadriceps femoris:* This four-headed muscle starts in the hip and attaches to the base of the patella via the quadriceps tendon. From there, the quadriceps tendon becomes the patellar ligament (see the earlier section "Hanging on with the ligaments" for more about this ligament). Contracting the quadriceps extends the knee.

- ✔ *Hamstring:* These muscles originate in the posterior part of the hip, and they flex the knee.

  - The *semitendinosus* inserts onto the medial superior part of the tibia.

  - The *semimembranosus* inserts onto the posterior portion of the medial tibial condyle.

  - The *biceps femoris* inserts onto the lateral side of the fibular head.

- ✔ *Tensor fasciae latae:* This muscle also originates in the hip. It inserts onto the lateral condyle of the tibia, and its function is to flex the thigh. It also helps stabilize an extended knee.

The *patellar reflex* (also called the *patellar tendon reflex*) is commonly tested to assess the patient for possible peripheral nerve damage (see Chapter 3 to find out more about the peripheral nervous system). It's performed by tapping the patellar ligament with a reflex hammer, which should cause the leg to extend with a bit of a kick. A decreased patellar reflex indicates a problem with the nerves that innervate the quadriceps muscle.

Aiming at the anterior compartment

The *anterior compartment* is located in front of the interosseus membrane and between the lateral part of the tibial shaft and the medial part of the fibular shaft. The muscles of the anterior compartment of the leg include the *tibialis anterior, extensor hallucis longus, extensor digitorum longus,* and the *fibularis (peroneus) tertius.* They all move the ankle and foot, so we discuss them all in Chapter 21.

Looking at the lateral compartment

The *lateral compartment* is defined as the area between the lateral portion of the fibula, the *intermuscular septa* (a sheet of connective tissue that divides the compartments), and the *deep fascia* (connective tissue covering the muscles) of the leg. Following are the main muscles here:

- The *fibularis (peroneus) longus* muscle originates on the head and superior part of the fibula.

- The *fibularis (peroneus) brevis* originates on the lower part of the fibula.

Both muscles insert onto the bones of the foot and help to evert the foot (move the sole of the foot outwards) and dorsiflex the ankle (bend the ankle to move the foot and toes upward). They're described further in Chapter 21.

Pondering the posterior compartment

The *posterior compartment* contains the calf muscles, which are divided into superficial and deep groups.

- **Superficial:** This group includes the gastrocnemius, soleus, and plantaris muscles, which are all described in Chapter 21 because they relate to the ankle and foot.

  - The *gastrocnemius* originates on the lateral and medial condyles of the femur.

  - The *soleus* muscle originates on the posterior part of the fibula and tibia.

  - The *plantaris* originates on the femur just superior to the lateral condyle.

  All three muscles insert onto the calcaneus (which you probably know better as the heel bone). The gastrocnemius is the only muscle of this group that helps flex the knee.

- **Deep:** The deep muscle group includes the *flexor hallucis longus, flexor digitorum longus,* and *tibialis posterior.* They plantarflex the ankle (bend the ankle so the toes point downward) and flex the toes, so they're covered in Chapter 21. Another deep muscle is the *popliteus* muscle, which originates on the lateral part of the lateral condyle and the lateral meniscus and inserts onto the posterior surface of the tibia. It helps to flex the knee.

Noticing the Nerves, Blood Vessels, and Lymphatics of the Knee and Leg

The knee and leg require nerve supply and circulation, which are provided by a number of nerves, blood vessels, and lymphatics (as you find out in the following sections). Most of them can be found in an area called the popliteal fossa.

The *popliteal fossa* is a diamond-shaped space posterior to the knee joint. It's bordered by several muscles (the biceps femoris, semimembranosus, semitendinosus, and gastrocnemius), skin, the *popliteal fascia* (connective tissue lining), the femur, and the joint capsule.

Noting the nerves

The following nerves of the popliteal fossa and leg can be seen in Figure 20-3:

- *Tibial nerve:* This nerve branches off the sciatic nerve (covered in Chapter 19) and runs down the midline of the popliteal fossa. It has branches that serve the muscles of the posterior compartment before moving down toward the ankle and foot (which we cover in detail in Chapter 21).

- *Common fibular (peroneal) nerve:* This nerve branches off the sciatic nerve in the popliteal fossa and runs along the biceps femoris and leaves the fossa to run around the head of the fibula and down the leg to the ankle.

- *Medial sural cutaneous nerve:* This nerve branches off the tibial nerve. It joins the *sural communicating branch* of the common fibular (peroneal) nerve to form the *sural nerve,* which innervates the skin on the posterior and lateral parts of the leg.

- *Lateral sural cutaneous nerve:* This nerve branches off the common fibular (peroneal) nerve to supply skin over the lateral part of the leg.

Fibular (peroneal) nerve dysfunction leads to loss of movement or sensation in the foot or the leg. It can happen after a one-time event such as a knee trauma, fractured fibula, or injury during knee surgery. Fibular (peroneal) nerve dysfunction can also occur after repetitive activities such as frequent sitting with one leg crossed over the other, after wearing tight, high boots, and from pressure from sleep positions. Treatment includes pain medication, corticosteroid injections, and surgery in severe cases.

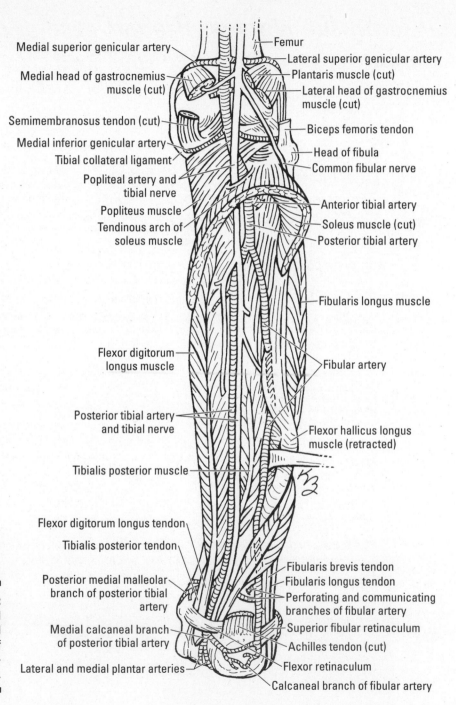

Medial superior genicular artery

Medial head of gastrocnemius muscle (cut)

Semimembranosus tendon (cut)

Medial inferior genicular artery

Tibial collateral ligament

Popliteal artery and tibial nerve

Popliteus muscle

Tendinous arch of soleus muscle

Femur

Lateral superior genicular artery

Plantaris muscle (cut)

Lateral head of gastrocnemius muscle (cut)

Biceps femoris tendon

Head of fibula

Common fibular nerve

Anterior tibial artery

Soleus muscle (cut)

Posterior tibial artery

Fibularis longus muscle

Flexor digitorum longus muscle

Fibular artery

Posterior tibial artery and tibial nerve

Flexor hallicus longus muscle (retracted)

Tibialis posterior muscle

Flexor digitorum longus tendon

Tibialis posterior tendon

Posterior medial malleolar branch of posterior tibial artery

Medial calcaneal branch of posterior tibial artery

Lateral and medial plantar arteries

Fibularis brevis tendon

Fibularis longus tendon

Perforating and communicating branches of fibular artery

Superior fibular retinaculum

Achilles tendon (cut)

Flexor retinaculum

Calcaneal branch of fibular artery

Figure 20-3:
Selected nerves and arteries of the leg (posterior view).

Analyzing the arteries and veins

The arteries that are found in the popliteal fossa provide blood to the structures of the knee, and they also take blood down to the ankle and foot (see Chapter 21). Following are the arteries that run through the popliteal fossa (refer to Figure 20-3):

- ✔ *Popliteal artery:* This artery continues from the femoral artery (see Chapter 19) at the *adductor hiatus,* which is a gap between the adductor magnus muscle of the thigh and the femur. It runs down into the popliteal fossa and divides into the tibial arteries.

- ✔ *Genicular arteries:* These arteries include the *superior lateral, superior medial, middle, inferior lateral,* and *inferior medial genicular arteries.* These arteries form the *genicular anastomosis,* which is a network of arteries surrounding the knee.

- ✔ *Anterior tibial artery:* This artery passes into the anterior compartment of the leg and continues to the ankle. It provides blood flow to the structures of the anterior compartment.

- ✔ *Posterior tibial artery:* This artery runs to the posterior compartment of the leg to provide blood to structures in the posterior and lateral compartments.

- ✔ *Fibular artery:* This artery branches off the posterior tibial artery and runs down to the posterior compartment of the leg. It also provides blood to the lateral and posterior compartments.

Blood that's finished delivering oxygen and nutrients to the knee, leg, and foot needs to return to the heart, and it does so via veins with corresponding names that accompany the arteries. The *popliteal vein* is the main vein located in the popliteal fossa. It starts from the *posterior tibial vein* and travels upward through the popliteal fossa, up into the thigh, and eventually becomes the femoral vein (see Chapter 19). Following are other veins that serve the knee and leg:

- ✔ *Lateral superior genicular vein:* Located superior to the lateral condyle of the femur; drains into the popliteal vein

- ✔ *Lateral inferior genicular vein:* Below the lateral condyle of the tibia; also drains into the popliteal vein

- ✔ *Great saphenous vein:* A superficial vein that travels from the foot, along the medial side of the knee, and all the way up to the hip

- ✔ *Small saphenous vein:* A superficial vein that travels along the lateral side of the ankle to the posterior leg and empties into the popliteal vein

Q angles, genu varum, and genu valgum

If you look at a picture of the body in the anatomical position (as shown in Chapter 2), you see that the femurs are somewhat diagonal as they run from the hip down to the knee, but the leg bones are more vertical. This relationship forms a *Q angle,* which is the angle formed by a line drawn from the anterior superior iliac spine of the hip bone (see Chapter 19) to the middle of the patella and another line

drawn from the middle of the patella to the tibial tubercle. Because women have wider pelvises, they usually have a larger Q angle than men.

Having too high of a Q angle can cause problems for the patella. One condition caused by increased Q angle is *genu valgum,* also known as having knock-knees. The opposite condition is called *genu varum,* also known as being bow-legged.

Listing the lymph nodes

The popliteal fossa also contains a few lymph nodes. *Popliteal lymph nodes* receive lymph from superficial and deep lymphatic vessels and the joint capsule. Superficial lymphatic vessels from the lateral side of the foot and leg accompany the small saphenous vein to the popliteal nodes. The deep lymphatic vessels follow along sides of the deep veins of the leg to the popliteal nodes. The lymph from these nodes flows in the deep lymphatic vessels of the thigh to the deep inguinal nodes (see Chapter 19).

Summing Up the Surface Landmarks

The knee is easy to find right between the leg and the thigh. You can visualize the popliteal fossa on the posterior aspect of the knee — it's a diamond-shaped area right over the part where the knee bends.

The popliteal artery can be palpated (medically examined) for a pulse, but it isn't always easy to find unless the patient is lying prone (on the stomach) with the knee bent. Press your fingers deeply into the popliteal fossa to feel the pulse.

Using the following clues, the bones are easy to find:

- ✔ The condyles of the femur and tibia give the knee its shape, and they're easy to palpate on either side of the knee; they're the largest bony prominences on either side of the knee above the articulation.

- ✔ The head of the fibula is located just inferior to the lateral condyles. It's the bony prominence on the lateral side, just inferior to the knee articulation.

- ✔ The patella is anterior to the knee joint and may be located by sight or palpation. It's the bony kneecap located anterior to the knee joint.

The leg gets its shape primarily from the superficial posterior muscles that form the calf. They may be visible under the skin, along with superficial veins.

Chapter 21

Finding the Ankle and the Foot

● ●

In This Chapter

▶ Boning up on the skeleton of the ankle and foot

▶ Constructing the joints and muscles

▶ Flowing with ankle and foot nerves, blood vessels, and lymphatics

▶ Examining the surface of the ankle and foot

● ●

*U*nderstanding the anatomy of the foot and ankle is important, to say
the least. Feet have to put up with a lot: walking, running, and maybe
wearing uncomfortable shoes, all of which put pressure on the arches (those
of you who regularly wear high heels or dress shoes know what we're talking
about!). Sprained ankles, fallen arches, and peripheral nerve damage require
examination of the ankles and the feet.

This chapter looks at the structures that make up the marvelous foot and
ankle. We start with the bones and joints and then move on to the muscles.
We also take a look at the circulation and nerves and, finally, peek at the
surface anatomy that helps you identify internal features.

Looking at the Framework of the Ankle and Foot

In some ways, the bones in your ankles and feet resemble the bones in your
wrist and hand (see Chapter 18), but instead of carpals and metacarpals,
you've got tarsals and metatarsals and phalanges in your toes. But your feet
certainly are shaped differently from hands because they have a different
purpose. Your feet are made for walking, running, standing, and climbing.

Find out about the different bones of the ankle and foot in the following
sections.

Aiming for the ankle bones

The ankle is the area where the leg attaches to the foot. The proximal parts (closer to the trunk) of the two bones of the lower leg, the tibia and fibula, are covered in Chapter 20. The distal ends of the tibia and fibula are part of the ankle. The tibia is the larger medial (toward the midline of the body) bone. It has a facet (smooth joint-forming surface) on the distal end that articulates (forms a joint) with the talus. The *medial malleolus* is a projection that you can palpate (medically examine by touch). It's the big bump on the medial part of the ankle. The *fibula* is the slender lateral (away from the midline) leg bone. The distal end enlarges to form the *lateral malleolus,* which is palpated as the large bump on the lateral side of the ankle. The shafts (long portions) of the tibia and fibula are connected by a thin sheet of connective tissue called the interosseous membrane.

One of the seven tarsal bones, the *talus,* meets up with the leg bones to form the ankle joint, which we talk about later on in this chapter.

The talus has three parts: The *head* is the distal part that articulates with the navicular bone, the *neck* is posterior to the head, and the *body* is cuboidal in shape and the posterior surface has two tubercles (medial and lateral). The top surface of the body is called the *trochlea of the talus*, which articulates with the malleoli of the tibia and fibula.

Assessing the architecture of the foot bones

The structure of the foot is made by the 6 remaining tarsal bones (other than the talus), the 5 metatarsals, and the 14 phalanges. We start by giving an overview of the tarsals:

✔ **Calcaneus bone:** The *calcaneus* is the heel bone, and it's the largest bone of the foot. The calcaneus comes in contact with the talus at the *sustentaculum tali* located at the superior (top) and medial part of the calcaneus (close to the midline of the body). The *fibular trochlea* is located on the lateral part of the calcaneus, and the *calcaneal tuberosity* is the posterior and inferior portion of the calcaneus (the part of the heel you stand on).

✔ **Navicular bone:** This boat-shaped bone is found in front of the head of the talus. It has a small tuberosity (projection, or bump) on its medial side that can be felt about 1 inch in front of and below the medial malleolus of the tibia.

> ✔ *Cuneiform bones:* These three bones sit anterior to the navicular bone.
>
> > • The *medial cuneiform* is on the medial side of the foot.
> >
> > • The *intermediate cuneiform* is in between the medial cuneiform and the *lateral cuneiform,* which is the most lateral.
>
> ✔ *Cuboid bone:* This bone is lateral to the navicular bone and the lateral cuneiform.

A row of five *metatarsal* bones sits between the tarsals and the bones of the toes (the phalanges). Each one has a head at the farthest (or distal) end, a shaft, and a base at the closer (or proximal) end. Their names are easy to remember because they're numbered. The first metatarsal is located on the medial side of the foot between the medial cuneiform and the bones of the big toe. Next are the second, third, fourth, and fifth metatarsals. The fifth metatarsal, which connects to the pinky-toe bones, has a tuberosity that sticks out over the cuboid bone.

The phalanges (singular: *phalanx*) form the toes. Each one has a base, a shaft, and a head, like the metatarsals, but the phalanges are smaller. The big toe has only two phalanges *(proximal* and *distal),* and the remaining toes each have three *(proximal, middle,* and *distal).*

Each of your feet has three *arches* formed by the bones of the foot that help absorb some of the shock of carrying you around all day. The *medial and lateral longitudinal arches* are between your heel and the ball of your foot, and the *transverse arch* runs from side to side and is made by the metatarsal, cuboid, and cuneiform bones.

Taking In the Ankle and Foot Joints

Your feet and ankles need to be sturdy, but they also need to be agile enough to adapt to slipping off a curb or doing some fancy footwork on the tennis court. Good thing they have as many joints as they do! Check out the following sections for all the details on ankle and foot joints.

Moving up and down: The ankle joint

The ankle joint is a synovial hinge joint (see Chapter 3 for more about types of joints), so you can *plantarflex* (point your toes down) and *dorsiflex* (move your foot and toes up). It allows a little wiggle from side to side, but most of the rest of the movement comes from the foot joints.

The ankle joint is made up of distal ends of the tibia and fibula, which form a socket that fits over the top portion of the talus (a metatarsal bone that we talk about in the earlier section "Aiming for the ankle bones"). The bones are held together by several ligaments (see Figure 21-1).

✔ **Medial (deltoid) ligament of the ankle:** This strong ligament attaches to the medial malleolus. It has four parts named for the bones (in addition to the tibia) that they attach to: the *tibionavicular,* the *tibiocalcaneal,* the *anterior tibiotalar,* and the *posterior tibiotalar.*

✔ **Lateral ligament of the ankle:** This ligament is made up of three bands that start at the *lateral malleolus* (again, these ligaments are named for the bones they attach to):

  • *Anterior talofibular ligament:* This ligament runs to the lateral surface of the talus.

  • *Calcaneofibular ligament:* This ligament runs to the lateral surface of the calcaneus.

  • *Posterior talofibular ligament:* This ligament runs to the lateral tubercle (small rounded eminence) of the talus.

If you've ever sprained an ankle, you injured one or more of the ligaments that hold the joint together. The lateral ligaments are damaged more often than the stronger medial ligament.

Supporting your weight: The foot and toe joints

The foot contains a number of joints, but two important joints are the subtalar and transverse tarsal joints. These two joints allow you to invert and evert the foot. (If you're wondering, *inversion* is when you move the bottom of your foot toward the midline of your body, and *eversion* is moving the bottom of your foot away from the midline of the body.)

✔ **Subtalar joint:** This joint is the posterior (back) joint formed between the talus and the calcaneus. It's a synovial joint (see Chapter 3 for more on different types of joints), and it's stabilized by *medial, lateral,* and *interosseous talocalcaneal ligaments* (refer to Figure 21-1).

✔ **Transverse tarsal joint:** The *transverse tarsal joint* is actually a combination of the following two joints:

  • *Talocalcaneonavicular joint:* This synovial joint is formed between the talus and the calcaneus and the navicular bones. It's stabilized by the *plantar calcaneonavicular ligament.*

• *Calcaneocuboid joint:* Another synovial joint, this one is formed between the front of the calcaneus and the posterior surface of the cuboid bone. It's stabilized by the *bifurcated ligament* on the top, the *long plantar ligament* on the bottom, and the *short plantar ligament*, which is deep to (located underneath) the long plantar ligament.

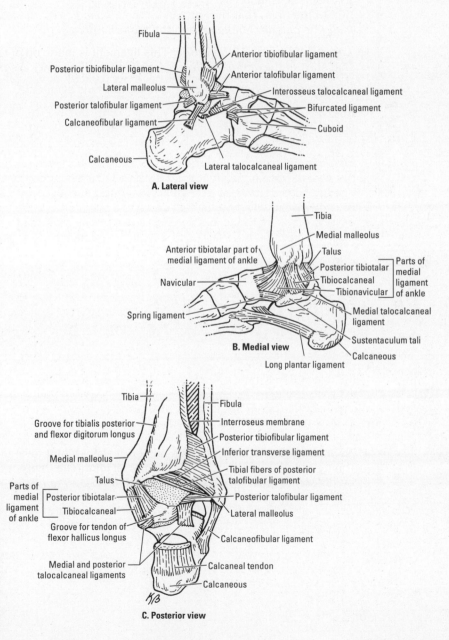

A. Lateral view

B. Medial view

C. Posterior view

Figure 21-1: Some ligaments and joints of the ankle and foot.

The remaining joints of the foot allow for a little movement of the foot and toes:

- *Cuneonavicular joint:* This synovial joint is formed between the navicular bone and the three cuneiform bones. It is supported by dorsal and plantar cuneonavicular ligaments. It allows for some gliding movement.

- *Cuboideonavicular joint:* This fibrous joint is between the cuboid and navicular bones. It's supported by dorsal, plantar, and interosseous ligaments.

- *Tarsometatarsal joints:* These synovial joints are formed between the tarsal bones and the bases of the metatarsal bones. These joints are strengthened by dorsal, plantar, and interosseus ligaments.

- *Intermetatarsal joints:* These synovial joints involve the bases of the metatarsal bones. All these joints are strengthened by dorsal, plantar, and interosseus ligaments.

- *Metatarsophalangeal joints:* These synovial joints are between the heads of the metatarsal bones and the bases of the proximal phalanges. They're supported by plantar and collateral ligaments. They allow you to flex and extend your toes as well as move them apart and closer together.

- *Interphalangeal joints:* These joints connect the phalanges. They're synovial joints strengthened by collateral and plantar ligaments, and they let you flex and extend your toes.

Delving into foot deformities

You may see a couple of different deformities affecting the feet:

- A *hammer toe* is a deformity of a toe, usually the second one. The toe becomes stuck in a claw-like position as the interphalangeal joints are constantly flexed. It may be congenital but is usually due to wearing shoes that are too short. Hammer toes can be painful, especially when a corn forms on the top of the toe or a callus forms on the sole of the foot, just under the metatarsal. Hammer toes may be treated by choosing roomier footwear, using shoe inserts to cushion the toe, taking pain relievers, using corticosteroid injections, or undergoing surgery.

- A *bunion* is a deformity of the first metatarsophalangeal joint. The bone becomes enlarged and forms a protuberance and may cause the big toe to become misaligned so that the big toe moves outward. The cause of bunions isn't clear, but they're more common in women. Bunions may cause no symptoms or they may be accompanied by redness, swelling, and pain. Bunions can be treated with rest, wider shoes, special exercises, and nonsteroidal anti-inflammatory medications.

Bending Your Ankle and Curling Your Toes: The Muscles

Many muscles do the work of moving the ankle and foot. As you find out in the following sections, some of the muscles that move the foot start higher up in the leg, and smaller muscles work right in the foot itself.

Turning to leg muscles that move the ankle and the foot

The leg is divided into compartments: the *anterior, lateral,* and *posterior compartments.* The muscles in these compartments help move the ankle and the foot:

- *Anterior compartment:* This compartment lies in front of the tibia and fibula (see Chapter 20) and is surrounded by fascia. The anterior muscles dorsiflex the foot at the ankle and extend the toes.

- *Lateral compartment:* The muscles here sit on the outer side of the leg and help evert the foot.

- *Posterior compartment:* This larger compartment is on the back of the leg. It has two layers of muscles, which are divided by a section of fascia called the *transverse intermuscular septum.* The posterior muscles plantarflex the ankle and flex the toes.

The following sections go into detail on the muscles of each compartment.

Anterior muscles

The tendons of the anterior dorsiflexors are held in place at the ankle by the thickened piece of fascia called the *superior* and *inferior extensor retinaculum.* These muscles are innervated (given nerve supply) by the deep fibular (peroneal) nerve (discussed later in this chapter):

- *Tibialis anterior:* This muscle originates on the lateral surface of the tibia and inserts on the medial cuneiform and base of the first metatarsal. It dorsiflexes the ankle and inverts the foot.

- *Extensor digitorum longus* and *extensor hallucis longus:* These muscles originate on the anterior surfaces of the shaft of the fibula and interosseous membrane. The extensor digitorum longus tendons insert on the middle and distal phalanges of the second, third, fourth, and fifth toes. The extensor hallucis longus inserts on the distal phalanx of the big toe. They dorsiflex the ankle and extend the toes.

✔ *Fibularis (peroneus) tertius:* This muscle originates on the anterior surface of the shaft of the fibula and inserts on the base of the fifth metatarsal bone. It dorsiflexes the ankle and everts the foot.

Lateral muscles

The lateral compartment contains two muscles: the *fibularis (peroneus) longus* and *fibularis (peroneus) brevis.* They originate on the lateral surface of the fibula. The fibularis longus inserts on the base of the first metatarsal and medial cuneiform, and the fibularis brevis inserts on the base of the fifth metatarsal. They're innervated by the superficial fibular (peroneal) nerve (which we describe later in this chapter) and help to plantarflex and evert the foot.

Posterior muscles

The posterior plantarflexors are innervated by the tibial nerve that we talk about later in this chapter. They are divided into superficial and deep layers. The tendons are held in place at the ankle by a thickened piece of fascia called the *flexor retinaculum.* (A fourth posterior compartment muscle, the popliteus, is covered in Chapter 20.)

The following superficial muscles, which plantarflex the ankle, have different origins, but they all merge into the *calcaneal tendon,* which inserts into the back of the calcaneus:

✔ *Gastrocnemius:* This muscle has two heads. The lateral head originates from the lateral condyle of the femur (see Chapter 20), and the medial head originates from the medial condyle.

✔ *Plantaris:* This muscle originates at the lateral supercondylar line of the femur.

✔ *Soleus:* This muscle originates on the shafts of the tibia and fibula.

Following are the deep muscles of the posterior compartment of the leg that plantarflex the ankle and flex the toes:

✔ *Flexor hallucis longus:* This muscle originates on the distal two-thirds of the posterior surface of the shaft of the fibula and inserts into the base of the distal phalanx of the big toe (see Figure 21-2). It plantarflexes the ankle and flexes the big toe.

✔ *Flexor digitorum longus:* This muscle originates on the posterior surface of the tibia, and the tendons insert into the bases of the distal phalanges of the lateral four toes (see Figure 21-2). It plantarflexes the ankle and flexes the lateral four toes.

✔ *Tibialis posterior:* This muscle originates on the posterior surfaces of the shafts of the tibia and fibula, and the interosseus membrane (see Chapter 20) and inserts on the tuberosity of the navicular bone. It plantarflexes the ankle and inverts the foot.

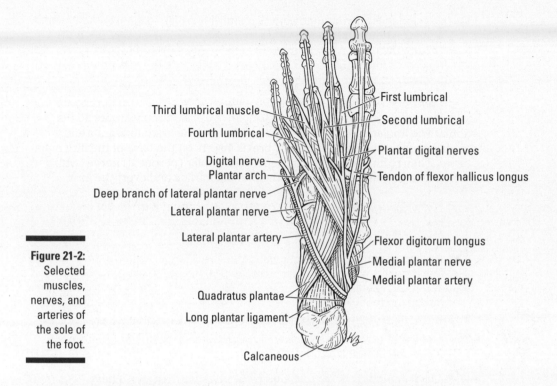

Third lumbrical muscle

Fourth lumbrical

Digital nerve

Plantar arch

Deep branch of lateral plantar nerve

Lateral plantar nerve

Lateral plantar artery

Quadratus plantae

Long plantar ligament

Calcaneous

First lumbrical

Second lumbrical

Plantar digital nerves

Tendon of flexor hallicus longus

Flexor digitorum longus

Medial plantar nerve

Medial plantar artery

Figure 21-2:
Selected
muscles,
nerves, and
arteries of
the sole of
the foot.

Minding the muscles of the foot

You can divide the foot muscles into groups based on their locations —
either in the sole of the foot (the bottom or plantar area) or the dorsum on
the top of the foot. Most of the muscles are in the sole. The muscles in the
sole of the foot are located in four layers. They don't work as intricately as
the small muscles in the hands (see Chapter 18); they mostly work together
to support the arches of the foot. They're innervated by the medial and lateral
plantar nerves that we talk about later in this chapter.

The muscles in the first layer originate on the calcaneus and insert on the toes:

✔ *Abductor hallucis:* Inserts on the proximal phalanx of the big toe;
abducts and flexes the big toe

✔ *Flexor digitorum brevis:* Inserts on the middle phalanges of the
lateral four toes; flexes the toes

✔ *Abductor digiti minimi:* Inserts on the lateral side of the proximal phalanx of the little toe; abducts and flexes the little toe

The second layer has the following two muscles (refer to Figure 21-2):

- ✔ *Quadratus plantae:* Originates on the calcaneus and inserts on the tendon of the flexor digitorum longus muscle (see the preceding section); helps the flexor digitorum longus flex the second through fifth toes

- ✔ *Lumbricals* **(numbered first through fourth):** Originate on the flexor digitorum longus tendons and insert on the proximal phalanges of the lateral four toes; flex the proximal phalanges and extend the middle and distal phalanges of toes two through five

The third layer has the following three muscles:

- ✔ *Flexor hallucis brevis:* Originates on the cuboid and lateral cuneiform and inserts on the proximal phalanx of the big toe; flexes the proximal phalanx of the big toe

- ✔ *Adductor hallucis:* Originates on the bases of the second, third, and fourth metatarsals and inserts on the proximal phalanx of the big toe; adducts the big toe (in other words, moves the big toe toward the midline of the foot)

- ✔ *Flexor digiti minimi brevis:* Originates on the base of the fifth metatarsal and inserts on the base of the proximal phalanx of the little toe; flexes the little toe

The fourth layer contains *plantar* and *dorsal interossei* that originate on the metatarsals and insert on the proximal phalanges. The plantar interossei adduct the toes, and the dorsal interossei abduct the toes (in other words, they move the toes away from the midline of the foot).

The muscles on the dorsum of the foot are the *extensor digitorum brevis* and *extensor hallucis brevis* (which actually form one muscle). They originate on the superolateral surface of the calcaneus and insert into the proximal phalanges of the toes (the hallucis brevis goes to the big toe). They extend the toes.

Getting Maintenance with Nerves, Blood Vessels, and Lymphatics

The joints and muscles that we describe earlier in this chapter need to be maintained properly. Nerves provide the ankle and foot with sensation and also tell the muscles when to contract and when to relax. Blood is carried into the ankle and foot via the arteries and returned to the heart in the veins. Lymphatic fluid is drained via the lymphatic vessels.

Naming the nerves

The ankle and foot require nerve supply to function properly. Here's a look at the nerves that keep the foot and ankle kicking.

- ✔ *Tibial nerve:* This nerve is a branch of the sciatic nerve (see Chapter 19). It runs down the leg, between the heads of the gastrocnemius, and passes under the soleus (see Chapter 20). It curves under the medial malleolus and continues into the foot. It innervates all the muscles in the posterior compartment of the leg.

- ✔ *Common fibular (peroneal) nerve:* This nerve branches off the sciatic nerve in the popliteal region (behind the knee). It travels posterior to the head of the fibula to enter the lateral compartment of the leg deep to the fibularis longus. Here it divides into the superficial and deep fibular nerves.

  - The *superficial fibular (peroneal) nerve* runs through the lateral compartment of the leg and innervates the muscles in the lateral compartment and the skin over the anterior portion of the ankle and the dorsum of the foot.

  - The *deep fibular (peroneal) nerve* runs through extensor digitorum longus and down the interosseous membrane. Then it crosses the tibia and enters the dorsum of the foot. It innervates the muscles in the anterior compartment of the leg and the dorsum of the foot. It also supplies a small region of skin between the first (big) and second toes.

- ✔ *Sural nerve:* This nerve (formed by the union of branches from both tibial and common fibular nerve) also runs between the heads of the gastrocnemius, but it runs under the lateral malleolus. It innervates the skin on the lateral side of the leg and foot.

- ✔ *Saphenous nerve:* This nerve is a branch of the femoral nerve and runs down the medial portion of the leg to the medial part of the foot and innervates the skin on the medial side of the ankle and foot.

- ✔ *Medial plantar nerve:* This branch of the tibial nerve runs between the abductor hallucis and flexor digitorum brevis in the foot. It innervates the skin of the medial side of the sole of the foot, and it's the nerve supply for the some of the foot muscles. (See this nerve for yourself in Figure 21-2.)

- ✔ *Lateral plantar nerve:* This nerve, also a branch of the tibial nerve, runs between the quadratus plantae and flexor digitorum brevis. It innervates the skin on the lateral part of the sole and several small muscles of the foot. (You can see this nerve in Figure 21-2.)

✔ *Plantar digital nerves:* These nerves branch off the medial and lateral planter nerves. They innervate the skin and nail beds of the toes. (Check out these nerves in Figure 21-2.)

✔ *Calcaneal branches of the tibial and sural nerve:* These branches run down to the posterior portion of the heel and innervate the skin of the heel.

Looking at blood vessels and lymphatics

The following arteries, which bring blood to the ankle and foot, include branches of the anterior and posterior tibial arteries. The anterior and posterior tibial arteries are the terminal branches of the popliteal artery located behind the knee (which we discuss in Chapter 20).

✔ *Anterior tibial artery:* This artery stems from the popliteal artery (see Chapter 20) and runs through the anterior compartment of the leg between the tibialis anterior and the extensor digitorum longus muscles. It supplies the anterior compartment of the leg and continues into the foot as the *dorsal pedis artery* (discussed later in this list).

✔ *Posterior tibial artery:* Starting at the popliteal artery, this artery runs through the posterior compartment of the leg down deep to the flexor retinaculum and continues into the sole of the foot, where it branches into the lateral and medial plantar arteries.

✔ *Fibular artery:* This artery branches off the proximal posterior tibial artery. It also runs down the posterior compartment of the leg behind the fibula. It supplies the posterior compartment and has perforating branches that supply the lateral compartment of the leg.

✔ *Dorsal pedis artery:* Coming from the anterior tibial artery, this artery runs along the dorsum of the foot. It passes through the first dorsal interosseous muscle as the *deep plantar artery* to the sole of the foot where it forms part of the *plantar arch* (deep plantar arch) with the *lateral plantar artery*. In the dorsum of the foot it gives off three branches: the *lateral tarsal artery,* the *arcuate artery,* and the *first dorsal metatarsal artery.* The *arcuate artery* gives off the *second, third,* and *fourth metatarsal arteries.*

✔ *Deep plantar artery:* This artery runs down into the sole of the foot and joins the lateral plantar artery to form the *plantar arch.*

✔ *Metatarsal arteries:* These arteries run down into the clefts between the toes and branch into digital arteries that supply the toes.

✔ *Lateral plantar artery:* Helping to form the plantar arch, this artery is a branch of the posterior tibial artery, located on the lateral side of the sole of the foot. (Check out this artery in Figure 21-2.)

✔ *Medial plantar artery:* This artery, another branch of the posterior tibial artery, is located on the medial side of the sole of the foot. (See this artery in Figure 21-2.)

✔ *Plantar metatarsal arteries:* The deep plantar arch gives off these arteries as well as many other branches that supply blood to the sole of the foot.

Deep veins drain blood from the foot, and they accompany the matching arteries. Superficial veins located on the dorsum drain most of the blood into *dorsal metatarsal veins,* which go on to form the *dorsal venous arch* and a *dorsal venous network.* A *plantar venous network* converges with the dorsal venous arch to form the great and small saphenous veins.

Lymph is collected in superficial and deep lymphatic vessels that follow the veins. The medial superficial lymphatic vessels drain into the superficial inguinal lymph nodes (see Chapter 19) and then into the deep inguinal nodes. Lateral superficial vessels and deep vessels drain into popliteal lymph nodes (see Chapter 20). (See Chapter 5 for more about the lymphatic system.)

Summing Up the Surface Landmarks of the Ankle and the Foot

The foot and ankle have very little fat, so spotting both the medial malleolus and the lateral malleolus is fairly easy; the medial malleolus is the big bump on the medial side of the ankle and the lateral malleolus is the big bump on the lateral side of the ankle. The foot and ankle have little to no hair. The toes are each topped off with a toenail.

You can palpate (medically examine by touch) the following bones in the foot:

✔ The head of the talus can be palpated just below the lateral malleolus when the foot is inverted (press your fingers into the flesh just distal to the malleolus while the sole of the foot is turned inward) or below the medial malleolous when the foot is everted (press into the flesh distal to the medial malleolus with the sole of the foot outward).

✔ The medial tubercle of the calcaneus can be palpated by grasping the heel and pressing your thumb into the flesh on the medial plantar surface of the heel. You may not feel much unless the patient has a heel spur (bony overgrowth).

✔ The tuberosity of the fifth metatarsal is palpable on the lateral side of the foot. It's the most prominent bump on the lateral side of the foot, about halfway between the heel and toes.

✔ The head of the first metatarsal forms a prominent bump on the medial portion of the foot — just at the base of the big toe. It may be inflamed and tender if the patient has a bunion.

The tendons of the extensor digitorum longus are usually visible (or at least palpable) where they run along the tops of the metatarsals. Just look for the tendons as they run along the dorsum of the foot from the toes to the ankle.

The great saphenous vein may be visible in a thin person, running just in front of the medial malleolus. The dorsal pedal artery may be palpated on the top of the dorsum of the foot. It can be found at the most prominent part of the dorsum, immediately lateral to the tendon of the extensor hallucis longus.

Part V
The Part of Tens

The 5th Wave   By Rich Tennant

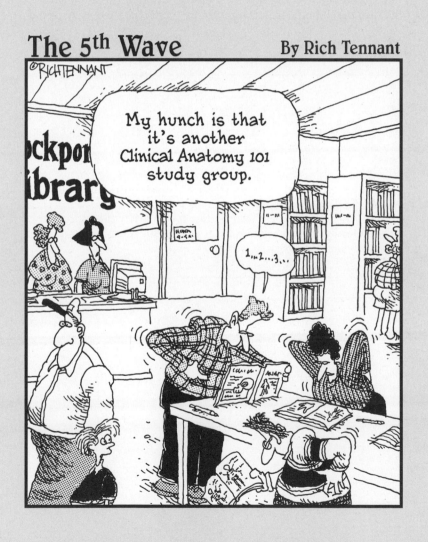

In this part . . .

Part V starts out with ten of our favorite mnemonics for remembering anatomy, including some ways to recall the bones of the head, the cranial nerves, the order of the intestinal tract, and which foot bone goes where. The final chapter of this part gives you an idea of how to look inside a body without cutting it open. We describe some radiological methods, ultrasonography, and a bunch of ways to use scopes.

Chapter 22

Ten Helpful Clinical Anatomy Mnemonics

● ●

In This Chapter

▶ Playing mind games to remember what's in your head

▶ Helping yourself remember bones of the wrist and ankle

● ●

Learning (and memorizing) the names and locations of anatomical structures isn't easy, so clinical anatomy students often develop mnemonics, or memory tricks, to make it a little easier. These mnemonics include acronyms, short poems, and silly (and frequently naughty) phrases that are quite effective for remembering parts of the body. In this chapter we show you ten of our favorite (G-rated) memory devices for different parts of the body, from the top to the bottom.

Thinking about the Cranial Bones

As you find out in Chapter 12, your skull has six cranial bones that form the cranial vault. You don't want to confuse them with the facial bones (see the next section), so you can remember them with this phrase:

PEST OF 6

Each letter stands for a cranial bone, and the number 6 reminds you that there are six of them:

- **P:** Parietal bone
- **E:** Ethmoid bone
- **S:** Sphenoid bone
- **T:** Temporal bone
- **O:** Occipital bone
- **F:** Frontal bone

Focusing on the Facial Bones

Your face is formed by eight facial bones (see Chapter 12). Here's a silly saying to help you remember them:

> **V**irgil **C**an **N**ot **M**ake **M**y **P**et **Z**ebra **L**augh.

The bold letters represent the facial bones:

- **V:** Vomer
- **C:** Conchae (inferior)
- **N:** Nasal bone
- **M:** Maxilla
- **M:** Mandible
- **P:** Palatine bone
- **Z:** Zygomatic bone
- **L:** Lacrimal bones

Memorizing the Cranial Nerves

The cranial nerves are described in Chapter 12. They each have a name and a number, so remembering which name goes with what number can be difficult. Use this little poem to remember:

> **O**n **O**ld **O**lympus's **T**owering **T**op, **A** **F**inn **A**nd **G**erman **V**iewed **S**ome **H**ops.

The bold letters each stand for a nerve:

- **O:** Cranial nerve I, olfactory nerve
- **O:** Cranial nerve II, optic nerve
- **O:** Cranial nerve III, oculomotor
- **T:** Cranial nerve IV, trochlear
- **T:** Cranial nerve V, trigeminal nerve
- **A:** Cranial nerve VI, abducent nerve

✔ **F:** Cranial nerve VII, facial nerve

✔ **A:** Cranial nerve VIII, auditory (or vestibulochochlear) nerve

✔ **G:** Cranial nerve IX, glossopharyngeal nerve

✔ **V:** Cranial nerve X, vagus nerve

✔ **S:** Cranial nerve XI, spinal accessory nerve

✔ **H:** Cranial nerve XII, hypoglossal

Summing Up the Heart-Valve Sequence

We describe the anatomy of the heart, including its chambers and valves, in Chapter 8. The following odd sentence helps you remember how blood flows through the heart by remembering the sequence of the valves:

TRy **PUL**ling **M**y **AORTA.**

The bold capital letters represent the valves, in order of blood flow:

✔ **TR:** Tricuspid valve

✔ **PUL:** Pulmonary valve

✔ **M:** Mitral valve

✔ **AORTA:** Aortic valve

Ordering the Abdominal Muscles

Our way of remembering the names of the abdominal muscles is to think of a spare tire, which is the nickname for the extra fat that can build up around a person's abdomen. The word **TIRE** stands for the four abdominal muscles found in Chapter 9.

✔ **T:** Transversus abdominis

✔ **I:** Internal abdominal oblique

✔ **R:** Rectus abdominis

✔ **E:** External abdominal oblique

Tracking the Intestinal Tract

The intestinal tract includes the small intestine, the colon, and the rectum (see Chapter 10 to review the parts). We get down to business with our phrase for remembering the parts of the intestinal tract and their sequence:

Dow **J**ones **I**ndustrial **C**limbing **A**verage **C**losing **S**tock **R**eport

The first three bold letters represent the three segments of the small intestine. The rest help you remember the colon and the rectum:

- ✔ **D:** Duodenum
- ✔ **J:** Jejunum
- ✔ **I:** Ileum
- ✔ **C:** Cecum
- ✔ **A:** Appendix
- ✔ **C:** Colon
- ✔ **S:** Sigmoid colon
- ✔ **R:** Rectum

Remembering the Rotator Cuff Muscles

Four rotator cuff muscles run from the scapula to the humerus and work together so you can rotate your arm (as you discover in Chapter 16). They're usually remembered by the acronym **SITS:**

- ✔ **S:** Supraspinatus
- ✔ **I:** Infraspinatus
- ✔ **T:** Teres minor
- ✔ **S:** Subscapularis

Concentrating on the Carpal Bones

Eight carpal bones form the wrist, as described in Chapter 18. They're arranged in two rows, with four bones in each row. Following is a phrase that can help you remember them:

She **L**ooks **T**oo **P**retty; **T**ry **T**o **C**atch **H**er.

The bold letters stand for each carpal bone. The first four form the *proximal* row (closer to the arm) starting *laterally* (thumb side). The second group of four make up the *distal* row (closer to the hand), also starting laterally:

- **S:** Scaphoid
- **L:** Lunate
- **T:** Triquetrum
- **P:** Pisiform
- **T:** Trapezium
- **T:** Trapezoid
- **C:** Capitate
- **H:** Hamate

Looking at the Lateral Rotator Muscles of the Hip

In Chapter 19, we describe the muscles of the hip. Six of them rotate the hip laterally. Following is a phrase that will help you remember them:

Piece **G**oods **O**ften **G**o **O**n **Q**uilts.

The bold letters represent the hip rotators, in order from most proximal to most distal:

- **P:** Piriformis
- **G:** Gemellus superior
- **O:** Obturator internus
- **G:** Gemellus inferior
- **O:** Obturator externus
- **Q:** Quadratus femoris

Taming the Tarsal Bones

Chapter 21 covers the bones of the foot and ankle, including seven tarsal bones. You can remember the tarsal bones with this sentence:

The **C**ircus **N**eeds **M**ore **I**nteresting **L**ittle **C**lowns.

The bold letters stand for the tarsal bones:

- **T:** Talus
- **C:** Calcaneus
- **N:** Navicular
- **M:** Medial cuneiform
- **I:** Intermediate cuneiform
- **L:** Lateral cuneiform
- **C:** Cuboid

Chapter 23

Ten Ways to Look into the Body without Cutting It Open

*Y*ou can tell a lot about the health of a person by examining the outside of the body, but sometimes you need to know what's happening on the inside, which is why clinical anatomy is more than skin deep. This chapter introduces ten ways to look inside the human body without cutting anything open. The techniques involve X-rays, digital imaging, and scoping.

Conventional Radiography

Conventional radiography is the fancier name for taking pictures of the inside parts of the body with X-rays. High-energy radiation (that's the X-ray part) is used to produce light and dark images on a piece of film called a *radiograph*. X-rays easily pass through air (like in your lungs), which shows up as dark areas on the radiograph, but the rays are blocked by dense tissues (like bones), which show up as white areas. Muscles, fat, and organs vary in their density, so they show up in different shades of gray.

Some types of X-rays include the use of a *contrast medium* like barium or iodine. The contrast medium helps a radiologist (a doctor who specializes in radiology) visualize certain structures, such as blood vessels or the digestive tract, that normally aren't easy to see on an X-ray.

X-rays are commonly used to detect problems with the bones, including fractures, arthritis, and bone cancer. They're also useful for detecting cavities in teeth. Chest X-rays may be taken to assess the lungs for signs of pneumonia or certain types of cancer or for signs of congestive heart failure.

Computerized Tomography

Computerized tomography (CT) is also known as a CAT scan, but no actual cats are involved in the procedure. A CT is a series of X-rays taken by a special X-ray machine. The X-rays are taken from different angles, which results in some very detailed cross-sectional images of the particular body part being examined.

The images can be viewed in sequence (think of them as slices of a loaf of bread) on a computer screen by a radiologist. They're commonly used to help diagnose cancerous and other types of tumors, vascular disease, blood clots, spinal problems, and other musculoskeletal damage.

Magnetic Resonance Imaging

Magnetic resonance imaging (MRI) uses a combination of a magnetic field and radio-wave energy to create digital images of organs and other body parts. It's often more detailed than X-rays or CT scans (both of which we cover earlier in this chapter). The images are similar to CTs in that they're taken from different angles and allow the radiologist to look at the body in sequential slices.

Magnetic resonance imaging may be used to detect a large array of problems including tumors, vascular disease, infection, bleeding, blockage, arthritis, bone marrow problems, torn ligaments and tendons, and damaged cartilage. One great benefit to this type of imaging is the lack of radiation exposure to the patient.

Positron Emission Tomography

Positron emission tomography (PET) is another type of imaging procedure. Patients undergoing a PET scan are given a radioactive substance by mouth or by injection. The radioactive material accumulates in areas where larger amounts of chemical activity are going on. These areas show up as bright spots on the scan and may be due to certain health conditions, including neurological problems, coronary artery (blood vessels that serve the heart) disease, and cancer.

Fluoroscopy

Fluoroscopy uses a continuous X-ray video used to look at the movement of a body part, and it usually involves the use of a contrast medium. For example, a patient may be instructed to swallow barium while the radiologist views the movement of the barium into and through the digestive tract. Fluoroscopy can also be used to study blood flow to various organs and to help guide the placement of *catheters* (hollow tubes that are inserted into blood vessels or body cavities or ducts).

Mammography

A *mammogram* is a specific type of image that uses X-rays to examine the breasts. It can be done as a conventional X-ray film or as a digital mammogram, which can be viewed on a computer screen.

Mammography is commonly used as a screening exam for early detection of breast cancer. It's routinely performed in women after the age of 40. It's also used for diagnosis of the disease in women who have breast lumps or other signs of breast cancer.

Ultrasonography

Ultrasonography is a type of imaging technique that involves the use of high-frequency sound waves called *ultrasound*. Echoes are produced when the sound waves bounce off organs and tissues in the body. The echoes are used to record and produce images and video.

Ultrasonography is used to assess the progress of a pregnancy, and it's often the first "picture" moms and dads have of their kids. Ultrasonography is also used to look for tumors in the ovaries, Fallopian tubes, and the uterus; to look for gallstones; and to assess the function of blood vessels.

Opthalmoscopy

Opthalmoscopy is looking into the eye to see the structures located on the fundus (the back portion of the interior eyeball). An instrument called an *opthalmoscope* is used to shine a light directly through the pupil of the eye, and the examiner looks through an eyepiece designed to visualize the retina. The opthalmoscope has different lenses so the examiner can see the eye at different levels of magnification and at different depths to get a clear view of the structures.

Opthalmoscopy is done to detect problems with the eye itself or to help diagnoses other diseases, such as diabetes mellitus, that can cause damage to the blood vessels on the retina. As an interesting note, the eye is the only place in the body where you can actually see arteries (without cutting anything open, of course).

Upper Endoscopy

Upper endoscopy, or *upper gastrointestinal endoscopy,* involves the use of an *endoscope,* which is a long tube with a light and a small camera on the end. The endoscope is inserted into the patient's mouth and moved carefully into the back of the throat, through the esophagus and into the stomach and duodenum. The camera transmits a video picture to a monitor so the doctor can see what the linings of the esophagus, stomach, and duodenum look like.

Upper endoscopy is used to help detect the causes of chest and abdominal pain or internal bleeding due to polyps, ulcers, cancer, or other abnormalities.

Colonoscopy

Colonoscopy is similar to an upper endoscopy (see the previous section) in that it involves the use of a light and camera attached to the end of a tube. Of course, this procedure is different because it's for the examination of the other end of the digestive tract. The colonoscope is inserted into the rectum and carefully moved into the colon (the colon is inflated with carbon dioxide to allow for a better view).

The camera transmits a video image to a camera screen so the examiner can view the walls of the rectum and colon for inflammation, polyps, and signs of cancer. Colonoscopy is used as a routine screening examination for people over the age of 50.

Index

• *B* •

• O •

• P •

Notes

Notes

Notes

Apple & Mac

iPad 2 For Dummies,
3rd Edition
978-1-118-17679-5

iPhone 4S For Dummies,
5th Edition
978-1-118-03671-6

iPod touch For Dummies,
3rd Edition
978-1-118-12960-9

Mac OS X Lion
For Dummies
978-1-118-02205-4

Blogging & Social Media

CityVille For Dummies
978-1-118-08337-6

Facebook For Dummies,
4th Edition
978-1-118-09562-1

Mom Blogging
For Dummies
978-1-118-03843-7

Twitter For Dummies,
2nd Edition
978-0-470-76879-2

WordPress For Dummies,
4th Edition
978-1-118-07342-1

Business

Cash Flow For Dummies
978-1-118-01850-7

Investing For Dummies,
6th Edition
978-0-470-90545-6

Job Searching with Social
Media For Dummies
978-0-470-93072-4

QuickBooks 2012
For Dummies
978-1-118-09120-3

Resumes For Dummies,
6th Edition
978-0-470-87361-8

Starting an Etsy Business
For Dummies
978-0-470-93067-0

Cooking & Entertaining

Cooking Basics
For Dummies, 4th Edition
978-0-470-91388-8

Wine For Dummies,
4th Edition
978-0-470-04579-4

Diet & Nutrition

Kettlebells For Dummies
978-0-470-59929-7

Nutrition For Dummies,
5th Edition
978-0-470-93231-5

Restaurant Calorie Counter
For Dummies,
2nd Edition
978-0-470-64405-8

Digital Photography

Digital SLR Cameras &
Photography For Dummies,
4th Edition
978-1-118-14489-3

Digital SLR Settings
& Shortcuts
For Dummies
978-0-470-91763-3

Photoshop Elements 10
For Dummies
978-1-118-10742-3

Gardening

Gardening Basics
For Dummies
978-0-470-03749-2

Vegetable Gardening
For Dummies,
2nd Edition
978-0-470-49870-5

Green/Sustainable

Raising Chickens
For Dummies
978-0-470-46544-8

Green Cleaning
For Dummies
978-0-470-39106-8

Health

Diabetes For Dummies,
3rd Edition
978-0-470-27086-8

Food Allergies
For Dummies
978-0-470-09584-3

Living Gluten-Free
For Dummies,
2nd Edition
978-0-470-58589-4

Hobbies

Beekeeping
For Dummies,
2nd Edition
978-0-470-43065-1

Chess For Dummies,
3rd Edition
978-1-118-01695-4

Drawing For Dummies,
2nd Edition
978-0-470-61842-4

eBay For Dummies,
7th Edition
978-1-118-09806-6

Knitting For Dummies,
2nd Edition
978-0-470-28747-7

Language &
Foreign Language

English Grammar
For Dummies,
2nd Edition
978-0-470-54664-2

French For Dummies,
2nd Edition
978-1-118-00464-7

German For Dummies,
2nd Edition
978-0-470-90101-4

Spanish Essentials
For Dummies
978-0-470-63751-7

Spanish For Dummies,
2nd Edition
978-0-470-87855-2

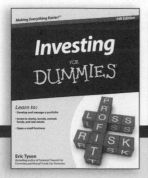

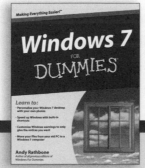

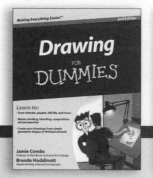

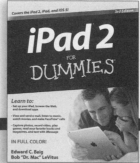

Math & Science

Algebra I For Dummies,
2nd Edition
978-0-470-55964-2

Biology For Dummies,
2nd Edition
978-0-470-59875-7

Chemistry For Dummies,
2nd Edition
978-1-1180-0730-3

Geometry For Dummies,
2nd Edition
978-0-470-08946-0

Pre-Algebra Essentials
For Dummies
978-0-470-61838-7

Microsoft Office

Excel 2010 For Dummies
978-0-470-48953-6

Office 2010 All-in-One
For Dummies
978-0-470-49748-7

Office 2011 for Mac
For Dummies
978-0-470-87869-9

Word 2010
For Dummies
978-0-470-48772-3

Music

Guitar For Dummies,
2nd Edition
978-0-7645-9904-0

Clarinet For Dummies
978-0-470-58477-4

iPod & iTunes
For Dummies,
9th Edition
978-1-118-13060-5

Pets

Cats For Dummies,
2nd Edition
978-0-7645-5275-5

Dogs All-in One
For Dummies
978-0470-52978-2

Saltwater Aquariums
For Dummies
978-0-470-06805-2

Religion & Inspiration

The Bible For Dummies
978-0-7645-5296-0

Catholicism For Dummies,
2nd Edition
978-1-118-07778-8

Spirituality For Dummies,
2nd Edition
978-0-470-19142-2

Self-Help & Relationships

Happiness For Dummies
978-0-470-28171-0

Overcoming Anxiety
For Dummies,
2nd Edition
978-0-470-57441-6

Seniors

Crosswords For Seniors
For Dummies
978-0-470-49157-7

iPad 2 For Seniors
For Dummies, 3rd Edition
978-1-118-17678-8

Laptops & Tablets
For Seniors For Dummies,
2nd Edition
978-1-118-09596-6

Smartphones & Tablets

BlackBerry For Dummies,
5th Edition
978-1-118-10035-6

Droid X2 For Dummies
978-1-118-14864-8

HTC ThunderBolt
For Dummies
978-1-118-07601-9

MOTOROLA XOOM
For Dummies
978-1-118-08835-7

Sports

Basketball For Dummies,
3rd Edition
978-1-118-07374-2

Football For Dummies,
2nd Edition
978-1-118-01261-1

Golf For Dummies,
4th Edition
978-0-470-88279-5

Test Prep

ACT For Dummies,
5th Edition
978-1-118-01259-8

ASVAB For Dummies,
3rd Edition
978-0-470-63760-9

The GRE Test For
Dummies, 7th Edition
978-0-470-00919-2

Police Officer Exam
For Dummies
978-0-470-88724-0

Series 7 Exam
For Dummies
978-0-470-09932-2

Web Development

HTML, CSS, & XHTML
For Dummies, 7th Edition
978-0-470-91659-9

Drupal For Dummies,
2nd Edition
978-1-118-08348-2

Windows 7

Windows 7
For Dummies
978-0-470-49743-2

Windows 7
For Dummies,
Book + DVD Bundle
978-0-470-52398-8

Windows 7 All-in-One
For Dummies
978-0-470-48763-1

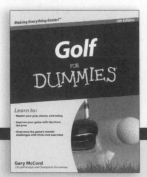
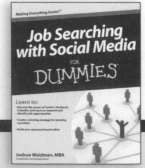
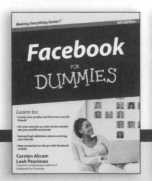
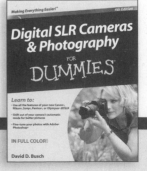